Medical and Healthcare Interactions

Presenting a series of empirical studies by scholars working with approaches from ethnomethodology and conversation analysis, *Medical and Healthcare Interactions* studies real-life work and training encounters among medical and healthcare professionals and trainees or between professionals and patients.

Using video analysis and detailed description, it considers the methods and procedures through which professionals, trainees, and patients produce actions and interpret those of others, exploring questions of member competence and socialization within situated courses of interaction.

The book offers fruitful contributions for training and education in the field of healthcare and will appeal to scholars in the human and social sciences with interests in interaction, ethnomethodology, and conversation analysis.

Sara Keel is a Senior Teaching and Research Assistant at the Institute of Education of the University of Zurich, Switzerland.

Directions in Ethnomethodology and Conversation Analysis

Series Editors:
Andrew Carlin, *University of Macau, Macau SAR, China*
K. Neil Jenkings, *Newcastle University, UK*

Ethnomethodology and Conversation Analysis are cognate approaches to the study of social action that together comprise a major perspective within the contemporary human sciences. Ethnomethodology focuses upon the production of situated and ordered social action of all kinds, whilst Conversation Analysis has a more specific focus on the production and organisation of talk-in-interaction. Of course, given that so much social action is conducted in and through talk, there are substantive as well theoretical continuities between the two approaches. Focusing on social activities as situated human productions, these approaches seek to analyse the intelligibility and accountability of social activities 'from within' those activities themselves, using methods that can be analysed and described. Such methods amount to aptitudes, skills, knowledge and competencies that members of society use, rely upon and take for granted in conducting their affairs across the whole range of social life.

As a result of the methodological rewards consequent upon their unique analytic approach and attention to the detailed orderliness of social life, Ethnomethodology and Conversation Analysis have ramified across a wide range of human science disciplines throughout the world, including anthropology, social psychology, linguistics, communication studies and social studies of science and technology.

This series is dedicated to publishing the latest work in these two fields, including research monographs, edited collections and theoretical treatises. As such, its volumes are essential reading for those concerned with the study of human conduct and aptitudes, the (re)production of social orderliness and the methods and aspirations of the social sciences.

Instructed and Instructive Actions
The Situated Production, Reproduction, and Subversion of Social Order
Edited by Michael Lynch and Oskar Lindwall

The Practical Accomplishment of Everyday Activities Without Sight
Edited by Brian L. Due

Medical and Healthcare Interactions
Members' Competence and Socialization
Edited by Sara Keel

For more information about this series, please visit: https://www.routledge.com/Directions-in-Ethnomethodology-and-Conversation-Analysis/book-series/ASHSER1190

Medical and Healthcare Interactions

Members' Competence and Socialization

Edited by Sara Keel

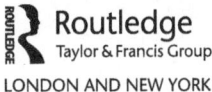
LONDON AND NEW YORK

First published 2024
by Routledge
4 Park Square, Milton Park, Abingdon, Oxon OX14 4RN

and by Routledge
605 Third Avenue, New York, NY 10158

Routledge is an imprint of the Taylor & Francis Group, an informa business

© 2024 selection and editorial matter, Sara Keel; individual chapters, the contributors

The right of Sara Keel to be identified as the author of the editorial material, and of the authors for their individual chapters, has been asserted in accordance with sections 77 and 78 of the Copyright, Designs and Patents Act 1988.

All rights reserved. No part of this book may be reprinted or reproduced or utilised in any form or by any electronic, mechanical, or other means, now known or hereafter invented, including photocopying and recording, or in any information storage or retrieval system, without permission in writing from the publishers.

Trademark notice: Product or corporate names may be trademarks or registered trademarks, and are used only for identification and explanation without intent to infringe.

British Library Cataloguing-in-Publication Data
A catalogue record for this book is available from the British Library

ISBN: 9781032320052 (hbk)
ISBN: 9781032320069 (pbk)
ISBN: 9781003312345 (ebk)

DOI: 10.4324/9781003312345

Typeset in Times New Roman
by Deanta Global Publishing Services, Chennai, India

Contents

List of figures		*vii*
List of contributors		*ix*
Introduction: Competence and socialization in medical and healthcare interactions		1
SARA KEEL		
Transcription conventions		22
1	**When neurologists solicit patients' treatment preferences: The relevance of talk as action for understanding why shared decision-making is so limited in practice**	24
	MERRAN TOERIEN	
2	**Working out interprofessional collaboration: Flight nurses' practical management of prehospital emergency care**	47
	NOZOMI IKEYA, SHINTARO MATSUNAGA, TATSUYA AKUTSU, SEIICHI TAKAHASHI, AND HIROKO NAKAZAWA	
3	**Senior staff member walks ahead, nursing intern follows: Mobility practices in hospital corridors**	73
	ESTHER GONZÁLEZ-MARTÍNEZ	
4	**Asking questions in the operating room**	102
	LORENZA MONDADA	
5	**Monitoring, coordinating, and correcting professional conduct: Soliciting absent requests during surgery**	130
	MIKAELA ÅBERG AND JONAS IVARSSON	

6   Teaching and learning how to identify an audible order in
     traffic: Street-crossing instructional sequences for the visually
     impaired   152
     MARC RELIEU

7   Instructing and socializing patients with aphasia to gaze at the
     therapist's mouth to produce speech sounds in language therapy   176
     SARA MERLINO

8   How to use a mobile app at home: Learning-by-doing
     introductions in physiotherapy consultations   207
     SARA KEEL, ANJA SCHMID, AND FABIENNE KELLER

9   Socialization and accountability: Instructional responses to peer
     feedback in healthcare simulation debriefing   239
     ELIN NORDENSTRÖM, GUSTAV LYMER, AND
     OSKAR LINDWALL

     Index   *259*

Figures

Chapter 2

1   Initial outpatient treatment being administered in the Emergency Medical Care unit at the hospital   53
2   Emergency prehospital treatment in the ambulance   53
3   (00:12) Ambulance crew members holding the patient down on the stretcher as the flight doctor enters the ambulance with a bag of equipment   55
4   (00:22) The flight nurse hanging a pack of lactate ringer solution on a hook as he enters the ambulance with two bags of medicine and equipment   57
5   (00:39) The flight nurse cuts small pieces of surgical tape from a roll and sticks each piece to the edge of the cupboard   58
6   (00:45) The flight nurse asks the ambulance crew member (CA) "Can you pull his arm up a little bit?" (1.34)   62
7   (00:58) The flight nurse tries to pull the patient's arm up "Wow extreme" (1.47)   62

Chapter 3

1   Clinic premises and recording set-up. The triangles represent the video cameras, the dots the wireless microphones, and the striped rectangle the rectangle/mixing/editing station. The area covered by the video cameras is represented in gray. Corridor A is 27.40 meters long, Corridor B (the section between A and C) 4.16 meters long, and Corridor C 31.50 meters long   75
2   Gloria, the observation intern, walking alone and with senior nursing staff. View of camera 4 except for 2.2, 2.4, and 2.5, which correspond to the view of camera 2   77
3   Coralie, the nursing intern, walking alone and with senior nursing staff. View of camera 2 except for 3.4, 3.5, and 3.6, which correspond to the view of camera 4   78
4   Ana, the senior nurse, walking alone and with senior nursing staff. View of camera 2 except for 4.2 and 4.3, which correspond to the view of camera 4   79

Chapter 5

1	Two related but parallel tasks	134
2	The operating room and participants' positions	134

Chapter 6

1	The orientation and mobility instructor and her student stand in close proximity to each other and to the roads	157
2	A two-way "T" crossing. The vehicles coming from the two-lane road, parallel to the walking direction of the pedestrian, can hit her/him when they turn into the one-way perpendicular road	158
3	If a pedestrian crosses while a vehicle moves next to her/him on the parallel road, then this vehicle prevents other cars from coming into the perpendicular road and hitting the pedestrian	158

Chapter 8

1	Video-recorded physiotherapy consultations	212
2	Activity structure of examined consultations	213
3	The app's functions and options	214
4	Instructional chains of introductions	232

Chapter 9

1	A debriefing room and a simulation room with a patient simulator. Picture from the data	243

Contributors

The editor

Sara Keel is a Senior Teaching and Research Assistant at the Institute of Education of the University of Zurich, Switzerland. Working within an ethnomethodological and conversation analytic perspective, she investigates members' understanding and embodied organization of ordinary, institutional, and professional practices. Her research projects focus on distinct settings, such as everyday family life, migrants' press conferences, interprofessional hospital meetings, and more recently physiotherapy consultations to address socialization, membership categorization, patient participation, or the use of digital tools in healthcare as a members' phenomenon. She has published in various international journals, her doctoral research, *Socialization: Parent-Child Interaction in Everyday Life*, has been published by Routledge (2016), she has co-edited a collection on institutional interactions and special issues, most recently on touch and closeness in naturally organized activities.

The contributors

Mikaela Åberg is a senior lecturer at the Department of Education, Communication, and Learning, where she also serves as the coordinator for the Faculty of Education Video Lab. In this role, she provides guidance and support to colleagues who are utilizing video-based methods and analysis in their research. Åberg's research interests focus on communication, instruction, and professional conduct, including topics such as classroom interaction and coordination between interdisciplinary professionals in institutional settings. Currently, she is investigating the impact of digital communication on teachers' work practices and professional conduct, specifically in regard to interactions between schools, students, and guardians.

Tatsuya Akutsu is a PhD candidate in library and information science at the Graduate School of Letters at Keio University in Tokyo. He studies the nature and concepts of information, health information services in libraries, and emergency medicine from an ethnomethodological perspective. His current research explores the possibility of ethnomethodological hybrid studies/disciplines of work in the field of library and information science. He is also interested in workplace studies, computer-supported cooperative work, and human–computer interaction. His work has been published in the journals *Library and Information Science* and *The Japanese Journal of Health and Medical Sociology*.

Esther González-Martínez is Full Professor of Sociology at the University of Fribourg, Switzerland. Her research adopts an ethnomethodological perspective and relies on conversation and multimodal analysis, supplemented by ethnographic fieldwork. She studies the situated organization of social interactions in institutional settings, analyzing them on the basis of audiovisual recordings. Her first studies centered around police and judicial interactions in France and the United States. More recently, she has conducted several projects on nurses' unscheduled interactions with co-workers in Swiss hospitals, with particular focus on telephone conversations, corridor interactions, mobility practices, and recruitment moves.

Nozomi Ikeya is a Professor of Humanities and Social Sciences at Keio University in Tokyo and holds a PhD in sociology from the University of Manchester. Her research interest is in examining the practices of people from their perspectives, following ethnomethodology's program. She has conducted ethnographic studies in various settings, including healthcare settings, IT project management, and the design and implementation of user services in libraries. By studying these settings, she has explored issues such as sharing knowledge and expertise in organizational settings, which has sometimes led her to inform professional communities about their practices and codesign their work.

Jonas Ivarsson is a Professor of Informatics with a background in communication studies and education. He has led multiple interdisciplinary research projects and is committed to advancing the use of video in ethnographic research. Ivarsson's research covers a range of topics, including assessment practices in higher education, the role of technology in architectural education, design research practices, and expertise and technology shifts in medical imaging. Currently, he is researching human-centered artificial intelligence and the interplay between humans and machines in the context of AI.

Fabienne Keller is currently part of the skills lab team at the medical faculty of the University of Zurich, Switzerland. Originally trained as a physical therapist, she also holds a master of science in Physiotherapy of the Zurich University of Applied Sciences. She has collaborated in various research projects on interprofessional collaboration and digitalization in healthcare regarding digital tools and remote physiotherapy at the School of Health Sciences (HESAV), HES-SO University of Applied Sciences and Arts Western Switzerland.

Oskar Lindwall is a Professor in Communication at the Department of Applied IT at the University of Gothenburg, Sweden. His major fields are ethnomethodology, conversation analysis, and the learning sciences. Lindwall has been the principal investigator in projects investigating dentist education, YouTube tutorials, surgical training, and feedback in higher education. He has also conducted research on conversational agents, lab work in science education, architect education, simulation training in medicine and maritime education, and the teaching and learning of craft. Recently (2023), he co-edited the volume *Instructions and Instructed Action: The Situated Production, Reproduction, and Subversion of Social Order* (Routledge).

Gustav Lymer is an Associate Professor at the Department of Education at Stockholm University, Sweden. He conducts research in the intersection between conversation analysis, ethnomethodology, and the learning sciences. He defended his PhD thesis (a study of design reviews in architectural education) in 2010, and has since been involved in various projects, including studies of dentistry education, professional radiology, participatory design, and workplace interaction and learning. The overarching theme of his research is the development, display, and communication of knowledge and expertise in interaction. Currently his research focuses on the delivery and reception of feedback in higher education.

Shintaro Matsunaga is an Associate Professor at Nagano University. He specializes in the sociology of work, labor process theory, and workplace studies. He has a long-standing interest in freelance workers' sustainability and coping practices in the Japanese animation industry. He is currently researching the labor process and communication of freelance workers in terms of the rhythms and temporality of their working lives. He is known as the author of *Workplace Studies on Freelance Animators in an Animation Studio* (Animeta wa dou hataraite irunoka: atsumatte hataraku furiransa tachino roudou syakaigaku, Nakanishiya Syuppan, 2020).

Sara Merlino is Assistant Professor at the University of Roma Tre. Her current research focuses on the organization of speech-language therapy for the treatment of aphasia as a form of social interaction and on the multimodal and multisensorial dimensions that underpin the therapeutic process. Her research is grounded in multimodal conversation analysis. Previously, she has investigated other institutional settings of communication (interpreter-mediated interactions, multilingual meetings, choral rehearsals), by exploring the interrelation between language and bodily resources in social interaction.

Lorenza Mondada is Professor for linguistics at the University of Basel. Working on social interaction in ordinary, professional, and institutional settings, from an ethnomethodological and conversation analytic perspective, she focuses on video analysis and multimodality. Her research is on how the situated and endogenous organization of social interaction draws on a diversity of multimodal resources, articulates language with gesture, gaze, body posture, body movements, and object manipulations as well as multisensorial practices involving vision, touch, taste, and smell. She has extensively published in the *Journal of Pragmatics, Discourse Studies, Language in Society, Research on Language and Social Interaction*, and the *Journal of Sociolinguistics* and has co-edited several collective books, as well as elaborated her approach to sensoriality in the book *Sensing in Social Interaction* (CUP, 2021).

Hiroko Nakazawa works in the emergency room (ER) as the Assistant Head Nurse of the Nursing Department at Yonemori Hospital in Kagoshima, Japan. She has 18 years of experience as a nurse in cardiovascular medicine, heart surgery, intensive care, and primary care. In addition, she has experienced over 650 dispatches as a flight nurse and is actively involved in research activities. Currently, she supports the research activities of flight nurses at her workplace. She was also part of the Japan Disaster Relief medical team deployed to Turkey for the February 2023 earthquake.

Elin Nordenström holds a PhD in education and works as a senior lecturer at the Department of Education, Communication and Learning at the University of Gothenburg, Sweden. She defended her PhD thesis in 2019, which was informed by ethnomethodology and conversation analysis and investigated feedback and instruction in simulation-based training for healthcare students. Since then, she has had a continuing interest in feedback and instruction in higher and professional education, particularly in technology-intense contexts. Currently she is involved in a project investigating simulation-based maritime education.

Marc Relieu is an Associate Professor at Telecom Paris. His work has focused on the organization of mediated interactions. In the 1990s, using video-recordings, he began studying the double embeddedness of text messages on mobile phones, concentrating on their sequential, remote context and the local sites in which they are co-produced and read. He has co-edited two special issues of the French journal *Réseaux* on the topic of mobile phones and video communication. More recently, he has developed a special interest in the organization of phone calls with "hidden" conversational agents and co-edited a special issue of *Réseaux* on the ethnography of conversational agents. His other research interests include orientation and mobility training for the visually impaired in public places. He has published several papers on how they interactionally learn to deploy perceptual and sensorial skills to walk, cross streets, and find their way using a cane.

Anja Schmid currently works as a project leader for digitization in an NPO for community interpreting, delving into her general interests in digital communication, talk on health-related issues, and multilingualism. She did her BA in French and sociology and her MA in "Language and Communication" at the University of Basel, Switzerland. Working mainly with the methods of conversation analysis, she wrote a master thesis on self-categorization in group discussions about mental illness and researched interprofessional collaboration, patient participation, and digitization in healthcare at the School of Health Sciences (HESAV), HES-SO University of Applied Sciences and Arts Western Switzerland.

Seiichi Takahashi has 24 years of experience as a nurse. He is currently the nurse manager at the Advanced Emergency Medical Service Center of

Saitama Medical Center, Saitama Medical University in Japan. The Advanced Emergency Medical Service Center provides initial treatment for and intensive care management of patients with severe trauma. In addition, he has 15 years of experience as a flight nurse with more than 700 activities and is committed to training novice flight nurses, researching effective training methods, and quantifying their practical skills for flight nurses.

Merran Toerien is a Professor in Sociology and the Director of the Centre for Advanced Studies in Language and Communication, at the University of York, UK. Her research has focused on interaction in a range of institutional settings, including beauty salons, recruitment to medical trials, UK jobcentres, and NHS neurology clinics. She is active in medical education and training researchers in the methods of conversation analysis (CA), around the UK and internationally (including in Brazil, China, the Netherlands, and South Africa). She has a particular interest in how patient choice is enacted in practice and the consequences of doing so.

Introduction

Competence and socialization in medical and healthcare interactions

Sara Keel

Introduction

Adopting ethnomethodology (EM) and conversation analysis (CA) to study medical/healthcare encounters, as they occur in real life, means focusing on the myriad ways they are produced, in an orderly and methodical fashion, through members' embodied and situated interactions and "provid[ing], through detailed analyses, that accountable phenomena [orderly organized interactions] are through and through practical accomplishments" (Garfinkel & Sacks, 1970, pp. 163–164). From its very beginning, the founders and earliest researchers of EMCA investigated the social organization of medical and healthcare interactions and provided original insight into the "[g]ood organizational reasons for 'bad' clinic records" and how "selection criteria ... in psychiatric outpatient clinics" are determined in practice (Garfinkel, 1967, pp. 186–207, 208–261); "[t]he social organization of dying" and how it reflects and constitutes social orders of kinship and friendship relations (Sudnow, 1967); the methods through which call-takers at a suicide prevention center try to find out callers' names, among other details, despite the callers' resistance to providing them (see Sacks, 1967; 1992, pp. 3–125); and how in an adolescents' group-therapy setting peers contribute to a newcomer's socialization (Sacks, 1992, pp. 136–203).

The initial interest has since developed rapidly to cover a wide array of issues with relevance for medical/healthcare research. Based on audio- or video-recordings, it has notably proven to be a highly productive area of empirical research on encounters among medical/healthcare professionals, between professionals and patients/clients, and/or between patients/clients and their relatives/caregivers. Beyond numerous articles and chapters, overviews, reviews, monographs, edited collections, and special issues addressing a particular topic have been published, see e.g., Heath (1986); Heritage and Maynard (2006a) on the interactive organization of primary-care consultations; ten Have (1995) for a selective overview of studies in medical ethnomethodology and the formulation of a future program in this field; Drew et al. (2001) on patient participation in doctor–patient encounters; Heath et al. (2003) and Hindmarsh et al. (2007) on how technology in healthcare and medical practice is handled in situ; Dalley et al. (2021) for a systematic review of CA studies on healthcare providers' and patients' management of telemedicine consultations; Pilnick et al. (2009) on healthcare settings beyond doctor–patient consultations; Gill and Roberts (2012) on hitherto focuses, developments, and future directions in the field; the introduction by Lindwall (2014) on the body in medical work and training; Mayor and Bietti (2017) for a scoping review on nurse–patient–relative encounters; Wilkinson et al. (2020) on "atypical interactions" in which at least one of the participants has a communicative impairment and the ways this impacts social interactions; Maynard and Turowetz (2022) for investigations on interactions involving individuals with autism; and Pilnick (frth) for a discussion of medical/healthcare studies' contribution to EMCA developments.

As pointed out by Gill and Roberts (2012, pp. 589–590), investigating the ways medical/healthcare encounters are socially organized is worth doing in its "own right." EMCA studies focus on the details of members' situated production of social order and the ways parties come to understand each other's contributions in interactions that are "naturally occurring," meaning not initiated or otherwise "orchestrated by researchers" (Mondada, 2006, p. 53). The attention to details that could easily be overlooked provides an in-depth understanding of how medical/healthcare interactions and work processes are achieved in situ. Moreover, it is argued that this critical insight constitutes a rich resource for contributions to medical/healthcare practices, policy, and education.

This introduction first discusses EMCA's approach to the volume's central topics: members' competence and socialization to competence in medical/healthcare work and training encounters. It then presents the nine empirical chapters and outlines how their contributors adopted distinct ways of collaborating with medical/healthcare members to address the volume's topics.

Members' competence in medical/healthcare interactions and EMCA's contribution to education

A central aim of EMCA research on medical/healthcare interactions is to reveal how the *minutia* of members' organization of interaction is relevant to the course of ongoing interaction and its outcome. Recently (but see Frankel, 1990), EMCA researchers have taken a growing interest in how exactly the insights on medical/healthcare encounters generated through their studies might inform practices, policy, and education and in turn contribute to their development.

Medical/healthcare encounters as interactive and situated achievements

Studies have focused on doctor–patient interactions and the ways distinct activities in the encounters, such as the opening, history-taking, physical examination, and treatment recommendations, are interactively achieved in situ (Robinson & Heritage, 2014). Investigations into pediatric consultations have for example focused on how a physical examination of a child is organized in the presence of the parent(s). They have revealed how pediatricians might use problem-oriented (versus non-problem-oriented) online commentary. Drawing on detailed analysis of this commentary, studies have deployed quantitative methods to show that the occurrence of problem-oriented commentary during physical examinations increases parents' questioning of subsequent treatment plans that do not include an antibiotic prescription (Heritage et al., 2010). It has also been revealed that parents' questioning of pediatricians' treatment plans is perceived by the latter as reflecting parents' expectations for antibiotics, resulting in an increase in inappropriate antibiotic prescriptions for viral infections in children (Mangione-Smith et al., 2006). Investigations on primary care have alternatively focused on the questions doctors ask patients at the end of a consultation: "do you have *some* [or *any*] other concerns?" (Heritage & Robinson, 2011). Studies have thus shown that a doctor's distinct choice of even one word might change the course of the interaction: the question "do you have *some* more questions?" is significantly more successful at eliciting unmet patient concerns than "do you have *any* more questions?" (Heritage et al., 2007; Robinson & Heritage, 2014).

Using audio- or video-recordings of naturally occurring interactions and detailed transcriptions of them to focus on the organization of an encounter as an interactive achievement, EMCA studies depart in crucial ways from other "education-oriented" research (Maynard & Heritage, 2005, pp. 433–434). While the former adopts an "interaction-focused ... approach" (Wilkinson, 2014, p. 221), other education research tends to focus on the conduct or experience of, for example, doctors and patients "separately" and on medical/healthcare professionals' conduct more specifically (Maynard & Heritage, 2005, p. 233). This involves, among other things, ignoring what lay members, such as patients and their relatives/caregivers, might contribute to the encounter at hand and how their conduct unavoidably impacts the course of interaction, the overall quality, and the effectiveness of the encounters (Parry & Land, 2013).

As stressed early on (see e.g., Maynard, 1991), instead of addressing features of medical/healthcare interactions that attract notice, such as asymmetrical power relations between doctors and patients or between distinct professionals (Gill & Roberts, 2012, p. 586), EMCA studies consider systematic and in-depth investigations on the interactive organization of medical/healthcare interaction as a prerequisite (Mayor & Bietti, 2017, p. 11). To contribute to medical/healthcare training, it is considered crucial to show how members accomplish social practices and specific tasks (e.g., Robinson & Heritage, 2014) and/or how the overall aims of medical/healthcare encounters, such as "patient-centeredness" and "shared decision-making" (e.g., de Kok et al., 2018, p. 27; Toerien et al., 2011), are, or are not, achieved in practice. For example, showing how neurologists' use of open rather than "traditional fact-oriented" questions solicit narratives with "diagnostically useful features" by patients constituted the basis for the development of a one-day intervention that helped doctors to change their ways of questioning during patients' problem presentations (Jenkins & Reuber, 2014).

Shedding light on how all parties to an encounter come to contribute to the task at hand (e.g., problem presentation) allows us also to understand *how* each party's talk and embodied conduct constitute an action that is at the same time "context shaped" and "context renewing" (Maynard & Heritage, 2005, p. 30). While the patients' narratives are shaped by the neurologists' way of soliciting a problem presentation from them, these narratives also provide doctors with resources for reaching a diagnosis and thus contribute to a renewal of the further course of the encounter.

Investigating members' perspectives

Beyond unpacking how each party's action contributes to the tasks at hand and impacts the course of interaction, EMCA's contributions to medical/healthcare training also aim to provide participants' own perspectives on the ongoing interaction (Heath et al., 2007). As pointed out by Maynard and Heritage (2005, p. 430), the "proof procedure" introduced by Sacks et al. (1974, p. 728) constitutes one method that makes it possible for members' actions to be analyzed from within. Parties to an interaction make sense of and mutually display their understanding of each other's actions before researchers analyze members' interactive accomplishment of it. In EMCA, each contribution to the interaction is understood as displaying (or in other words "proofing") members' understanding of the immediately previous contribution (Heritage, 1984).

Drawing on the programmatic study by Schegloff et al. (1977) on how ordinary members treat interactional problems and manage to repair them, Ivarsson and Åberg (2020) focus on a surgical team's deployment of repair practices. The repairs concern turns-at-talk that address some problem related to the ongoing talk. Either the person that is currently talking initiates and/or produces repair (in which case the method involves "self-repair") or another party to the conversation indicates a problem of speaking, hearing, and/or understanding and in this case this other person initiates or produces an "other-repair" (Schegloff et al., 1977). By focusing on instances that are treated by members as repair-worthy and thus problematic for the ongoing surgery, the study reveals how repair practices serve the surgical team to prevent delays from occurring at delicate points in controlled apnea episodes (Ivarsson & Åberg, 2020). It shows how "repairs are central in establishing a joint understanding" between members of the surgical team, as they make it possible to fix (among other things) the "flexibility," "versatility," and "vagueness" inherent to language use in surgical practices and thus to increase patients' safety (Ivarsson & Åberg, 2020, p. 6).

Based on their findings, the authors suggest that recommendations, for example the use of systematic pre-requests, could remove ambiguity from the situation and inform members' training and practice. Moreover, revealing members' situated repair actions and their perspective on problematic instances of interprofessional collaboration involves highlighting what they do methodically and competently instead of focusing and dwelling on their deficiencies.

Spotlight on medical/healthcare tasks and members' displayed competences

In line with Garfinkel's fundamental criticism of the way that the predominant social and human theory tends to construe the "man-in-the-sociologist's-society" as a "cultural dope" who simply "produces the stable features of the society by acting in compliance with pre-established and legitimate alternatives of action that the common culture provides" (Garfinkel, 1967, p. 68), EMCA studies have a programmatic interest in members' competences (Heritage, 1984). Medical/healthcare studies are no exception to this. From their beginning, they have shone a light on competent conduct that professional and lay members bring to bear, and thus display, to accomplish tasks conjointly. In the programmatic collection *Interaction Competence* edited by Psathas (1990a), Frankel (1990) investigates physicians' and patients' displayed dispreference for patient-initiated questions. Based on a corpus of audio-recorded, naturally occurring physician–patient encounters, Frankel's study reveals that in contrast to ordinary conversations, both physicians and patients organize their talk in a way that minimizes the occurrence of patient-initiated questions. Instead of treating this asymmetrical distribution as reflecting a problematic power relationship, the author discusses it in terms of members' displays of competence. By minimizing patient-initiated questions, both physicians and patients contribute to the management of tasks, such as history-taking, clinical examination, and the reaching of a diagnosis, while taking into account the in situ constraints inherent to a given task: physicians *must* ask patients numerous questions and the patients in turn *must* answer them, all within a limited period of time.

In his conclusion, Frankel (1990, p. 255) suggests that, in addition to highlighting members' competences, studies examining the interactive organization of medical encounters should also increasingly inform medical training. Adopting the proof procedure as a method of investigation is a way to provide evidence from within of how medical/healthcare members (including patients) orient to and, at the same time, accomplish their interactions in an intelligible way and how they treat each other's actions as contributing competently to the accomplishment of the specific tasks at hand. In contrast, a lack of attention to and understanding from within of members' conjoint achievement of in situ interaction has led to recommendations and guidelines that fail to consider the whole picture, which includes the complexity involved in simultaneously achieving specific medical/healthcare tasks/activities and overall aims, for example regarding "patient-centered care" (see Pilnick & Dingwall, 2011) and/or "shared decision-making" (see de Kok et al., 2018; Toerien et al., 2011), in real-life consultations.

In the abovementioned collection (Psathas, 1990a), Psathas (1990b) investigated a medical history interview conducted by a student in optometry. Basing his analysis on video-recordings, the author reveals how the student deploys gaze to direct the patient's own gaze to activities or other features available in the setting that allow the ongoing talk to be intelligible. Psathas's examination of the embodied organization of the interview task makes it possible to account for the presence of silences as displaying the student's embodied competences instead of portraying them as evidencing the student's inexperience in conducting medical history interviews and/or a lack of competence in ensuring its steady progression.

Analyzing brief calls that newly graduated nurses make to other hospital professionals, González-Martínez and Bulliard (2018) show how these anodyne phone calls are key for organizing patients' smooth discharge from the hospital and come to a conclusion that is in line with Psathas's (1990b) observation. The authors stress that "focusing on the competences of young nurses, particularly with regard to the global vision of patient situations, the organization of the health system and interprofessional work" (González-Martínez & Bulliard, 2018, p. 33 my translation), makes it possible to gain important insights on interprofessional coordination work and communication occurring outside of formal interprofessional meetings, thereby suggesting that the findings could be used to inform healthcare professionals' vocational training and the integration of newcomers in the clinical work space.

The studies by Psathas (1990b) and González-Martínez and Bulliard (2018) are in line with Garfinkel et al.'s proposal of the late 1960s and early 1970s (1982) to "respecify" socialization research on children (see Keel, 2016, p. 30ff. for a thorough discussion). This brings us to the second topic of the volume.

Medical/healthcare education/socialization as a member's phenomenon

As pointed out by Lindwall (2014), it is not enough to look at members' competent organization and coordination of interactions and highlight how parties rely on expertise, competence, skills, and a large amount of knowledge to achieve tasks at hand conjointly. Putting the spotlight on the myriad ways required competences and skills are taught and acquired in training and work settings in the first place is critical for understanding what it takes to interact competently in medical/healthcare settings. Furthermore, investigating in detail how teaching and learning are conjointly achieved constitutes a perspicuous setting for education research because how it is done is relevant for members of the field, for instance medical/healthcare educators, senior and junior professionals, students, patients, and patients' relatives/caregivers, before it ever becomes relevant for researchers.

Over the past two decades, studies have increasingly investigated medical/healthcare education settings as a member's phenomenon in its own right. They have focused on distinct formal medical/healthcare education and on-the-job training settings, such as simulation training in which dentistry students use a simulator to practice manual skills (Hindmarsh et al., 2014), dental clinics in which students work on patients under the supervision of tutors (Hindmarsh, 2010; Hindmarsh et al., 2011), and bedside teaching activities for medical students in which the students attend to patients (Elsey et al., 2017). The operating room has also been investigated as an "ecology for instruction" (Sanchez Svensson et al., 2009, p. 892): studies reveal how instructions are not only used to collaboratively accomplish the ongoing operations, but also to provide trainees with learning opportunities in the middle of an operation (Koschmann et al., 2011; Sanchez Svensson et al., 2009; Zemel & Koschmann, 2014). Moreover, when operations are broadcast to advanced trainees and experts on a large screen in an adjacent room, trainees can watch the ongoing operation and the chief surgeon's demonstrations of critical aspects in real time (Mondada, 2003, 2014).

These studies have also examined educational settings in which the addressee is not a future medical/healthcare professional but a patient/client to be educated (Halpin et al., 2021). Studies have, for example, looked at how, during ultrasound examinations, midwives instruct and guide expectant mothers through touch and other means so that they can understand the ultrasound images that are processed and/or feel their fetus with their own hands (Nishizaka, 2014, 2020). Other topics of focus include an instructor teaching a person with visual impairment to safely cross busy streets in Paris during their locomotion and orientation training (Relieu, 1994); physiotherapists supervising, instructing, and correcting a patient who is learning to perform therapeutic exercises to support the rehabilitation process (Martin & Sahlström, 2010; Parry, 2005); and speech therapists instructing and supporting persons with aphasia in performing exercises to reacquire speech competences after a stroke (Merlino, 2018; Merlino, 2020).

Shifting focus from deficiency to members' contribution to socialization

In contrast to other medical/healthcare and patient-education research, the primary aim of EMCA studies on members' accomplishment of medical/healthcare training or patient education is not a critical focus (Hindmarsh et al., 2014 and Pilnick et al., 2018). Quite the contrary, as advocated by Garfinkel et al. (1982) and early studies on young children's socialization, it involves (first) refraining from adopting a normative approach to socialization by moving away from a "deficiency model" (Mackay, 1975, p. 181), whose adoption generates explications of the to-be-socialized's conduct as "naturally, normally, obviously, objectively, really and observably" deficient compared to adults'/teachers' conduct (Garfinkel et al., 1982, p. 4).

When the focus is shifted from "deficiency" to "competence" (Mackay, 1975, p. 184), the conduct of students, trainees, novices, or lay members is no longer *by default* understood as "faulty" compared to the conduct of more senior professionals, experts, or instructors (Garfinkel et al., 1982, p. 4). Instead, EMCA studies highlight competences that novices, trainees, students, or lay members bring to bear to achieve education-oriented activities in medical/healthcare settings. They have for example shown how patients' embodied accommodations allow dental students to follow tutors' instructions while attending to them during clinical training (Hindmarsh, 2010); how, over time, patients in physiotherapy gradually develop practices to repair their exercise performance themselves, instead of leaving it to the supervising physiotherapist (alone) to initiate and repair it (Martin & Sahlström, 2010); and how students watching an endodontic surgery remotely address questions about the broadcasted surgical procedures to the co-present instructor and thus display their competence in identifying "instructable observabilities," i.e., what can be observed and questioned in the broadcasted operation and further elaborated upon by the co-present tutor (Lindwall & Lymer, 2014, p. 271). Students thereby contribute to their own socialization to the practice of surgery.

In line with EMCA's interest in members' interactive deployment of ordinary sense-making methods (Garfinkel, 1967, p. 10), such studies refrain from using the ordinary sense-making device – teachers/experts are competent while students/lay members are incompetent (or not-yet-fully-competent) – as a "resource" for scientific explications (Mackay, 1975, p. 181). Instead, they adopt Garfinkel et al.'s (1982) proposition to respecify the study of socialization and approach education

8 *Sara Keel*

in medical/healthcare as a "members' phenomenon" that requires investigation in its own right (Mackay, 1975, p. 181). They thus provide empirical grounds for deepening our understanding of how teaching and learning are achieved in situ during medical/healthcare work and training interactions.

Spotlight on not-yet-fully-competent versus competent members

Describing members' competence in accomplishing education activities, independently of their being not-yet-fully-competent *or* experts in their field, does not mean ignoring members' possibly incompetent conduct altogether. Quite the contrary, before revealing how members' accomplishment of educational tasks requires specific competences by *all* involved parties, this type of approach focuses on how members' competence or lack thereof is treated from within. In doing so, it seeks to answer the question: how do members orient to and constitute each other distinctively as fully, or to the contrary not-yet-fully competent?

The studies reveal how parties to the interaction treat the tutor, senior surgeon, supervisor, instructor, or professional as being responsible for monitoring and identifying features of not-yet-fully-competent conduct *and* for providing, for example, overt or ostensible demonstrations and instructions in the middle of a surgery for advanced trainees to recognize anatomical features and understand critical moments of a surgical procedure (Koschmann et al., 2011; Mondada, 2003; Sanchez Svensson et al., 2009). Alternatively, they may analyze how in routine interventions students are instructed to perform parts of the operation and that if addressed to a medical student (versus to a resident), the attendee's instructions and student's instructed action are accomplished incrementally, meaning that "each demonstrative action by the attending is followed by an enactment" by the medical student (Zemel & Koschmann, 2014, p. 177). They furthermore demonstrate how tutors "embed" their corrections of students' instructed action "within the context of clinical work to reveal the reasoned character of skilled performance" (Hindmarsh et al., 2014, p. 261); or how corrective instructions regarding the way a visually impaired student should hold their cane during locomotion and orientation training are serially organized by participants (Relieu, 1994); or how speech production by a person with aphasia during labeling exercises in speech therapy is scaffolded through speech therapists' deployment of touch and other embodied means (Merlino, 2020).

They thus provide detailed descriptions of the ways parties to medical/healthcare settings accomplish typical educational devices (Lindwall et al., 2015), such as the classic three-part pedagogical I-R-E device (Mehan, 1979). While focusing on the ways that experts produce embodied demonstrations and instructions (I), how these are turned into a course of action, or in other words are responded to by students/patients (R), and finally how in turn this instructed course of action is received, positively evaluated, or corrected by tutors (E), the studies put the spotlight on how socialization of the not-yet-fully competent is interactively achieved. In contrast to research on "instructions," used "as a more general term for 'directives' or 'requests'," which "have to do with divisions of labour rather than differences in knowledge – as in the fluent cooperation between a surgeon and an assistant" (Lindwall, 2014, p. 128), EMCA studies on educational medical/healthcare settings thus show how the trainees, students, or lay members turn embodied instructions, demonstrations, scaffolding, or corrections into a course of action that is treated by experts and students as an apprenticeship-in-interaction in which students learn the embodied skills and relevant knowledge.

Contributing to medical/healthcare education research from within

Investigating members' collaborative accomplishment of educational tasks from within (Macbeth, 2004), EMCA researchers aim to gain an "endogenous comprehensiveness" and to provide "non-ironic"/"non-competitive" (Watson, 1992, p. 261) descriptions and explications of members' in situ educational interaction. Focusing on the members' distinction between not-yet-fully versus fully competent conduct and the ways not-yet-fully-competent members are supervised, instructed, evaluated, and corrected so that they may acquire the required skills and competences, researchers "share in their [tutors, experts, novices, students, trainees, lay members'] 'weak sense' of unique adequacy," and engage in "recognizing how it is their [members'] task, first" to teach and learn medical/healthcare skills, procedures, and knowledge, before it becomes a phenomenon of scientific investigation (Macbeth, 2014, p. 297) and critical discussion (Macbeth, 2003). Refraining from (critically) judging members' conduct from an outside perspective (Lindwall et al., 2015), the studies thus contrast in a significant way with other educational research, thereby serving as a striking reminder of EM's and CA's "shared fundamentals" (Watson, 1992, p. 262).

Members' socialization to competence constitutes a member's focus first. Its detailed analysis provides relevant insight for involved practitioners and lay members before it does so for education research. Yet, it has been pointed out that overall research in medical/healthcare education makes only limited use of the insight gained by EMCA studies (Halpin et al., 2021; Mayor and Bietti, 2017). Reviews have for example revealed that most studies concerning patient education do not account for naturally occurring talk and interaction (75–90%) and that only 1% of publications also consider relatives and caregivers of patients (Halpin et al., 2021, p. 1). Instead, interviews followed by surveys still constitute the usual method of investigation (Halpin et al., 2021, p. 2). Although EMCA studies contribute to a better understanding of "actual interaction" instead of merely being a "memory of experiences" (Mayor & Bietti, 2017, p. 9), the approach is overall still underutilized in medical/healthcare research and EMCA studies have so far gained little acknowledgment and resonance in "policy, education and practice" (Parry & Land, 2013, p. 3).

In the following section, I first give an overview of the nine empirical studies in this volume. Next, I outline how the adopted approach involves distinct ways of collaborating with the members of the medical/healthcare work and training fields to achieve a good understanding of the phenomenon under study and to provide for insights that are relevant for them.

Overview of the volume

The volume adopts a broad view of medical/healthcare interactions. The nine empirical studies that are presented investigate the organization of situated and embodied interactions as they occur in a wide array of bilateral and multi-party medical/healthcare work and training encounters in which professional and lay members orient to matters of illness, health, and rehabilitation (ten Have, 1995, p. 246). Their investigative scope thus goes "beyond" (Gill & Roberts, 2012, pp. 579–580; Pilnick, fth; Pilnick et al., 2009) the well-studied doctor–patient interaction in primary care (Collins et al., 2005; Heath, 1986; Heritage & Maynard, 2006a, 2006b). As the chapters provide detailed insight on the accomplishment of distinct work and training practices, they allow us to delve into the volume's topic: competence and socialization to competence as displayed, treated, and achieved by members in everyday medical and healthcare interactions. In doing this, we can begin to comprehend how a more thorough understanding of these practices constitutes a rich resource for education and training in this field.

In the first chapter, "When neurologists solicit patients' treatment preferences: the relevance of talk as action for understanding why shared decision-making is so limited in practice," Merran Toerien examines shared decision-making (SDM) in outpatient neurology consultations. Based on a collection of 149 cases, Toerien examines two recurrent sequential positions in which the neurologists deploy patient view elicitors (PVE): after the neurologist makes a recommendation or as a preliminary to doing so. Taking the view that to talk is to do something, she reveals how, in both locations, neurologists' PVEs and patients' responses are being used to achieve other social actions than SDM. Although PVEs enact the requirement to solicit patients' preferences, neurologists' deployment of PVEs may thus work against the ideal of SDM. By examining their talk as social action rather than approaching it as a kind of "pure" exchange of views, as assumed by SDM models, Toerien allows readers to understand why, despite a long history of educational efforts to implement SDM in clinical practice, there is still such a tenacious gap between the SDM ideal and decision-making in real-life medical/healthcare encounters.

Chapters 2–5 address members' competence and socialization in interprofessional or multi-party work settings.

In the second chapter, "Working out interprofessional collaboration: Flight nurses' practical management of prehospital emergency care," Nozomi Ikeya, Shintaro Matsunaga, Tatsuya Akutsu, Seiichi Takahashi, and Hiroko Nakazawa describe triage practices as a study of work. The context of their example is prehospital care provided to seriously injured or sick patients in an ambulance before they are transferred to a hospital by helicopter. Pointing out that little opportunity exists for flight doctors and nurses to learn the competences involved in managing prehospital care, the researchers based their study on video-recordings made by flight nurses during interventions. Having conducted the study in close collaboration with members of the field, they discuss first how flight doctors and nurses collaborate with the ambulance crew within various constraints that differ from the ones they face in their usual work in a hospital emergency care unit. They then unpack what flight doctors and nurses know at each moment of their collaboration with the ambulance crew and thus propose another way of approaching issues of interprofessional collaboration and training in prehospital care.

The third chapter, "Senior staff member walks ahead, nursing intern follows: Mobility practices in hospital corridors," by Esther González-Martínez, invites the reader to focus on embodied walking practices occurring in the corridors of a hospital outpatient clinic and to discover that nursing interns systematically walk behind senior nursing staff. By grounding the study on a corpus of video-recordings, supplemented by ethnographic material, she first presents some basic features of the intern's moves in the clinic's corridors when walking alone, in a pair, or in a group. She then describes four mobility practices through which interns *and* nurses or senior nurses contribute to establishing and maintain the observed serial order of "senior member walks ahead, intern follows." Finally, she accounts for this by referring to the internal organization of the observed configuration in contrast to an external system such as deference rules based on status. The interns are interactionally included in the clinic's activities in a specific spatial and interactional configuration (behind senior members) that orients their potential contributions.

The fourth chapter, "Asking questions in the operating room," by Lorenza Mondada, is a systematic study of how asking questions, as a classical device for learning and instructing, is collectively accomplished in the middle of a minimally invasive key-hole surgery. Mondada examines how, in real time, surgeons and remote video-connected experts watching the broadcast operation highlight specific environments for questions, while, with the aid of the camera team, they indicate which questions are relevant at that point of the ongoing operation. These practices provide experts with opportunities to ask questions themselves in addition to instructing advanced trainees, who like the experts are remotely connected, to address their questions to the surgeon. By revealing how trainees are remotely instructed and enabled to ask questions and how they actually ask questions and participate in and learn about the ongoing work, the study casts light on the ways questions are treated by members as a crucial vehicle for professional socialization in the middle of the investigated operations.

In the fifth chapter, "Monitoring, coordinating, and correcting professional conduct: Soliciting absent requests during surgery," by Mikaela Åberg and Jonas Ivarsson, a common vascular surgery procedure is examined. It is based on a collection of 115 video-recorded instances in which a team of vascular surgeons, anesthesiologists, radiologists, and nurses jointly perform digital subtraction angiographies. In preparation for the angiography, the surgeon regularly requests the nurse anesthetist to put the anesthetized patient's breathing on hold so as to temporarily induce apnea. Whenever this is done, breathing must be promptly resumed to secure the patient's health and safety. The first part of their analysis reveals the usual grounds for this routine coordinative practice. In the remaining sections they address instances in which members treat the practice of resuming the patient's breathing as problematic. It reveals that episodes in which requests to resume the patient's breathing are not only treated as officially absent but may also become professionally accountable and thus constitute a perspicuous phenomenon for addressing members' mutual socialization as it occurs during an operation.

Chapters 6–9 address socialization to specific competences as they are oriented to and accomplished in circumscribed patient/client education (Chapters 6–8) or interprofessional simulation training tasks (Chapter 9).

The sixth chapter, "Teaching and learning how to identify an audible order in traffic: Street-crossing instructional sequences for the visually impaired," by Marc Relieu, is based on a close examination of a video-recorded lesson in which a sighted professional provides orientation and locomotion training to a visually impaired student. The single-case analysis examines how the two participants orient to audible, moving features of urban settings in order to learn and teach, through repetition of simulated attempts, how to safely cross a street and how the learner develops specific listening skills to make sense of the instructions the teacher is giving her. Focusing on instructional sequences in and through which the participants (1) initiate a reconfiguration of their location and bodily arrangements, (2) orient to the sounds that make the ongoing trajectories of various categories of motor vehicles accountable, and (3) simulate a "safe" street crossing, Relieu reveals how, through an embodied apprenticeship, visually impaired students develop a new set of skills that transform them into competent pedestrians.

In the seventh chapter, "Instructing and socializing patients with aphasia to gaze at the therapist's mouth to produce speech sounds in language therapy," Sara Merlino investigates the instructional dimension of speech-language therapy for people diagnosed with aphasia. It focuses on the way the patient is instructed in the communicative dynamics of the therapy as a specific form of social interaction and, more particularly, in a specific therapeutic scaffolding technique that consists of gazing at the therapist's mouth to make use of audio-visual cues (such as mouth position). Merlino's contribution reveals how this technique, which is observed during the accomplishment of labeling activities, can help the patient solve difficulties in the production of target words and speech sounds, while also requiring precise bodily coordination and gaze control. Through an analysis of a corpus of video-recorded sessions with the same patient that were recorded over the first weeks of early recovery in a hospital setting, Merlino explores how speech therapists instruct and socialize the patient to this specific institutional and therapeutic form of communication.

In the eighth chapter, "How to use a mobile app at home: Learning-by-doing introductions in physiotherapy consultations," Sara Keel, Anja Schmid, and Fabienne Keller focus on face-to-face physiotherapy consultations in which a mobile eHealth tool (hereafter "the app") is introduced to the patient. Their analysis reveals how physiotherapists and patients organize the introduction through serially linked instructional sequences that provide participants with situated teaching and learning opportunities. The examination of the instructional sequences, which involve operating the app on the patient's smartphone, reveals that these sequences are constantly adapted to contingencies, such as time constraints inherent to physiotherapy consultations, technological affordances, and patients' claimed or displayed understanding of the app. Achieving these sequences in a time-efficient way, although expansions on issues that participants consider relevant for using the app to support the therapeutic process remain possible at any time, the participants treat the patient's socialization to eHealth literacy as sufficient for all practical purposes at hand.

In the ninth and final chapter, "Socialization and accountability: Instructional responses to peer feedback in healthcare simulation debriefing," Elin Nordenström, Gustav Lymer, and Oskar Lindwall explore the organization of feedback in simulation-based team training for healthcare students at a Swedish university. The students in the investigated setting conduct team-training scenarios based on a patient simulator, after which their simulation performance is jointly discussed and critiqued. The researchers examine two feedback sequences in which instructors respond to prior critical feedback students have given to their peers. Prior studies show that peer feedback tends to be locally oriented and characterized by hedging and mitigation, whereas feedback from instructors embodies a generalized stance that reframes local events in terms of professional considerations. The study builds on these, and the analyzed sequences, to show how socialization in this healthcare setting not only includes the learning of different modes of conduct but also operates at the level of accountability, addressing how the social and professional significance of conduct is constructed in accounts.

Studying medical/healthcare interactions while collaborating with members of the field

EMCA investigations based on recordings of real-time medical/healthcare interactions have given rise to fruitful collaboration between researchers and members of the field in developing recommendations and designing education-oriented interventions. The sometimes year-long collaboration between EMCA researchers and the studied professionals/lay persons and other stakeholders (see e.g., Vom Lehn & Heath, 2022) have thus proved important for developing training interventions that are considered relevant by the target populations. Moreover, basing research on recordings of interactions makes it possible to involve the studied parties in the research process from the outset and throughout the intervention process. For example, Wilkinson (2014) reports on how he involved individuals suffering from aphasia and their relatives in his study from the very beginning: he asked them to record their daily interactions, to identify conversational activities that they oriented to as problematic (p. 224), and thus to contribute to decision-making concerning what the intervention would target and eventually to evaluate their effects throughout the intervention process (Wilkinson, 2014, p. 223).

Through this type of collaboration with the members involved, researchers conducting intervention-oriented EMCA studies ensure that their investigation is in accordance with what is relevant to the members (Harwood et al., 2018; Parry et al., 2022; Pilnick et al., 2018; Schoeb et al., 2015; Wilkinson, 2014). Moreover, the use of "real-life video clips" is described by participants as contributing significantly to the high quality and relevance (Harwood et al., 2018, p. viii) and acceptability of the suggested interventions for the target populations and the effectiveness in improving medical/healthcare practices (de Kok et al., 2018, p. 23; Parry et al., 2022; Pilnick et al., 2018). It has also been identified as a feature that enables the design of educational interventions that aim to encourage professionals to reflect upon their own practices with a view to improving them from within when deemed necessary from the members' point of view (Schoeb et al., 2015).

Conducting detailed investigations of members' management of work and training practices to inform medical/healthcare practice, education, or policy is commonly considered to belong to the realm of "applied" research (see e.g., González-Martínez et al., 2016; Halpin et al., 2021; Parry et al., 2016; Robinson & Heritage, 2014). In contrast, Ikeya (2020) discusses her study of an emergency call center at a Japanese hospital with respect to the practical management of what Garfinkel (2002) called "hybrid study of work." Although Ikeya (2020, pp. 33–34) points out that when the study was conducted, "it was not that the researcher attempted to follow the set of criteria Garfinkel presented for hybrid studies of work," she provides a stimulating discussion of the concrete research methods/practices that were deployed in the scope of her study and reveals how they can retrospectively be appreciated as contributing to the achievement of the "criterial properties" (Garfinkel, 2020, pp. 100–103) involved in conducting a hybrid study of work.

In doing so, she makes available to readers how "ethnomethodological indifference" (Ikeya, 2020, p. 35) requires researchers to investigate social practices that are of "topical relevance" to members of the field under study before they become relevant for the researchers (p. 35), and how the "unique adequacy requirement" means that researchers must acquire at least a "weak sense" (pp. 23, 33–34, 36) of the practices under investigation if the study is to offer "descriptions" of the "problems" and "solutions" involved in members' achievement of the practices under investigation that have a "praxeological validity" for members of the field (p. 38). Moreover, she also provides the reader with a first-hand account that evidences how achieving set criteria of hybrid studies of work does not constitute a distinct ethnomethodological end in itself. Instead, she discusses pursuing set criteria in practice as powerful constituents of the very foundation upon which solutions for improving the studied practices (or members' education) can be conjointly envisaged, appreciated, reflected upon, and successfully implemented.

Apart from the chapter by Ikeya et al., the studies presented in this volume were not conducted to satisfy criteria of hybrid studies of work from the outset. However, basing them on video-recordings unavoidably required the contributors to *collaborate with* the directorate or managers of the institutions, professionals or future professionals, educators, and lay members under study, even if "only" to obtain the video-recordings produced by the members of the studied field (Ikeya et al.; Mondada), gain access, get permission, and set the cameras/microphones up (González-Martínez; Merlino; Mondada; Nordenström et al.; Toerien), record the screens of digital tools used by practitioners (Åberg & Ivarsson; Keel et al.), or follow the studied training setting with a hand-held camera (Relieu) in a non-obstructive way, and obtain the members' trust and informed consent to be filmed (see also Parry et al., 2016).

Moreover, by outlining for example how the researcher used a hand-held camera to capture participants' orientation to critical features of mobile training practices (Relieu), how a complex recording configuration made it possible to capture and examine (novice and experienced) nurses' mobile practices as they occur naturally in the hospital corridor (González-Martínez), and how recording the screens of digital tools used by participants provides an additional invaluable resource for addressing members' perspective of complex surgery procedures (Arberg & Ivarsson; Mondada) and/or of remote education of advanced trainees (Mondada), the chapters reveal how a whole array of practices involved in filming naturally occurring interactions, much like transcribing/describing[1] them, provided contributors with precious opportunities to *delve deep* into the minute details of the embodied methods through which members organize and accomplish them.

As such, collecting recordings, although time- and resource-consuming (see e.g., Parry et al., 2016),[2] constitutes an invaluable opportunity for researchers to collaborate with members of the field and gain new insight into the studied practices, and thus to contribute to their own socialization as EMCA researchers, while getting a step closer to satisfying the unique adequacy requirement, at least in its weak sense.

Finally, the contributors to this volume highlight that from the outset their studies were jointly designed and financing was jointly obtained by researchers and members of the studied training field (Nordenström et al.), and/or that researchers closely collaborated with the studied medical/healthcare providers, educators, and/or lay members throughout the research process (Åberg & Ivarsson; Keel et al.; Merlino; Nordenström et al.; Toerien). While some contributions stress that the collaboration was driven by the aim of ensuring that the investigated phenomena and the educational interventions (Åberg & Ivarsson; Keel et al.; Nordenström; Toerien) were relevant for the work and training practices from a member's point of view, meaning that they were "topically relevant to the parties in the actual empirical lived workplace occasions of the work [they] describe" (Garfinkel, 2002, p. 100; see also Parry, 2016, p. 1283), others point out that collaborative encounters emerged out of the long-lasting collaboration between the researcher and the members of the field (Merlino), and were from the outset organized as part of the medical/healthcare practitioners' ongoing training (Aberg & Ivarsson), as aiming to contribute to it (Ikeya et al.; Keel, et al.), and/or to invite practitioners of the field (Aberg & Ivarsson; Ikeya et al.; Nordenström et al.; Toerien) to "bring their expertise to bear upon the quality, insightfulness and rigour of analytic insights and findings" (see Heath et al., 2007, p. 114).

The distinction between "applied" and "hybrid" studies of medical/healthcare settings is fraught with difficulties and worthy of a book-length study itself. It is neither the purpose of this collection nor the goal of its introduction to explore this matter in any detail. However, in contrast to criticisms made of the meaning and relevance of conducting hybrid studies from an EM point of view (see Sormani, 2019), it is argued here that outlining how contributors to the volume collaborated closely with the studied professionals and lay members to conduct their research yields a good understanding of the practices under investigation, and informs practice and education. This then allows for insight that is relevant for the development of applied studies, EMCA research, and the medical/healthcare work and training fields alike.

Conclusion

This volume encompasses studies on a wide array of medical/healthcare work and training encounters and includes contributions that adopt distinct EMCA approaches (see e.g., Luff et al., 2000; Schegloff, 1987; Sormani, 2019) and ways of collaborating with the studied work and training field for the purpose of addressing, examining, and describing members' competences and socialization in medical/healthcare interactions and of contributing to medical/healthcare education and research.

Yet, the nine investigations all present to readers how to discover "a phenomenon in a noisy practical field" (Lynch & Eisenmann, 2022, p. 107) and reveal "'seen but unnoticed,' expected, background features of everyday [working and training] scenes" (Garfinkel, 1967, p. 36). In its scope, the volume provides new insights into the ways social interactions are organized and made intelligible in the wild: how medical/healthcare members constantly and competently adapt their actions to emerging working and training problems and how solutions are in turn discovered, evaluated, and corrected as situated and embodied practical accomplishments.

The volume thus invites readers to *practice EMCA investigation* "in and as its constitutive multiplicity, both from within and across, if not against its major strands" (Sormani, 2019, p. 15). All of its contributors took care to provide "careful descriptions" of the studied work and training practices, i.e., descriptions that are "written in natural language, which can be read in alternate ways depending on the occasion; that is, as descriptions, as instructions, or as actions produced in response to those instructions, 'without absurd errors and other incongruities'" (Garfinkel, 2002, p. 101, quoted in Ikeya, 2020, p. 27). It is hoped that readers will be able to discover or rediscover the wealth of competences that members of medical/healthcare work and training settings display to accomplish their tasks and will in turn be inspired to engage in collaborative EMCA investigations of medical/healthcare interactions with a view to informing practices, education, or policy.

Notes

1 Note that although they adopt distinct methods to describe members' situated and embodied organization of interactions, all of the contributions in this volume include excerpts and/or figures of sequences of filmed interactions that adopt or draw on EMCA transcription conventions developed by Jefferson (2004) and Mondada (2018). An overview of these conventions appears after this introduction.
2 The paper by Parry et al. (2016) discusses the challenges involved in getting access to and filming in medical/healthcare, in which informed patient consent and ethical issues are of paramount importance. It provides a literature review and recommendations on video research in medical/healthcare settings.

References

Collins, S., Drew, P., Watt, I., & Entwistle, V. (2005). 'Unilateral' and 'bilateral' practitioner approaches in decision-making about treatment. *Social Science and Medicine*, *61*(12), 2611–2627. https://doi.org/10.1016/j.socscimed.2005.04.047

Dalley, D., Rahman, R., & Ivaldi, A. (2021). Health care professionals' and patients' management of the interactional practices in telemedicine videoconferencing: A conversation analytic and discursive systematic review. *Qualitative Health Research*, *31*(4). https://doi.org/10.1177/1049732320942346

de Kok, B. C., Widdicombe, S., Pilnick, A., & Laurier, E. (2018). Doing patient-centredness versus achieving public health targets: A critical review of interactional dilemmas in ART adherence support. *Social Science and Medicine*, *205*, 17–25. https://doi.org/10.1016/j.socscimed.2018.03.030

Drew, P., Chatwin, J., & Collins, S. (2001). Conversation analysis: A method for research into interactions between patients and health-care professionals. *Health Expectations*, *4*(1), 58–70. http://onlinelibrary.wiley.com/store/10.1046/j.1369-6513.2001.00125.x/asset/j.1369-6513.2001.00125.x.pdf?v=1&t=i5p0vv4d&s=9cd25109697af2460ca42fcbd1a3f6c43fff750c

Elsey, C., Challinor, A., & Monrouxe, L. V. (2017). Patients embodied and as-a-body within bedside teaching encounters: A video ethnographic study. *Advances in Health Sciences Education*, *22*(1), 123–146. https://doi.org/10.1007/s10459-016-9688-3

Frankel, R. M. (1990). Talking in interviews: A dispreference for patient-initiated questions in physician-patient encounters. In G. Psathas (Ed.), *Interaction competence* (pp. 231–262). International Institute for Ethnomethodology and Conversation Analysis & University Press of America.

Garfinkel, H. (1967). *Studies in ethnomethodology*. Prentice-Hall.

Garfinkel, H. (2002). *Ethnomethodology's program: Durkheim's aphorisme*. Rowman & Littlefield Publishers, Inc.

Garfinkel, H., Girton, G., Livingston, E., & Sacks, H. (1982). *Studies of Kids' Culture and Kids' Talk*. unpublished research project. University of California.

Garfinkel, H., & Sacks, H. (1970). On formal structures of practical action. In J. McKinney & E. A. Tiryakian (Eds.), *Theoretical sociology* (pp. 337–366). Appleton Century Crofts.

Gill, T. V., & Roberts, F. (2012). Conversation analysis in medicine. In J. Sidnell & T. Stivers (Eds.), *The handbook of conversation analysis* (pp. 575–592). Balckwell Publishing Ltd.

González-Martínez, E., Bangerter, A., Le Van, K., & Navarro, C. (2016). Hospital staff corridor conversations: Work in passing. *Journal of Advanced Nursing*, *72*(3), 521–532. https://doi.org/10.1111/jan.12842

González-Martínez, E., & Bulliard, C. (2018). Collaboration interprofessionnelle jeune infirmière diplômée-assistante sociale : Appels téléphoniques de préparation de la sortie de l'hôpital. *Recherche en Soins Infirmiers*, *133*(2), 15–36.

Halpin, S. N., Konomos, M., & Roulson, K. (2021). Using applied conversation analysis in patient education. *Global Qualitative Nursing Research*, *8*, 23333936211012990. https://doi.org/10.1177/23333936211012990

Harwood, R. H., O'Brien, R., Goldberg, S. E., Allwood, R., Pilnick, A., Beeke, S., Thomson, L., Murray, M., Parry, R., Kearney, F., Baxendale, B., Sartain, K., & Schneider, J. (2018). A staff training intervention to improve communication between people living with dementia and health-care professionals in hospital: The VOICE mixed-methods development and evaluation study. *Health Services and Delivery Research*, *6*(41), 1–134.

Heath, C. (1986). *Body movement and speech in medical interaction*. Cambridge University Press.

Heath, C., Luff, P., & Svensson, M. S. (2003). Technology and medical practice. *Sociology of Health and Illness*, *25*(3), 75–96.

Heath, C., Luff, P., & Svensson, M. S. (2007). Video and qualitative research: Analysing medical practice and interaction. *Medical Education*, *41*(1), 109–116. https://doi.org/10.1111/j.1365-2929.2006.02641.x

Heritage, J. (1984). *Garfinkel and ethnomethodology*. Polity Press.

Heritage, J., Elliott, M. N., Stivers, T., Richardson, A., & Mangione-Smith, R. (2010). Reducing inappropriate antibiotics prescribing: The role of online commentary on physical examination findings. *Patient Education and Counseling*, *811*(1), 119–125. https://doi.org/10.1016/j.pec.2009.12.005

Heritage, J., & Maynard, D. W. (Eds.). (2006a). *Communication in medical care interaction between primary care physicians and patients*. Cambridge University Press.

Heritage, J., & Maynard, D. W. (2006b). Problems and prospects in the study of physician-patient interaction: 30 years of research. *Annual Revue of Sociology*, *32*(1), 351–374.

Heritage, J., & Robinson, J. D. (2011). 'Some' versus 'any' medical issues: Encouraging patients to reveal their unmet concerns. In C. Antaki (Ed.), *Applied conversation analysis. Palgrave advances in linguistics* (pp. 15–31). Palgrave Macmillan. https://doi.org/10.1057/9780230316874_2

Heritage, J., Robinson, J. D., Elliott, M. N., & Beckett, M. (2007). Reducing patients' unmet concerns in primary care: The difference one word can make. *Journal of General Internal Medicine*, *22*(10), 1429–1433. http://www.ncbi.nlm.nih.gov/pmc/articles/PMC2305862/pdf/11606_2007_Article_279.pdf

Hindmarsh, J. (2010). Peripherality, participation and communities of practice: Examining the patient in dental training. In N. Llewellyn & J. Hindmarsh (Eds.), *Organisation, interaction and practice* (pp. 218–239). Cambridge University Press.

Hindmarsh, J., Hyland, L., & Banerjee, A. (2014). Work to make simulation work: 'Realism', instructional correction and the body in training. *Discourse Studies*, *16*(2), 247–269. https://doi.org/10.1177/1461445613514670

Hindmarsh, J., Jenkings, K. N., & Rapley, T. (2007). Introduction to healthcare technologies in practice. *Health Informatics Journal*, *13*(1), 5–8. https://doi.org/10.1177/1460458207073642

Hindmarsh, J., Reynolds, P., & Dunne, S. (2011). Exhibiting understanding: The body in apprenticeship. *Journal of Pragmatics*, *43*(2), 489–503. https://doi.org/10.1016/j.pragma.2009.09.008

Ikeya, N. (2020). Hybridity of hybrid studies of work: Examination of informing practitioners in practice. *Ethnographic Studies*, *17*, 22–40. https://doi.org/10.5281/zenodo.405053

Ivarsson, J., & Åberg, M. (2020). Role of requests and communication breakdowns in the coordination of teamwork: A video-based observational study of hybrid operating rooms. *BMJ Open*, *10*(5), e035194. https://doi.org/10.1136/bmjopen-2019-035194

Jenkins, L., & Reuber, M. (2014). A conversation analytic intervention to help neurologists identify diagnostically relevant linguistic features in seizure patients' talk. *Research on Language and Social Interaction*, *47*(3), 266–279.

Keel, S. (2016). *Socialization: Parent-child interaction in everyday life*. Routledge.

Koschmann, T., LeBaron, C., Goodwin, C., & Feltovich, P. (2011). "Can you see the cystic artery yet?" A simple matter of trust. *Journal of Pragmatics*, *43*(2), 521–541. https://doi.org/10.1016/j.pragma.2009.09.009

Lindwall, O. (2014). The body in medical work and medical training: An introduction. *Discourse Studies*, *16*(2), 125–129. https://doi.org/10.1177/1461445613514671

Lindwall, O., & Lymer, G. (2014). Inquiries of the body: Novice questions and the instructable observability of endodontic scenes. *Discourse Studies*, *16*(2), 271–294. https://doi.org/10.1177/1461445613514672

Lindwall, O., Lymer, G., & Greiffenhagen, C. (2015). The sequential analysis of instruction. In N. Markee (Ed.), *The handbook of classroom discourse and interaction* (pp. 142–157). John Wiley & Sons, Inc.

Luff, P., Hindmarsh, J., & Heath, C. (Eds.). (2000). *Workplace studies: Recovering work practice and informing system design*. Cambridge University Press.

Lynch, M., & Eisenmann, C. (2022). Transposing Gestalt phenomena from visual fields to practical and interactional work: Garfinkel's and Sacks' social praxeology. *Philosophia Scientiae*, *26*(3), 95–122. https://doi.org/10.4000/philosophiascientiae.3619

Macbeth, D. (2003). Hugh Meha''s "learning lessons" reconsidered: On the differences between the naturalistic and critical analysis of classroom discourse. *Research in Language and Social Interaction*, *40*, 239–280.

Macbeth, D. (2004). The relevance of repair for classroom correction. *Language in Society*, *33*(5), 703–736.

Macbeth, D. (2014). Studies of work, instructed action, and the promise of granularity: A commentary. *Discourse Studies*, *16*(2), 295–308. https://doi.org/10.1177/1461445613514676

Mackay, R. (1975). Conceptions and models of socialization. In R. Turner (Ed.), *Ethnomethodology* (pp. 180–193). Penguin Books

Mangione-Smith, R., Elliott, M. N., Stivers, T., McDonald, L., & Heritage, J. (2006). Ruling out the need for antibiotics: Are we sending the right message? *Archives of Pediatric and Adolescent Medicine*, *160*(9), 945–952.

Martin, C., & Sahlström, F. (2010). Learning as longitudinal interactional change: From other-repair to self-repair in physiotherapy treatment. *Discourse Processes*, *47*(8), 668–697. https://doi.org/10.1080/01638531003628965

Maynard, D. (1991). Interaction and asymmetry in clinical discourse. *American Journal of Sociology*, *97*(2), 448–495.

Maynard, D. W., & Heritage, J. (2005). Conversation analysis, doctor-patient interaction and medical communication. *Medical Education*, *39*(4), 428–435. https://doi.org/10.1111/j.1365-2929.2005.02111.x

Maynard, D. W., & Turowetz, J. J. (2022). Ethnomethodology and atypical interaction: The case of autism. In D. W. Maynard & J. Heritage (Eds.), *The ethnomethodology program: Legacies and prospects* (pp. 442–475). Oxford University Press.

Mayor, E., & Bietti, L. (2017). Ethnomethodological studies of nurse-patient and nurse-relative interactions: A scoping review. *International Journal of Nursing Studies*, *70*, 46–57. https://doi.org/10.1016/j.ijnurstu.2017.01.015

Merlino, S. (2018). Assisting the client in aphasia speech therapy: A sequential and multimodal analysis of cueing practices. *Hacettepe University Journal of Education*, 1–24. https://doi.org/10.16986/huje.2018038810

Merlino, S. (2020). Professional touch in speech and language therapy for the treatment of post-stroke aphasia. In A. Cekaite & L. Mondada (Eds.), *Touch in social interaction. Touch, language, and body* (pp. 197–223). Routledge.

Mondada, L. (2003). Working with video: How surgeons produce video records of their actions. *Visual Studies*, *18*(1), 58–73. https://doi.org/10.1080/1472586032000100083

Mondada, L. (2006). Video recording as the reflexive preservation and configuration of phenomenal features for analysis. In H. Knoblauch, B. Schnettler, J. Raab, & H.-G. Soeffner (Eds.), *Video analysis: Methodology and methods* (pp. 52–67). Peter Lang.

Mondada, L. (2014). Instructions in the operating room: How the surgeon directs their assistant's hands. *Discourse Studies*, *16*(2), 131–161. https://doi.org/10.1177/1461445613515325

Parry, R. (2005). A video analysis of how physiotherapists communicate with patients about errors of performance: Insights for practice and policy. *Physiotherapy*, *91*(4), 204–214. https://doi.org/10.1016/j.physio.2005.05.004

Parry, R., & Land, V. (2013). Systematically reviewing and synthesizing evidence from conversation analytic and related discursive research to inform healthcare communication practice and policy: An illustrated guide. *BMC Medical Research Methodology*, *13*(69), 1–13.

Parry, R., Pino, M., Faull, C., & Feathers, L. (2016). Acceptability and design of video-based research on healthcare communication: Evidence and recommendations. *Patient Education and Counseling*, *99*(8), 1271–1284. https://doi.org/10.1016/j.pec.2016.03.013

Parry, R., Whittaker, B., Pino, M., Jenkins, L., Worthington, E., & Faull, C. (2022). RealTalk evidence-based communication training resources: Development of conversation analysis-based materials to support training in end-of-life-related health and social care conversations. *BMC Medical Education*, *22*(1). https://doi.org/10.1186/s12909-022-03641-y

Pilnick, A. (fth). Medicine and healthcare. In A. Carlin, A. Dennis, O. Lindwall, M. Mair, & K. N. Jenkings (Eds.), *Routledge international handbook of ethnomethodology & conversation analysis*. Routledge.

Pilnick, A., & Dingwall, R. (2011). On the remarkable persistence of asymmetry in doctor/patient interaction: A critical review. *Social Science and Medicine*, *72*(8), 1374–1382. https://doi.org/10.1016/j.socscimed.2011.02.033

Pilnick, A., Hindmarsh, J., & Gill, T. V. (2009). Beyond 'doctor and patient': Developments in the study of healthcare interactions. *Sociology of Health and Illness*, *31*(6), 787–802.

Pilnick, A., Trusson, D., Beeke, S., O'Brien, R., Goldberg, S., & Harwood, R. H. (2018). Using conversation analysis to inform role play and simulated interaction in communications skills training for healthcare professionals: Identifying avenues for further development through a scoping review. *BMC Medical Education*, *18*(1). https://doi.org/10.1186/s12909-018-1381-1

Psathas, G. (Ed.). (1990a). *Interaction competence*. International Institute for Ethnomethodology and Conversation Analysis & University Press of America.

Psathas, G. (1990b). The organization of talk, gaze, and activity in a medical interview. In G. Psathas (Ed.), *Interaction competence* (pp. 206–230). International Institute for Ethnomethodology and Conversation Analysis & University Press of America.

Relieu, M. (1994). Les catégories dans l'action. L'apprentissage des traversées de rue par des nonvoyants. In B. Fradin, L. Quéré, & J. Widmer (Eds.), *L'enquête sur les catégories. De Durkheim à Sacks* (pp. 185–218). Editions de l'école des hautes études en sciences sociales.

Robinson, J. D., & Heritage, J. (2014). Intervening with conversation analysis: The case of medicine. *Research on Language and Social Interaction*, *47*(3), 201–218.

Sacks, H. (1967). The search for help: No one to turn to. In E. S. Schneidman (Ed.), *Essays in self-destruction* (pp. 203–223). Science House Publishers.

Sacks, H. (1992). *Lectures on conversation* (Vol. (I+II)). Blackwell Publishers.

Sacks, H., Schegloff, E., & Jefferson, G. (1974). A simplest systematics for the organization of turn taking for conversation. *Language, 50*(4), 696–735.

Sanchez Svensson, M. S., Luff, P., & Heath, C. (2009). Embedding instruction in practice: Contingency and collaboration during surgical training. *Sociology of Health and Illness, 31*(6), 889–906. https://doi.org/10.1111/j.1467-9566.2009.01195.x

Schegloff, E. (1987). Analyzing single episodes of interaction: An exercise in conversation analysis. *American Sociological Association, 50*(2), 101–114.

Schegloff, E., Jefferson, G., & Sacks, H. (1977). The preference for self-correction in the organization of repair in conversation. *Language, 53*(2), 361–382. https://doi.org/10.1353/lan.1977.0041

Schoeb, V., Hartmeier, A., & Keel, S. (2015). Reflexion als Sprungbrett für Veränderungen im Praxisalltag. *Schweizerische Ärztezeitung, 96*(5), 132–135. https://www.researchgate.net/publication/271509194_Reflexion_als_Sprungbrett_fur_Veranderungen_im_Praxisalltag

Sormani, P. (2019). Ethnomethodological analysis. In P. Atkinson, S. Delamont, A. Cernat, J. W. Sakshaug, & R. A. Williams (Eds.), *Sage Research methods foundations* (Sage ed.). https://doi.org/10.4135/9781526421036788330

Sudnow, D. (1967). *Passing on: The social organization of dying.* Prentice Hall.

Ten Have, P. (1995). Medical ethnomethodology: An overview. *Human Studies, 18*(2–3), 245–261.

Toerien, M., Shaw, R., Duncan, R., & Reuber, M. (2011). Offering patients choices: A pilot study of interactions in the seizure clinic. *Epilepsy and Behavior, 20*(2), 312–320. https://doi.org/10.1016/j.yebeh.2010.11.004

Vom Lehn, D., & Heath, C. (2022). Embedding impact in research: Addressing the interactional production of workplace activities. *British Journal of Management, 33*(2), 539–552. https://doi.org/10.1111/1467-8551.12468

Watson, R. (1992). Ethnometodology, conversation analysis and education: An overview. *International Review of Education, 38*(3), 257–274.

Wilkinson, R. (2014). Intervening with conversation analysis in speech and language therapy: Improving aphasic conversation. *Research on Language and Social Interaction, 47*(3), 219–238. https://doi.org/10.1080/08351813.2014.925659

Wilkinson, R., Rae, J., & Rasmussen, G. (Eds.) (2020). *Atypical interaction. The impact of communicative impairments within everyday talk.* Palgrave Macmillan.

Zemel, A., & Koschmann, T. (2014). 'Put your fingers right in here': Learnability and instructed experience. *Discourse Studies*, 16(2), 163–183.

Transcription conventions

Transcription conventions for talk-in-interaction developed by Gail Jefferson (2004, pp. 24–31)

[	A left bracket indicates the beginning of overlapping talk.
]	A right bracket indicates the end of overlapping talk.
=	Equal signs indicate no break or gap (latching talk). A pair of equal signs, one at the end of one line and one at the beginning of a next, indicate no break between the two lines.
(1.0)	Numbers in parentheses indicate a timed pause (measured in tenths of seconds) within or between utterances.
(.)	A dot in parentheses indicates a brief interval (+/– a tenth of a second) within or between utterances.
YES	Upper case indicates extra loud sounds relative to the surrounding talk.
yes	Underscoring indicates some stress, via pitch and/or amplitude.
°yes°	Degree signs bracketing an utterance or parts of it indicate that the sounds are softer than the surrounding talk. The more degree signs there are, the softer the sound.
>yes<	Right/left carats bracketing an utterance or utterance part indicate that the bracketed material is sped up compared to the surrounding talk.
((smile))	Double parentheses contain transcriber's descriptions.:: Colons indicate prolongation of the immediately prior sound. The longer the row of colons, the longer the prolongation.
par-	A dash indicates a cut-off.
.h	A dot-prefixed row of h's indicates an in-breath. Without the dot, the h's indicate an out-breath.
xxxxx	A row of x's indicates that the transcriber was unable to grasp what was said. The number of x's reflects the length of the missing talk.
(a little)	Parenthesized words indicate a guess at the talk.
(( ))	Doubled parentheses contain transcriber's descriptions.
?	A question mark indicates upward intonation.
.	A dot indicates a downward intonation.
,	A comma indicates a continuing intonation.

Transcription conventions for embodied actions developed by Lorenza Mondada (2018, p. 106)[1]

* *	Descriptions of embodied movements are delimited between
+ +	two identical symbols (one symbol per participant's line of action) and are synchronized with corresponding stretches of talk/lapses of time.
*--->	The action described continues across subsequent lines
---->*	until the same symbol is reached.
>>	The action described begins before the extract's beginning.
--->>	The action described continues after the extract's end.
.....	Preparation.
----	Full extension of the movement is reached and maintained.
,,,,,	Retraction.
ava	Participant doing the embodied action is identified when (s)he is not the speaker.
fig #	The exact moment at which a screen shot has been taken is indicated with a symbol showing its temporal position within turn at talk/segments of time.

Note

1 For a more detailed version see also: https://www.lorenzamondada.net/_files/ugd/ ba0dbb_3978d2a34cf44376adb7a341975d23aa.pdf

References

Jefferson, G. (2004). Glossary of transcript symbols with an introduction. In G. H. Lerner (Ed.), *Conversation Analysis: Studies from the first generation* (pp. 13–31). Benjamins. https://doi.org/10.1075/pbns.125.02jef

Mondada, L. (2018). Multiple temporalities of language and body in interaction: Challenges for transcribing multimodality. *Research on Language and Social Interaction*, 51, 85–106. https://doi.org/10.1080/08351813.2018.1413878

1 When neurologists solicit patients' treatment preferences

The relevance of talk as action for understanding why shared decision-making is so limited in practice

Merran Toerien

Introduction

Shared decision-making (SDM) is now accepted as an ideal within many healthcare systems around the world – including the UK's National Health Service (NHS), where the present study was conducted. Although there is a range of definitions (for reviews, see Bomhof-Roordink et al., 2019; Makoul & Clayman, 2006; Moumjid et al., 2007), SDM can be described, most simply, as patients and clinicians working together to decide on the best care plan for the individual (Rake et al., 2022). Core to this process is eliciting the patient's "personal perspective on their health, based on the individual's context, values, and preferences" (Rake et al., 2022, p. 2860). Although this may sound straightforward, a recent systematic review found low levels of "personal perspective elicitation" across almost 100 empirical studies of decision-making in clinical practice (Rake et al., 2022, p. 2860). Such studies are important for highlighting the gap between SDM as an ideal and what happens in real decision-making interactions. However, this entails largely a focus on failure. We can read this focus – in line with the theme of this edited collection – as a concern about the failure of long-standing attempts to (re)socialise clinicians from a more "paternalistic" approach to a more "collaborative" one. This concern is significant, given the moral case for SDM (see Stiggelbout et al., 2015). However, the focus on failure leaves us with a very important question: what happens, interactionally, when clinicians *do* enact one or more of the elements of SDM? In this chapter, I address this question with respect to eliciting patients' views. I argue that, by seeing what talk about patients' views is used to do, "in the wild," we gain a much better understanding of why the ideal of SDM is so difficult to implement consistently in practice.

I take a conversation analytic (CA) approach, which means that I start from the understanding of talk as social action; in other words, talk is a means to do things. This contrasts starkly with the widespread model of talk as a mechanism for information exchange (see Drew, 2005; Schegloff, 1996). The latter perspective maintains a focus on *what* gets said. For instance, Rake et al.'s (2022) systematic review also found that, on the rare occasions when patients' perspectives were elicited, clinicians asked only about physical health, leaving social or psychological matters unaddressed. Moreover, they seldom went on to integrate what was discussed into the patient's care plan. Again, then, we have some important insights into failures to enact the ideal of SDM. What we do not know, is what clinicians and patients are *doing* when they do talk about the patient's views.

The analysis presented in this chapter builds on a rare exception in the literature. Using CA, Landmark et al. (2017) investigated how clinicians in a Norwegian teaching hospital talked about patients' treatment preferences. They identified an interactional practice that involves the clinician formulating a hypothesis about the patient's preference and then making a treatment option contingent on that preference (i.e., "If you think X + we/you can do Y") (p. 2081). These hypotheses could be framed in different ways, but, in all cases, the hypotheses were used in a sequential context where the patient had already indicated some resistance to a recommended option. The practice was thus typically used to try to secure acceptance of what the clinician thought was best. Positively framed hypotheses were used to promote the clinician's already stated recommendation, e.g., "If you have a bit of patience and could wait..." (p. 2084), followed by another version of the original recommendation. Negative framing was used to present an alternative to the recommended treatment, but in such a way as to discourage the patient from choosing it, e.g., "If you are very impatient then..." (p. 2084), followed by an option that was presented as less optimal than the recommended option. Even the more neutrally framed hypotheses could be embedded in a complex turn that was tilted toward acceptance of the clinician's recommendation. "The effect", Landmark et al. argue, "is a communicative 'double bind'" (p. 2086): even as the clinicians were ostensibly offering a choice, they were simultaneously presenting the patient's (resistant) position as sub-optimal relative to their own.

Landmark et al.'s (2017) study exemplifies what is to be gained by studying decision-making "in the wild." By focusing on the situated practice of talk about patients' perspectives, they go beyond the binary question of whether or not such talk occurs. By understanding talk as action, they show how, even when it does occur, such talk may not have the effect of truly enacting the SDM ideal. In this chapter, I take up their call for more fine-grained analysis of how patients' views are discussed in practice. Also using conversation analysis – but with a much larger dataset – I show that patients' views may be elicited in two recurrent sequential locations: (i) in post-recommendation position (i.e., after a treatment recommendation has already been made); and (ii) in pre-recommendation position (i.e., just prior to a recommendation that is projected to be forthcoming). The first of these accords with Landmark et al.'s findings: I show how a patient view elicitor (PVE), when it comes after a recommendation, may be heard as pursuing the *clinician's* preferred option. The second of these offers some novel insights: I show how, by seeking to establish the patient's preferences as a first step in the decision-making process, clinicians can avoid the double bind that Landmark et al. highlighted.

However, I also show how PVEs used in pre-recommendation position have their own limitations with respect to enacting the SDM ideal. I conclude by discussing an evidence-based solution to these challenges and by reflecting on what the idea of talk as action can contribute to our understanding of why SDM is so hard to enact in practice.

Data, methods, and defining "patient view elicitors"

The analysis reported in this chapter arises out of a wider, collaborative study, funded by a grant from the UK's National Institute for Health and Care Research. Our team recorded 223 neurology consultations in two large neuroscience centers in the UK in 2012. The primary aim of the study was inductive: we employed conversation analysis to identify the practices used by neurologists to offer patients choice and the interactional consequences thereof. Following our foundational CA work, we coded for the interactional practices we had identified. This allowed for statistical claims about their relative use across our dataset (for our project reports, see Reuber et al., 2015; Reuber et al., 2018).

Our team included conversation analysts and neurologists, working in close collaboration. Thus, although our starting point was always the recorded interactions, our focus was guided, from the start, by what practitioners themselves experienced as challenging in their day-to-day encounters with patients. This drew our attention to their experience of dual demands, which are not always easy to reconcile: on the one hand, neurologists are expected to use their expertise to make patients better (or at least better able to cope with chronic conditions); on the other hand, they are also expected to empower patients to make their own decisions about their care. Our focus on how "patient choice" plays out in real decision-making sequences thus arises out of the lived experience of practitioners, rather than an abstract interest. At the same time, our specific findings have emerged from what's observably happening in the give-and-take of real decision-making sequences, captured "in the wild" (see Ikeya, 2020, for more on this "hybrid" approach to ethnomethodological work).

The neurologists in our dataset oriented to patients' right to choose in a variety of ways. We coined the umbrella term "patient view elicitor" (PVE) to capture a range of turn designs that we identified, inductively, within our recordings. What holds them together is that they serve to *explicitly invite* the patient to express a preference, their thoughts or feelings about a treatment, medical investigation, or referral option. These include open formats (e.g., "What do you think of that") and closed formats (e.g., "D'you want to try some steroids"). The term PVE is akin to what Rake et al. (2022) call "personal perspective elicitation," which they define as:

> The disclosure (either elicited by the clinician or spontaneously expressed by the patient) of information related to the patient's preferences, values, and/or context, that are potentially relevant to the process of decision-making.
> (p. 2861)

Like Rake et al. (2022), I recognize that patients' perspectives can be woven into the decision-making in a host of subtle ways, not all of which depend on the clinician's active solicitation. For instance, in their CA study of how clinicians broach whether to undertake cardiopulmonary resuscitation (CPR) with older patients admitted to a Swiss-francophone hospital, Sterie et al. (2022) showed how even pronouncements (Stivers et al., 2017), strongly in favor of CPR, can be done in a way that "highlight[s] the role of the patient in the decision process" (p. 889). This accords with a long-standing line of research in CA showing how patients can influence decision-making even through passive resistance (see Stivers, 2005; Koenig, 2011). I agree entirely with these important observations. However, if we are to understand what happens when clinicians demonstrably enact elements of SDM, then there's value in distinguishing between *recommending* and *patient view eliciting* as approaches to decision-making. While different recommendation formats will certainly encode varying degrees of pressure for the patient to accept what the clinician thinks is best, recommendations set up a slot in which acceptance of the clinician's treatment preference is the interactionally preferred response. By contrast, patient view elicitors set up a slot in which the decision is explicitly made contingent on the patient's preference (Toerien, 2021). Thus, I would not code pronouncements like "so uh ... if there's a problem with uh: the heart or something general ... we resuscitate you" (Sterie et al., 2022, p. 998) as a patient view elicitor, even though I agree with Sterie et al.'s (2022) analysis that such a turn requires the patient's validation. Similarly, this chapter will retain our term – "patient view elicitor" – to avoid broadening our focus to the spontaneous disclosure of a preference by the patient, as captured by Rake et al.'s (2022) term. Our focus, in other words, is firmly on what happens when clinicians actively seek to solicit patients' views.

In line with studies using other methodologies, we found that the neurologists in our dataset were far more likely to recommend a treatment than to offer the patient a choice. Nevertheless, from 623 instances that we coded as decision-points about a treatment, referral, or investigation, we were able to build a collection of 149 turns that met our definition for a patient view elicitor (Chappell et al., 2018). It is this collection that I draw on in the present chapter. In the two analytic sections, below, I focus on two recurrent locations where these PVEs occurred: in post-recommendation and pre-recommendation position.

Analysis

Soliciting the patient's treatment preference in post-recommendation position: A means to pursue acceptance

One recurrent position in which neurologists sought patients' treatment preferences in our dataset was *after* they had made a recommendation. Unavoidably, due to their sequential placement, PVEs in post-recommendation position can only be understood by reference to the (often extensive) decision-making sequence that comes before them. It is thus only practical to work through a single, illustrative case in this section. For clarity, I have divided the example into three consecutive parts (shown in Extracts 1a–c[1]). These map onto three key moments in how the neurologist directs the decision-making, which can be summarized as follows:

1. The neurologist initiates the decision with an option-list, laying out a choice between two alternatives (Extract 1a);
2. He then shifts to a recommendation, indicating his preference for the first option (Extract 1b);
3. Having failed to secure the patient's acceptance of his recommended treatment, he pursues with another recommendation (Extract 1c).

In the rest of this analytic section, I will track these key moments, showing that the patient does reveal her treatment preference and the neurologist does explicitly seek her views. Thus, some of the "machinery" of shared decision-making can be seen in operation in this example. However, by examining how this "machinery" works in practice, we can see how the discussion of the patient's preferences is being done in the service of other social actions: resisting the neurologist's recommended option and pursuing the patient's acceptance of that option.

The patient in our example has possible multiple sclerosis (MS) and has described some difficulty with climbing stairs. Just before Extract 1a, the neurologist has reminded the patient of some recent test results, sent to her by post. These suggest she is at risk of further inflammation, but the diagnosis is not yet definite. The test results thus lay the groundwork for decision-making, but do not indicate a definitive next step with respect to treatment. We join the consultation as the neurologist indicates that there is, rather, a choice: "two ways of dealing with this" (l. 1). Using an approach that we have called option-listing (Toerien et al., 2013; Toerien et al., 2018), he lays out two possibilities: she can take a short-term course of oral steroids, which can help MS patients to recover more quickly following a period when their symptoms have worsened; or she can be referred to an MS specialist who may be able to recommend other forms of treatment. By setting up the decision with an option-list, the neurologist appears to be opening a slot for the patient to consider which of these alternatives she may prefer. This is evident also in how he makes the steroid option contingent on her *self*-assessment of her current condition (l. 2–6), using the same format identified by Landmark et al. (2017): "If you think X + we/you can do Y" (p. 2081). By the end of Extract 1a, then, the neurologist has laid a foundation for discussing the patient's preferences, as many SDM models suggest should occur.

Please note that, in all the transcripts, "Neu" refers to the neurologist and "Pat" to the patient. The code for each extract indicates the location of recording ("S" for site 1, "G" for site 2), the unique patient ID (first three digits), and the unique neurologist ID (last two digits).

Extract 1a (G01805)

```
01 Neu:  And there's two: ways of dealing with this,
02       (0.2) If you: don't feel that things are (1.2)
03       absolutely back to normal,=if you still feel
04       that you're inhibited a wee bit (0.2) in this:.
05       .hh then I can (0.3) give you some (0.3)
06       steroid treatment for a short while,
07 Pat:  Mhm,
08       (0.9)
09 Neu:  .tchhh and we could see how you (1.0) do after tha:t,
10 Pat:  Yeah.
11       (0.7)
12 Neu:  Alternatively I could arrange for you to be seen by one
13       of our (0.5) MS specialists.
14 Pat:  Uhuh,
15       (0.4)
16 Neu:  Er get them to see you and see if they think that the
17       (2.1) inflammation=the cha::nge in the signal. (.)
18       would benefit from some (0.5) other forms of treatment.
19       (0.4)
20 Pat:  Mhm.
```

Throughout Extract 1a, the patient only produces minimal responses (see turns in boldface). There is good evidence from the prior literature that minimal responses are typically understood as a form of passive resistance in response to treatment recommendations (Koenig, 2011; Stivers, 2005). However, I would caution against assuming that the same applies in response to option-lists. Not only would it be premature for the patient to accept the first option before hearing the second (e.g., at l. 7), but we found that, when options were listed, patients generally waited for an explicit slot to voice their views – even when they went on to choose without any interactional trouble (Reuber et al., 2018). This slot was created with a patient view elicitor. In Extract 1a, this could have come at line 19 or after the minimal turn at line 20. However, as Extract 1b shows, this neurologist changes tack. Having started with an option-list, he now makes a recommendation for the first option: steroids (l. 21–24). He justifies this based on the patient's prior report of a symptom: "having difficulty with the< stai::rs," (l. 23-24). This recasts the optionality introduced in Extract 1a (l. 2–6) as something that he has already assessed: she is not "absolutely back to normal" and thus treatment "make[s] sense" to *him* (l. 24). There is, then, a shift from foregrounding the relevance of the patient's preference (in Extract 1a) to foregrounding his own (in Extract 1b).

Extract 1b (G01805)

```
21 Neu: Rec  →  .Hhhh Now no matter what happens (0.3) I think
22            →  a short course of steroids may well be helpful=
23            →  >If you're having difficulty with the< stai::rs,
24            →  .hh that would make sense to me.
25              (0.5)
```

```
26  Neu:  Pur →  Is that absolutely essential, no it's not.
27              (0.5)
28         →    But I think if you're tellin' me that you
29         →    h've problems on the stai::rs,=
30  Pat:        =It's j's:t (.) you fee:l the tingles more
31              (0.1) [doctor.
32  Neu:              [ (Mm)
33  Neu:        °Oka[y,°
34  Pat:            [Um: (0.5) and obviously if I'm carrying=
35              which I always am carrying heavy bags 'cos
36              (of-) (.) I work security so .hh I've also
37              got the horses .hh so I've always got a big
38              bag with me with either my uniform in it,
39              (0.2) or my,
40  Neu:        Mhm,
41  Pat:        horsey clothes in it, .hhh so if I'm carrying
42              bags of shoppin' I just (0.2) by the time I get
43              up (0.2) to (the top) flight of stairs I'm startin'
44              to (0.4) feel the pre:ssure a wee bit, (0.2) but
45              I mean it's no: (1.0) cripplin' or sto:ppin' me or
46              anything but-
47  Neu:        °Right.°
48  Pat:        I'm awa:re of it, put it that way.
49  Neu:        °Okay.° .h[hh
50  Pat:                  [I'm aware of it.
```

The patient makes no immediate vocal response to the recommendation (l. 25). Since she declined permission to video record, we cannot tell if there was a non-vocal response. However, we can see the neurologist treating this as passive resistance through his pursuit of acceptance (Stivers & Timmermans, 2020). Although he retains the optionality of treatment (l. 26), he works to persuade the patient, again drawing on her reported symptom (l. 28–29). The patient now responds, resisting the treatment recommendation in two ways. First, she minimizes the symptom, both with the use of "j's:t" and by formulating the symptom as one of "fee:l((ing)) the tingles more" (l. 30). This downgrades the trouble from a practical limitation (struggling to climb stairs) to a sensory experience – and a mild one at that (suggested by the word "tingles"). Second, she normalizes her experience: the stairs present challenges because she's "carrying heavy bags" (l. 35), implying that the problem is one that anybody might experience and thus is not treatment-relevant. She also further minimizes the symptom: it is only when she "get((s)) up (0.2) to (the top) flight of stairs" that she feels anything untoward; even then, she's only "startin' to (0.4) feel the pre:ssure a wee bit" (l. 43–44). Like "tingles", "pressure" does not index pain. Finally, she explicates the lack of impact on her daily routine: "it's no: (1.0) cripplin' or sto:ppin' me or anything" (l. 45–46) (see Toerien, 2021).

Here, then, we have evidence of an exchange of preferences: the neurologist is in favor of steroids while the patient appears not to be. However, to think of this only as an exchange of *information* is to neuter it of its interactional import. The neurologist's preference has been articulated as a recommendation for treatment, with persuasive work done to tilt the recommendation quite strongly in favor of acceptance (l. 21–29). The patient, likewise, is doing interactional work across her extended telling at lines 30–50. By detailing her experience of climbing stairs, she is countering the neurologist's assessment that steroids are indicated. Subtly, without any outright disagreement, she is resisting the neurologist's recommendation. What we have here is not a "pure" exchange of views. This is better understood as a pair of social actions: recommending and resisting treatment (see Stivers, 2005).

Extract 1c shows how the neurologist handles this resistance. At first it seems as if he's going to seek the patient's view of some proposed plan (projected by the "How about" at the start of his turn). However, he self-repairs (note the use of ">I mean" on line 51), the effect of which is to shift back into doing recommending: again, where he first seemed set on foregrounding the relevance of the patient's view, he instead shifts to foreground his own. While he continues to orient to the option of doing nothing (l. 56), thereby implicitly acknowledging the patient's apparent preference, he counters this with a repeated justification for steroids. He also tilts this second recommendation in favor of acceptance by further minimizing what's involved: the option of "some (0.3) steroid treatment for a short while" (l. 5–6, Extract 1a) is transformed into merely "*a wee trial* of a >short course of steroids<" (l. 57–58, Extract 1c, emphasis added). He self-labels his action as providing his "take on this" (l. 55) – as opposed, say, to issuing a directive to the patient (Enfield & Sidnell, 2017). While this suggests an openness to the patient's "take," in its sequential context, this contrasts with what the patient has already said (l. 30–50). He is, then, voicing a contrastive position with the patient's normalizing of her experience on the stairs. The work being done here is thus to (further) pursue acceptance of his prior recommendation for steroids. What's relevant at line 59, then, is the acceptance that has thus far been absent. When the patient does produce a response (l. 60), it is only to make a minimal acknowledgment. In this sequential context – where a treatment recommendation has been pursued with persuasive work by the neurologist – such a response is inadequate for acceptance and is thus understood as a form of passive resistance (Koenig, 2011; Stivers, 2005).

Extract 1c (G01805)

```
51 Neu:        How about (0.9) (uh-)/(I-) >I mean I< (m-)
52              think that whether or not you're seen by the
53        Rec→  MS specialist,=I think if that, (.) if the- if
54          →  these are affecting you, if these are affecting
55          →  what you're doing:. my take on this would be:
56          →  (0.2) could we leave it alone, yeah we could.
57          →  .hh But I think a wee trial of a >short course
58          →  of steroids< would >make a bit of< sense to me:.
59              (0.4)
60 Pat:        Mhm,
61              (0.4)
62 Neu:  PVE→  How d'you feel about that,
63              (1.0)
```

```
64  Pat:         Yeah,
65               (0.2)
66  Pat:         (mhh.)
67               (0.3)
68  Neu:         °Okay.°
69  Pat:         I think,
```

And so, we finally come to our target turn: the patient view elicitor at line 62. A binary, check-list appraisal of the neurologist's practice might simply note that he has indeed sought her preferences; he has even done so with an open-ended question: "How d'you feel about that,". However, the work being done here would be misconstrued without taking account of the longer decision-making sequence that has come before: the option-list and recommendation, the patient's resistant narrative (about the stairs), and the neurologist's pursuit with another version of his recommendation. It is against this backdrop that we must understand the work that the patient view elicitor is doing: further pursuit of the patient's still missing acceptance. The neurologist is creating another slot for her to respond in the context of a prior response that was too minimal to allow him to treat the decision-making as closed (see Stivers, 2005). In overtly seeking the patient's feelings about steroids, the neurologist is not neutrally creating a slot for her to voice an as-yet not known in common treatment preference. He has already displayed an understanding that she'd prefer not to take steroids and has sought to persuade her otherwise. What he is seeking, then, is a *change* in her stated preference.

This helps us to understand the patient's apparently unfitted response to the PVE (l. 64). The delayed "yeah" does not align with the action agenda conveyed by the question's design (Boyd & Heritage, 2006); she does not (now) reveal her feelings about treatment. Instead, what this turn does is to (finally) grant the neurologist his pursued acceptance. Thus, the patient displays her understanding that, in this sequential position, the PVE is no "neutral" question, designed purely to solicit her treatment preferences. Following the lengthy delay (l. 63), her acceptance is hearably reluctant, and is further cast as uncertain, with the increment "I think," (l. 69). Nevertheless, the neurologist treats this as adequate, going on to explain that he will write to the patient's GP, who will then prescribe a specific tablet (data not shown). This reflects the system in the UK's NHS, where the GP typically manages the patient's treatment, even if they are receiving input from a secondary care consultant (such as a neurologist). It is worth noting that they also agree that she will be referred to a specialist (data not shown) – thus, what began as an apparently either/or choice between steroids or a referral becomes a yes/no decision with respect to each of the two options.

This was a lengthy case to work through; I hope that the way I have broken it down has helped to clarify what we gain from understanding both parties' interactional moves in their wider sequential context. To sum up, I have tried to show how talk about patients' treatment preferences – a key element of many models of shared decision-making – may be done in the service of other social actions. If we think of the patient view elicitor from this interactional perspective, then we see how it can sometimes serve less as a mechanism for sharing a decision, and more as a tool for pursuing the neurologist's preferred option.

This is not meant to imply that the neurologist is doing anything wrong. While the patient may be seeking to avoid a treatment she does not want, the neurologist has a duty of care to ensure she understands its potential value. This is part of his institutional role – arguably, even more prominently so than the expectation that he enact SDM (see Pilnick & Dingwall, 2011). My point is not that the neurologist necessarily ought to have done otherwise. Rather, this kind of analysis highlights why it may be profoundly *difficult* to do otherwise, even after decades of clear guidance on the principles of SDM. There is a mismatch between the inevitable abstraction of such guidance and the doing of real interactional work. When seeking patients' preferences "in the wild," clinicians are not doing so in the abstract; they are doing so in the service of trying to accomplish the project of medicine: treating the patient (see also Pilnick, 2022). As our example illustrates, the PVE can work, in post-recommendation position, to secure acceptance of a treatment option that has been previously resisted. The PVE can be understood, then, as an effective tool for pursuing the neurologist's duty of care even if it is not so effective, in this context, for enacting SDM.

Soliciting the patient's treatment preference in pre-recommendation position: "Testing the water"

One implication of the prior section is that sequence really matters. As we saw, a patient view elicitor may be heard as a pursuit of acceptance if it is positioned *after* a recommendation. So, what happens if it is used *before* any recommendation is uttered? In this section, I explore examples from our dataset where neurologists initiated the decision-making sequence by seeking patients' preferences – as a first step.

Extract 2[2] provides a clear example. This patient has already been seen by another neurologist for her headaches, which they believe to be migraines. However, because she has another neurological condition, the two neurologists have consulted each other. As the neurologist explains to the patient near the start of the recorded appointment: "we had a chat and I said 'well just in case something's brewing, one of us ought to see her again.'" In other words, this consultation is at the neurologist's invitation rather than the patient's request, and the main priority is diagnostic: to ensure that her headaches are only migraines, rather than an indication of something more serious.

As it turns out, the neurologist agrees with her colleague that the patient experiences migraines. The question then arises of what to do about them. Although preventative treatments are available, whether they're worth taking is generally deemed to be a preference-sensitive decision because they can have side effects and typically only reduce the number of migraines experienced, rather than controlling them entirely. In our dataset, it was thus usual for neurologists to offer patients a range of possible migraine treatments – often using extensive option-lists. What distinguishes the decision in Extract 2 is that the neurologist launches the entire decision with a patient view elicitor. Before introducing any treatment information, she asks a question that seeks the patient's treatment preference (l. 9–11). The question also gives a basis for deciding: symptom frequency (l. 9–10). This is akin to the first offer of steroids in Extract 1a (l. 2–6) in that the option is made contingent on the patient's self-assessment. However, it differs both in its design and sequential placement. As we have seen, the offer of steroids was initially part of an option-list, making it reasonable for the patient to wait for the second option before expressing a view. The offer of steroids was also designed using an "if-then" declarative format (i.e., more like informing than a request for her views). In Extract 2, by contrast, the patient is asked to consider just one option, and this is presented using an interrogative format. There is, then, substantially more interactional pressure on the patient in Extract 2 to produce an immediate response regarding whether she wants to try treatment (see Stivers & Rossano, 2010). Although displaying some hesitancy, she indicates a preference for treatment at line 13.

Extract 2 (S08504)

```
01  Neu:       Um a::nd you know e:::r some people find it's:: (.)
02             certain (mex-) .hh if they're in that sort of (0.3) f::::
03             I'm gonna get (0.1) a bit of a migraine and then you eat
04             choc[olate then you get one=or
05  Pat:           [Mm:
06  Neu:       cheese:=um .hh but other people it- it- not true at a:ll
07             but certainly that sounds very typical
08  Pat:       Nyuh::
09  Neu: PVE→  for a migraine aura, .hhhh a:re these >kind of< often
10         →  enough that you would be wanting to try:: (0.6) a drug
11         →  to try and redu:ce how (.) often it's happening.
12             (0.3)
13  Pat:       .thhh U:m:: (1.1) .t (0.4) yes: I (sp-) <yeah.
14  Neu:       Yeah.
15             (0.1)
16  Neu:       U::m how did=you get on with Amitriptyline before?
17  Pat:       .thhh I lost the feeling in: e::r (0.1) my arms and
18             my le:gs:.
19  Neu:       So it didn't suit you at all did it,=
20  Pat:       =No:. [I wasn't- I wasn't on it for very lon::g.
21  Neu:             [Okay
```

In contrast to the case in Extracts 1a–c, this patient's treatment preference has been sought *before* the neurologist has articulated a recommendation. Thus, instead of reaching back across the sequence – to try to secure the patient's acceptance of a treatment that the neurologist has already endorsed – here the PVE is prospective in nature. It projects a forthcoming recommendation but makes this contingent on the patient's perspective. It is thus hearable as a preliminary (Schegloff, 2007). Barnes (2018) has shown how GPs' requests for information about patients' prior use of medications (e.g., "what've you tried taking," p. 1369) are understood as pre-recommendations when they occur after a diagnosis has been made. In Extract 2, we see an example of this at line 16. Rather than directly recommending amitriptyline, the neurologist seeks the patient's experience of using that drug in the past. As Barnes notes, this more cautious approach enables clinicians to "test the water" (p. 1367) before making a recommendation. They can then deal with any barriers to acceptance that the pre-sequence may reveal (such as seen in lines 17–21). The query about the patient's treatment preference (l. 9–11) functions in the same way. It projects the possibility of a recommendation for "a drug to try and redu:ce how (.) often it's happening" (l. 10–11) but makes this dependent on the patient's response.

Broadly, recipients of preliminaries have three options when responding: they can give the go-ahead, block, or hedge (Barnes, 2018; Schegloff, 2007). If we recognize the turn as a preliminary, we know that this has implications for what's to come next. To take a familiar example, a friend may ask if I'm driving past her house the next morning. At face value, this is a request for information. However, if we think of this in action terms, it is understandable as a pre-request – as preliminary to a projected request for a lift. I am thus well advised to respond with that projected request in mind. If I say "yes" but do not wish to grant the request, it becomes harder to then decline it (most of us have experience of doing things we wish not to do because we could not come up with an "excuse" in time!). Thus, just as a response to a post-recommendation PVE is made in light of what has already occurred, a response to a pre-recommendation PVE is made in light of what is projected to be coming.

This is well illustrated by cases in which patients hedge in response to a pre-recommendation. Extracts 3 and 4 show examples of this. Structurally, they are akin to Extract 2. In all three extracts, the PVEs (see arrowed lines) follow a discussion about a symptom the patient is experiencing. In Extract 3, we see the tail-end of a history-taking sequence about the patient's memory problems, which could affect her work (l. 1–5), although thus far she's benefited from her employers being "understanding" (l. 1–2). Just prior to Extract 4, the patient has reported "getting like an electric shock," which an MS nurse has explained to her as being "li:ke mixed- mixed messages" from the brain (l. 1). Just like in Extract 2, then, here we see PVEs being used to *initiate* the treatment decision-making.

Extract 3 (S08304)

```
01  Pat:         … and I just think I've been right lucky with
02               that, I thi[nk they're (right) understanding.
03  Neu:                    [Okay,  s o  t h a t ' s-
04               that's- that's >good<.
05  Pat:         (.hhhh) But yeah i- it [could- it could.
06  Neu: PVE→                           [Is- is it enough that
07       →       you would like (e) to see:: a psychologist.
08               (0.9)
09  Pat:         hh. U:::m well if it'd (0.1) help, I suppose
10               cos:: I- (1.1) I don't know=would i::t.
11               (0.1)
12  Pat:         Wh- what [would that
13  Neu:                  [Well >I- I- I-< I think there're two
14               ways of (.) helping with kind of memory problems'
```

Extract 4 (S06204)

```
01  Pat:          It's probably just li:ke mixed- mixed messages.
02                (0.4)
03  Neu:          Ye[ah.
04  Pat:             [(You kno:[:w)
05  Neu: Pre→               [Ba:d enough to want to take tablets,
05                (0.[7)
06  Pat:              [((Visible in-breath during this silence))
07  Pat:          Phhhhh.hhu. E:r what kind of tablets.
08                (0.5)
09  Neu:          Well (.) the sorts of drugs that work for this
```

Just like in Extract 2, the PVEs in Extracts 3 and 4 seek the patient's treatment preference, making treatment contingent on their self-assessment. Coming after the expression of trouble, these questions are hearably done in the service of another action: recommending a solution (see Shaw et al., 2015, on advice-implicative interrogatives). If they indicate a preference for treatment, then, the patients are giving the go-ahead for a more specific recommendation to be made. The patients are clearly alert to the implications of where these sequences are headed. They each respond with a hedge, which makes their go-ahead contingent on further information (see boldface turns, above). In Extract 3, the patient produces a conditional acceptance: "if it'd (0.1) help," (l. 9). She thereby displays herself to understand what is meant by "see:: a psychologist" (l. 7), that she is willing to do so, but is uncertain about the *efficacy* of such treatment. She seeks further information as a basis for producing a fully fitted response, first countering (see Schegloff, 2007) the neurologist's yes/no question with her own (l. 10). In the absence of an immediate answer (l. 11), she reformulates her question to an open-ended one. This seems to be seeking information, either about what the treatment would achieve or what it would involve (l. 12). In response, the neurologist starts to provide further information about treatment options. Extract 4 shows a more extreme hedge in that the patient does not express even tentative acceptance (l. 7). Rather, she produces a repair initiator, targeting the neurologist's general reference to "tablets" (l. 5). The patient treats this as inadequate for expressing a preference. Like in Extract 3, she shows herself to require more information in order to produce the response made relevant by the PVE (Schegloff, 2007).

These examples indicate a challenge for patients in articulating their treatment preferences so early in a decision-making sequence. If they say "yes," they know that a recommendation is almost certainly going to be forthcoming. However, with such limited information about what the neurologist may be offering them, it can be difficult to know whether they want the treatment. Moreover, because the neurologist has also sought their self-assessment of whether treatment is warranted by their lived experience of the symptom, if they give the go-ahead, subsequent refusal of a recommended treatment risks seeming perverse. Thus, giving the go-ahead sets up a trajectory in which refusal may be particularly hard to do. Hedging addresses this challenge and has the advantage of opening up discussion by seeking further information from the neurologist. This can lead to (a more informed) acceptance or refusal of treatment (as it does in Extracts 3 and 4, respectively, data not shown due to space constraints).

The risk, however, is that the patient might block the relevance of such a discussion. Extract 5 shows an example. The patient has been referred to the neurologist because she's planning a gap year trip to Peru. Her GP wants a specialist opinion about the patient's headaches before writing a letter for her insurance provider (l. 21–25). There is, then, a similarity here with Extract 2: in both cases the primary goal is to rule out a more worrying underlying explanation for the headaches; treatment is a secondary consideration. The neurologist decides to order a scan but makes it clear that this is for reassurance – he strongly suspects that she has nothing more serious than migraines (data not shown). We join the consultation immediately after the neurologist has told the patient about his own experience in Peru. At line 1, he brings them back to the business of the consultation, initiating decision-making about treatment. Like we have seen in Extracts 2–4, he uses a PVE to seek the patient's preference (l. 4) – as a very first step in the decision-making. In this case, the relevance of the projected treatment recommendation is soundly blocked (see patient's extended response, in boldface).

Extract 5 (G08704)

```
01 Neu:       Erm Okay (0.4) Er right what do we do
02            about this.
03            (0.7)
04 Neu: PVE→  D'you want this treated,
05            (1.1)!
06 Pat:       .HHH (0.2) If (it /er) I mean it does
07            sound like it's probably just a migraine
08            I get in the night I mean I know that I
09            can um generally ways of ('s) like staving
10            off (m-) migraines is just make sure that I
11            stay calm,
12 Neu:       [Mm.
13 Pat:       [Um (0.5) with my exams right now it's a
14            wee bit stressful 'cos like uni depends on
15            them right now but- um I know how to deal
16            with migraines but I didn't know what these
17            were, so if I know that these- th- pretty much
18            are migraines (in the night), I, I know how I
19            can then counteract th[at.
20 Neu:                             [Yeah.
21 Pat:       We were just checking that it wasn't, she
22            seemed to think, w- there is, like (I) said
23            "if it is something more serious then I
24            can't obviously write you this
25            [letter. So we just need to [check it out"
26 Neu:       [Mm.                        [Mm.
27 Pat:       But if- (1.4) the pl: most plausible thing
```

```
28                is, is a migraine in the night, I think I
29                know how can I deal with that. [Pretty much.
30   Neu:                                        [Alright.
31   Neu:         (Now) that's up to you.
32                (0.5)
33   Neu:         Okay. (C- there-) I mean you don't have to
34                treat this. You [can you know (you) can
35   Pat:                         [Yeah
36   Neu:         tolerate it if you- if you must
37   Pat:         Yeah.
```

The patient's block is produced in three ways: first, by indicating that she already knows how to deal with her migraines (l. 8–11 and l. 18–19), second, by orienting to her current situation as exceptional (l. 13–15), and third, by indicating that the reason for the consultation was primarily diagnostic (l. 16–17). She expands on the third point after the neurologist's minimal response (l. 20), formulating the consultation as "just [to] check" that her symptom was not "something more serious" (l. 21–25) and primarily for bureaucratic purposes. Since the "check" has already been handled by the neurologist's recommendation to scan, the purpose of the visit, from the patient's perspective, has been fulfilled. She completes her turn with a version of how she began: if the diagnosis is migraines, then she already knows how to handle her condition (l. 27–29).

Having tested the water with a turn that made the decision entirely contingent on the patient's treatment preference ("D'you want this treated," l. 4), the neurologist now has no interactional basis for making a recommendation. As Landmark et al. (2017) note, clinicians may make recommendations even in such inauspicious sequential environments. However, in this case, he does not. He maintains the preference-sensitive nature of the decision – "that's up to you." (l. 31) – and only hints at an alternative view through the way he formulates the option of not treating (l. 33–36). This is suggestive of the advantages of treatment (not having to "tolerate" the headaches) and the use of "must" seems to imply a kind of perversity to the patient's stance, given that treatment is available. However, he does not produce a recommendation for treatment. It seems likely that this approach to the decision is (subtly) oriented to the unsolicited revelation, during the history-taking, that the patient "doesn't like taking medication" (data not shown). This was announced by the accompanying other (possibly, the patient's mum), as an account for the patient's use only of paracetamol, which the neurologist characterizes as "not taking anything for it really". Explaining that this is due to a bad experience in hospital, the patient uses an extreme case formulation (Pomerantz, 1986): "I don't like taking pills unless it's absolutely necessary. And I'm like dying or something". Thus, the patient's preference against treatment has been "in the air" since before the possibility of prescribing was broached by the neurologist (see also Britten et al., 2004). The PVE, used in pre-recommendation position, is thus well fitted to handling the treatment decision-making in this case; it offers a means to approach the decision cautiously, demonstrating that the neurologist has paid attention to the patient's general preference against medication.

The neurologist goes on to remind the patient that she can see him again if she changes her mind (data not shown). However, no further treatment information is provided. The absence of any attempt to persuade the patient to consider treatment is in line with her right to decline treatment, with the preference-sensitive nature of this decision (there is no research evidence to suggest that migraines are associated with damage to the brain), and with the primary, diagnostic purpose of this consultation. However, since her block has effectively shut down the discussion, it remains unclear as to whether the patient is aware of the wide range of treatment options available for migraines. While she may have made a more autonomous decision than the patient in Extracts 1a–c – since she is not revealing her preference *in response* to the neurologist's – here it is not possible to judge whether the decision is an informed one (see also Sterie et al., 2022).

To sum up, this section has explored what happens when patient view elicitors are used to initiate a decision-making sequence. Just as we saw with respect to post-recommendation PVEs, these pre-recommendation PVEs are being used in the service of another social action. In this preliminary position – like Barnes's (2018) preliminary questions about the prior use of medicines – they can serve to "test the water" for a potential recommendation. This overcomes one possible barrier to shared decision-making. Since clinicians are typically oriented to as having greater knowledge in the medical domain (Heritage, 2005; Landmark et al., 2017), clinician and patient do not exchange views from a level "playing field." Thus, if a patient's views are sought after a treatment recommendation, they are in a particularly challenging position if they wish to refuse treatment: not only is it generally interactionally delicate to disagree (Clayman, 2002), but this is compounded by their respective institutional roles. To disagree in post-recommendation position, the (lay) patient must go against an expert's opinion. PVEs in pre-recommendation position give the patient a slot to indicate their preference at the very first opportunity. They may be seen, therefore, as a tool to support shared decision-making (see also Barnes, 2018). As this section has shown, however, the use of PVEs in this pre-recommendation position also carries risks. Not only is the patient having to voice a view at a point where they may know little about the treatment option(s), but if they block the relevance of a recommendation, they may leave without really knowing what it is they have turned down.

Discussion

Addressing the recurrent finding of a gap between practice and the widespread ideal of shared decision-making, this chapter has argued for the value of examining decision-making "in the wild." Taking a CA approach, we go beyond the binary question of whether or not some element of SDM has been enacted in a consultation, to the interactional question of what happens when it is enacted. In this chapter, I showed that the neurologists in my dataset actively elicited patients' views in two sequential locations: following a recommendation and as a preliminary to making a recommendation. In line with Landmark et al. (2017), I showed how clinicians' recommendations may "interfere with the SDM process" (p. 2086).

Even as they appeared to be enacting a core principle of SDM – by discussing patients' treatment preferences – they were actually doing other interactional work: they were trying to secure acceptance of their own preferred option. Thus, post-recommendation PVEs may achieve a goal that is important for doing medicine: securing the patient's acceptance of a recommended treatment. However, this may come at the expense of doing SDM. Using a PVE prior to making any recommendation offers a solution to this problem as the patient's views are sought right from the start of the decision-making sequence. As I have shown, this approach is not trouble-free either, as the patient may lack the resources needed to formulate an informed view.

My analysis of PVEs in these two naturally occurring locations thus raises a dilemma for communication training in how to seek patients' treatment preferences. If we advise clinicians to provide information about the option(s) first (as in Extracts 1a–c), the risk is that they do so in a way that conveys their own view. Patients will then be responding in a sequential slot where they must take account of that view. If their views differ, they will have to handle the delicate task of disagreeing with an expert. If we propose – as the solution to this – that the clinician should seek the patient's views first (as in Extracts 2–5), then patients may not be able to engage in informed decision-making (see also Reuber et al., 2015).

Grappling with this dilemma, I came to see full-form option-listing as a good solution. This is an approach to decision-making that also occurred naturally in our dataset – although rarely (Chappell et al., 2018). It involves three key steps, which I have summarized in our training for clinicians using the acronym ALF:

- <u>A</u>nnounce that there's a decision to be made.
- <u>L</u>ist the options and relevant information about each (e.g., pros and cons).
- <u>F</u>ind out what the patient thinks about the options (to access the training, see NICE, 2021 or contact the author).

These steps address the pitfalls, for achieving SDM, identified in the present chapter with respect to using PVEs. The initial announcement that there are legitimate options not only indicates that the decision has yet to be made (thus holding choice open), but also creates space for doing information provision in its own right. For instance, in one of our clearest cases, the neurologist initiates an option-list as follows: "Possibilities. (0.9) .tch Okay let me talk through these." (Toerien et al., 2018, p. 1254). In so doing, he not only projects a list of options, but explicitly formulates what is to come *as informing* rather than recommending. Having set up the activity in this way, the list of options then allows the clinician to give the patient information. In so doing, the patient gains an evidence base for formulating a treatment preference – the very thing that may be lacking if a clinician seeks the patient's views first. By following the list immediately with a patient view elicitor, clinicians can explicitly seek the patient's views *before* articulating their own. In this way, they can decrease the pressure on the patient to align with an expert opinion, the problem that we saw so clearly illustrated in Extracts 1a–c.

Full-form option-listing, then, has the potential to resolve the dilemma outlined above (Reuber et al., 2015).

My initial plan for writing this chapter was simply to set up the dilemma and then propose full-form option-listing as the solution. However, as I engaged more closely with the theoretical SDM literature on patients' preferences, I was troubled by just how similar this solution is to Stiggelbout et al.'s (2015) four-step model of SDM:

1. The professional informs the patient that a decision is to be made and that the patient's opinion is important;
2. The professional explains the options and the pros and cons of each relevant option;
3. The professional and patient discuss the patient's preferences; the professional supports the patient in deliberation;
4. The professional and patient discuss the patient's decisional role preference, make or defer the decision, and discuss possible follow-up (p. 1173).

Although some elements of their model were largely absent from our dataset (e.g., the neurologists seldom explained the importance of the patient's opinion or discussed whether they wished to make the decision), our inductive discovery of full-form option-listing accords closely with their four steps. Also in line with our findings, Stiggelbout et al. (2015) concluded that there is only limited evidence of their model occurring in practice. Thus, they provide detailed explanation of the steps, along with suggested phrases that may be used to implement them. The intended audience is practitioners themselves, the aim being to reduce the gap between the SDM ideal and observed practice.

As a conversation analyst, I have been socialized to be skeptical about "communication propositions" (Stiggelbout et al., 2015, p. 1174) that arise out of models rather than close analysis of how interaction works in practice. Thus, Stiggelbout et al.'s (excellent) paper made uncomfortable reading for me. While, by definition, any model must be "abstracted" from the nitty-gritty of specific moments of talk-in-interaction, SDM theorists tend to take account of two crucial features of how interaction works: that precisely *how* and *when* a turn is produced in a sequence of talk really matters. It matters for how the turn is understood (e.g., as a choice or not, see Toerien et al., 2018), and it matters for what subsequently happens in the interaction, including, for instance, whether the patient ultimately leaves with a prescription despite indicating that they do not want one (Toerien, 2021). This twin recognition is built into Stiggelbout et al.'s model, not only in their detailed examples, but in their insistence on a particular conversational sequence for achieving SDM – hence a set of numbered steps. They also offer more fine-grained advice on sequencing. For instance, they tell clinicians to "*first* mention the options explicitly" (p. 1175, emphasis added) before discussing patients' preferences.

In effect, we had reached similar conclusions by different routes. My team started with what actually happened in a set of clinical encounters and then derived training implications from our analysis of how "choice" played out. Stiggelbout et al. (2015) started with a model of SDM and then assessed the extent to which it is implemented. That we came to similar conclusions about how to advise clinicians is perhaps cause for celebration – at least, we achieved triangulation! However, I had spent long hours figuring out, inductively, that neurologists were (sometimes) enacting a kind of reduced version of SDM in their interactions with patients. I was left wondering: what (if anything) is the added value of our approach? The answer, I think, lies in CA's understanding of talk as action.

If we think about PVEs in terms of *social action*, then we can see these as functional for engaging in a larger activity that is central to clinical practice: deciding on treatment. This activity is integral to achieving the overarching project of many medical consultations: addressing the patient's presenting problem (Robinson, 2003). In a nutshell, that is what the doctor is typically there to do. When clinicians seek patients' preferences, they are not doing so in order to achieve some sort of "pure" exchange of views. They are doing so in the service of accomplishing that project. If they have a clear opinion on what is best for the patient – but the patient thinks otherwise – they might use a PVE to pursue acceptance, while maintaining an orientation to the patient's (legal and moral) right to choose. If they have reason to approach a recommendation cautiously, they might use a PVE to test the water, a practice which can help avoid resistance altogether (Barnes, 2018). In short, these uses of PVEs make sense as part of doing the work of doctoring (see also Pilnick, 2022).

Likewise, in both sequential locations, patients are also doing interactional work when they reveal a preference. Following a recommendation, they may be working to secure some alternative or compromise. Before a projected recommendation, they may be working to avoid an unwanted recommendation altogether. Again, these make sense in the context of doing the work of being a (reasonable) patient. As we have seen, patients are observably balancing an orientation to the clinician's expertise with any wish they may have not to receive a particular prescription or referral. Revealing a preference that contra-indicates a treatment option can allow the patient to resist (either retrospectively or prospectively) based on "knowledge to which they are entitled" (Gill et al., 2010, p. 16) – their own lived experience of symptoms and prior treatments.

This understanding of the interactional work that talk about patients' views is being used to do helps explain, I would argue, why SDM is so difficult to implement routinely. It is not just that clinicians fail to remember to enact a particular set of guidelines. As this chapter has shown, even when they do enact them – e.g., by eliciting patients' views – this is not done in some sort of abstract way. To talk is always to do something. When doctors elicit patients' views, and patients reveal their views, they are doing so in the service of (sometimes conflicting) interactional goals, and the goal may sometimes be at odds with SDM; for instance, the clinician may be prioritizing a duty of care (by pursuing acceptance of a recommended option) over the ideal of patient choice (Reuber et al., 2015). Models of SDM, however sophisticated, fail to recognize this. They assume a kind of "pure" exchange of information between clinician and patient. From that perspective, it is impossible to understand why clinicians – after decades of effort to try to (re)socialize them into taking a shared approach to decision-making – are still failing to do so (see also Pilnick, 2022). After all, asking patients about their preferences sounds like such a simple thing to do. If we understand talk as action, however, we see that it is far from simple. To get clinicians to *do* SDM on a regular basis, they do not just need to believe it is a good thing and know how to do it. They need to fully reconceptualize what they are *doing* in the activity of treatment decision-making: shifting the emphasis from delivering on what they think is best to facilitating the patient's ability to make up their own mind.

Pilnick and Dingwall (2011) have drawn similar conclusions in relation to the notion of "patient-centered" care. In their controversial, and compelling, critical review of CA studies of doctor–patient interaction, they argue that "asymmetry lies at the heart of the medical enterprise" (p. 1374). Thus, they propose, while communication training may enable doctors to exercise their authority "in more civil ways," it is misguided to think that patient-led medical practice can be achieved "without some major shift in the social function of officially sanctioned medical practice" (p. 1374). I find myself somewhat more optimistic about the implementation of SDM than Pilnick and Dingwall (2011) were about reforming medical authority more broadly. This is because, while the latter is diffuse, SDM models articulate a set of defined, skills-based interactional practices; and these are already occurring in clinical practice to some extent (as our inductive identification of option-listing shows). I believe, then, that it is viable for SDM to occur more regularly, at least. However, for it to become *routine*, I think Pilnick and Dingwall are right: we would need to see a shift in the institutional goals of medicine. At present, the evidence strongly suggests that clinicians are prioritizing the goal of trying to "fix" the patient – even if that conflicts with the patient's preferences. For SDM to become routine, it would need to become the over-riding goal instead. Whether that is in our collective best interests, however, is the real question. As Pilnick (2022) rightly concludes, the careful study of real medical interaction reveals that we need a broader rethink of what we – as a society – want from the institution of medicine.

Acknowledgments and statement of ethical approval

This chapter arises out of a wider project funded by the UK's National Institute for Health and Care Research (NIHR), Health and Social Care Delivery Research (HS&DR) programme. Project numbers 10/2000/61 and 14/19/43. The views and opinions expressed in this paper are the authors' and do not necessarily reflect those of the NHS, NIHR, MRC, CCF, NETSCC, Health Services and Delivery Research program, or Department of Health.

I acknowledge the invaluable contributions of the full project team: Markus Reuber (Chief Investigator) and, in alphabetical order, Paul Chappell, Rod Duncan, Clare Jackson, Rebecca Shaw (co-applicants), and Zoe Gallant and Fiona Smith (research assistants responsible for recruitment and data collection). Special thanks to the patients and neurologists who made this study possible.

All potential participants received a written information sheet in advance of the consultation and gave written consent to a research assistant who explained the study and answered questions. Ethical approval was granted by the NRES Committee for Yorkshire and the Humber (South Yorkshire) on 11 October 2011.

I would like to thank Sara Keel and an anonymous reviewer for their enormously helpful feedback on an earlier version of this chapter.

With thanks also to Elsevier for granting permission to reprint Extracts 1a, 1b, 1c.

Notes

1 Extracts 1a–c have been presented and discussed, for different analytic purposes, in Reuber et al. (2018, pp. 26–28) and in Toerien (2021, pp. 19–21).
2 Extract 2 has been presented and discussed, for different analytic purposes, in Reuber et al. (2015, p. 101).

References

Barnes, R. K. (2018). Preliminaries to treatment recommendations in UK primary care: A vehicle for shared decision making? *Health Communication*, *33*(11), 1366–1376. https://doi.org/10.1080/10410236.2017.1350915

Bomhof-Roordink, H., Gärtner, F. R., Stiggelbout, A. M., & Pieterse, A. H. (2019). Key components of shared decision making models: A systematic review. *BMJ Open*, *9*(12). https://doi.org/10.1136/bmjopen-2019-031763

Boyd, E., & Heritage, J. (2006). Taking the history: Questioning during comprehensive history-taking. In J. Heritage & D. Maynard (Eds.), *Communication in medical care: Interaction between primary care physicians and patients* (Studies in Interactional Sociolinguistics, pp. 151–184). Cambridge: Cambridge University Press. https://doi.org/10.1017/CBO9780511607172.008

Britten, N., Stevenson, F., Gafaranga, J., Barry, C., & Bradley, C. (2004). The expression of aversion to medicines in general practice consultations. *Social Science and Medicine*, *59*(7), 1495–1503. https://doi.org/10.1016/j.socscimed.2004.01.019

Chappell, P., Toerien, M., Jackson, C., & Reuber, M. (2018). Following the patient's orders? Recommending vs. offering choice in neurology outpatient consultations. *Social Science and Medicine*, *205*, 8–16. https://doi.org/10.1016/j.socscimed.2018.03.036

Clayman, S. E. (2002). Sequence and solidarity. *Advances in Group Processes*, *19*, 229–253. https://doi.org/10.1016/S0882-6145(02)19009-6

Drew, P. (2005). Conversation analysis. In K. L. Fitch & R. E. Sanders (Eds.), *Handbook of language & social interaction* (pp. 71–101). Mahwah, NJ: Lawrence Erlbaum.

Enfield, N., & Sidnell, J. (2017). On the concept of action in the study of interaction. *Discourse Studies*, *19*(5), 515–535. https://doi.org/10.1177/1461445617730235

Gill, V. T., Pomerantz, A., & Denvir, P. (2010). Pre-emptive resistance: Patients' participation in diagnostic sense-making activities. *Sociology of Health and Illness*, *32*(1), 1–20. https://doi.org/10.1111/j.1467-9566.2009.01208.x

Heritage, J. (2005). Revisiting authority in physician-patient interaction. In J. F. Duchan & D. Kovarsky (Eds.), *Diagnosis as cultural practice* (pp. 83–102). Berlin: Mouton de Gruyter

Ikeya, N. (2020). Hybridity of hybrid studies of work: Examination of informing practitioners in practice. *Ethnographic Studies*, *17*, 22–40. https://doi.org/10.5281/zenodo.405053

Koenig, C. J. (2011). Patient resistance as agency in treatment decisions. *Social Science and Medicine*, *72*(7), 1105–1114.

Landmark, A. M. D., Ofstad, E. H., & Svennevig, J. (2017). Eliciting patient preferences in shared decision-making (SDM): Comparing conversation analysis and SDM measurements. *Patient Education and Counseling*, *100*(11), 2081–2087. https://doi.org/10.1016/j.pec.2017.05.018

Makoul, G., & Clayman, M. L. (2006). An integrative model of shared decision making in medical encounters. *Patient Education and Counseling*, *60*(3), 301–312. https://doi.org/10.1016/j.pec.2005.06.010

Moumjid, N., Gafni, A., Brémond, A., & Carrère, M.-O. (2007). Shared decision making in the medical encounter: Are we all talking about the same thing? *Medical Decision Making*, *27*(5), 539–546. https://doi.org/10.1177/0272989X07306779

NICE. (2021). Consultation skills. Shared decision making learning package. https://www.nice.org.uk/guidance/ng197/resources/shared-decision-making-learning-package-9142488109

Pilnick, A. (2022). *Reconsidering patient centred care : Between autonomy and abandonment*. Emerald Publishing Limited.

Pilnick, A., & Dingwall, R. (2011). On the remarkable persistence of asymmetry in doctor/patient interaction: A critical review. *Social Science and Medicine*, *72*(8), 1374–1382. https://doi.org/10.1016/j.socscimed.2011.02.033

Pomerantz, A. (1986). Extreme case formulations: A way of legitimizing claims. *Human Studies*, *9*(2), 219–229. https://doi.org/10.1007/BF00148128

Rake, E. A., Box, I. C. H., Dreesens, D., Meinders, M. J., Kremer, J. A. M., Aarts, J. W. M., & Elwyn, G. (2022). Bringing personal perspective elicitation to the heart of shared decision-making: A scoping review. *Patient Education and Counseling*, *105*(9), 2860–2870. https://doi.org/10.1016/j.pec.2022.05.009

Reuber, M., Chappell, P., Jackson, C., & Toerien, M. (2018). Evaluating nuanced practices for initiating decision-making in neurology clinics: A mixed-methods study. *Health Services and Delivery Research*, *6*(34), 1–148. https://doi.org/10.3310/hsdr06340

Reuber, M., Toerien, M., Shaw, R., & Duncan, R. (2015). Delivering patient choice in clinical practice: A conversation analytic study of communication practices used in neurology clinics to involve patients in decision-making. *Health Services and Delivery Research*, *3*(7), 1–170. https://doi.org/10.3310/hsdr03070

Robinson, J. D. (2003). An interactional structure of medical activities during acute visits and its implications for patients' participation. *Health Communication*, *15*(1), 27–59. https://doi.org/10.1207/S15327027HC1501_2

Schelgoff, E. A. (1996). Confirming allusions: Toward an empirical account of action. *American Journal of Sociology*, *104*(1), 161–216. https://doi.org/10.1086/230911

Schegloff, E. A. (2007). *Sequence organization in interaction: A primer in conversation analysis* (Vol. 1). Cambridge University Press. https://doi.org/10.1017/CBO9780511791208

Shaw, C., Potter, J., & Hepburn, A. (2015). Advice-implicative actions: Using interrogatives and assessments to deliver advice in mundane conversation. *Discourse Studies*, *17*(3), 317–342

Sterie, A.-C., Weber, O., Jox, R. J., & Rubli Truchard, E. (2022). 'Do you want us to try to resuscitate?': Conversational practices generating patient decisions regarding cardiopulmonary resuscitation. *Patient Education and Counseling, 105*(4), 887–894. https://doi.org/10.1016/j.pec.2021.07.042

Stiggelbout, A. M., Pieterse, A. H., & De Haes, J. C. J. M. (2015). Shared decision making: Concepts, evidence, and practice. *Patient Education and Counseling, 98*(10), 1172–1179. https://doi.org/10.1016/j.pec.2015.06.022

Stivers, T. (2005). Parent resistance to physicians' treatment recommendations: One resource for initiating a negotiation of the treatment decision. *Health Communication, 18*(1), 41–74. https://doi.org/10.1207/s15327027hc1801_3

Stivers, T., Heritage, J., Barnes, R. K., McCabe, R., Thompson, L., & Toerien, M. (2017). Treatment recommendations as actions. *Health Communication, 33*(11), 1335–1344. https://doi.org/10.1080/10410236.2017.1350913

Stivers, T., & Rossano, F. (2010). Mobilizing response. *Research on Language and Social Interaction, 43*(1), 3–31. https://doi.org/10.1080/08351810903471258

Stivers, T., & Timmermans, S. (2020). Medical authority under siege: How clinicians transform patient resistance into acceptance. *Journal of Health and Social Behavior, 61*(1), 60–78. https://doi.org/10.1177/0022146520902740

Toerien, M. (2021). When do patients exercise their right to refuse treatment? A conversation analytic study of decision-making trajectories in UK neurology outpatient consultations. *Social Science and Medicine, 290*, 114278. https://doi.org/10.1016/j.socscimed.2021.114278

Toerien, M., Reuber, M., Shaw, R., & Duncan, R. (2018). Generating the perception of choice: The remarkable malleability of option-listing. *Sociology of Health and Illness, 40*(7), 1250–1267. https://doi.org/10.1111/1467-9566.12766

Toerien, M., Shaw, R., & Reuber, M. (2013). Initiating decision-making in neurology consultations: 'Recommending' versus 'option-listing' and the implications for medical authority. *Sociology of Health and Illness, 35*(6), 873–890. https://doi.org/10.1111/1467-9566.12000

2 Working out interprofessional collaboration

Flight nurses' practical management of prehospital emergency care

*Nozomi Ikeya, Shintaro Matsunaga,
Tatsuya Akutsu, Seiichi Takahashi and
Hiroko Nakazawa*

Introduction

As part of emergency medicine, prehospital care is provided to seriously sick or injured patients who need treatment before they are transferred to a hospital. A flight doctor and a flight nurse normally administer prehospital care to these patients by flying to a rendezvous point to which an ambulance crew brings the patient. Appropriate prehospital care must be provided in a short period of time so that the patient can be safely transferred. This includes a physical assessment of the patient, on the basis of which necessary treatment is provided, such as intravenous catheterization for the administration of drugs and intratracheal intubation to maintain an open airway. Flight doctors and flight nurses must work within various constraints differing from those they face in their usual work in a hospital Emergency Medical Unit in terms of staff numbers, devices for testing, and types of medicine.

According to the rules established by the Flight Nurse Committee of the Japan Society for Aeromedical Services, a medical professional must have at least five years of nursing experience in addition to a minimum of three years of experience in the emergency department before he or she can qualify to enter the program for flight nurses (Japan Society for Aeromedical Services, 2017). As is evident in the definition of "flight nurse" below, flight nurses play a vital role in the prehospital setting:

> [...] a nurse, who is dispatched by helicopter to provide nursing to both seriously ill or injured patients whose emergency is high and transfer them by ambulance or helicopter while continuing the provision of the initial treatment and nursing to the patient.
> (Japan Society for Aeromedical Services, 2017, p. 2)

Textbooks on flight nursing often stress that nurses in training to become flight nurses must be aware of the differences between working in the prehospital setting and working in the Emergency Medical Unit at a hospital (Japanese Association for Emergency Nursing, 2018). However, as one flight nurse normally works with one doctor in the prehospital setting, and only a limited number of individuals can fly in a helicopter at the same time, flight nurses do not have opportunities to work with other flight nurses

DOI: 10.4324/9781003312345-4

in the actual prehospital setting. It is therefore not easy for them to learn the competences involved in the practical management of prehospital care through socialization.

To solve this problem, experienced flight nurses (certified instructors in charge of training new flight nurses) introduced a video camera into this setting to record their activities for training purposes. These video recordings allow the nurses to reflect on their own activities during prehospital care and receive feedback from instructors. The instructors also conducted research using the recorded data. For example, an analysis was carried out on the number and content of utterances made by newly trained nurses compared with those made by experienced flight nurses. The analysis showed that more utterances made by experienced flight nurses led to conversations with others, while those made by newly trained nurses were treated as instances of "talking to oneself" (Takahashi, et al., 2018, p. 435). In another study, they presented an indicator of proficiency through the application of machine learning to changes in the entropy of recorded prehospital activities (Tsuchiya et al., 2021).

While these studies deal with flight nurses' competences in different ways, the *range* of what is known to flight nurses in the prehospital setting, and *how* they carry out their activities in response to different emergency situations each time, have yet to be examined. One aim of this paper is to present the competences of flight nurses that are involved in the practical management of prehospital care activities. To put it differently, through examining moment-by-moment interaction among a flight doctor, a flight nurse, and emergency crew members, we aim to capture what is known to the members at each moment, including what is taken for granted by the members and thus not explicitly expressed in words but nevertheless known to them (Garfinkel, 1986; 2002). By doing so, we intend to provide some material that may help facilitate the training of flight nurses, who have only limited opportunities for socialization by working with other flight nurses.

Prehospital care activities are a form of interprofessional collaboration. Studies on interprofessional collaboration in healthcare settings, with some exceptions in the areas of ethnomethodology and conversation analysis, have focused mainly on an aspect of communication, especially horizontal communication among different professionals with different backgrounds (Schot et al., 2020). The rationale behind this focus is likely linked to assumptions that horizontal communication is effective in terms of information-sharing and responsiveness to the development of situations. This chapter, instead of focusing on the mode of communication, will study prehospital care activities from the members' point of view of accomplishing a series of tasks for the achievement of prehospital care. By focusing on cases in which experienced flight nurses are involved, we aim to present their competence, i.e., their "solutions" to the problem of working with other professionals, in part through working out the division of labor under which each professional operates in accomplishing the prehospital care (what Anderson et al. (1990, p. 242) call division of labor as "transcendental presence").

Flight nurses in the prehospital care setting: Textbooks, guidelines, and studies

A flight nurse, together with a flight doctor, fly to the rendezvous point to provide prehospital care to patients being transported by an ambulance crew before the patients are moved to a hospital for further treatment. In doing so, the flight nurse is expected to coordinate closely with the doctor. Furthermore, they need to work in an ambulance, which has more constraints in terms of space and available devices than a hospital, where they normally work. For example, without image examination results, which they normally use in a hospital, they need to base their judgment mostly on information they gather from the emergency crews and their own observations of the patient while responding to moment-by-moment changes.

The set of guidelines called *Japan Nursing for Trauma Evaluation and Care (JNTEC)* includes a chapter, "JNTEC and Its Reality," that explains that the flight nurse must (1) be aware of the differences between prehospital care and initial care in the Emergency Medical Unit at the hospital and (2) be able to observe and anticipate the procedures to be performed by the physician (Japanese Association for Emergency Nursing, 2018).

The abovementioned textbook and guidelines both suggest that flight nurses on an ad hoc team (or an "instant team") formed on a case-by-case basis should act differently than they would in their usual work in the Emergency Medical Unit. In other words, the prehospital care setting is a *reconfigured* setting.

As Braithwaite and Steele (2020) have highlighted, identifying what constitutes flight nurses' competences has long been an issue for educational purposes, as well as for establishing the foundations of their own specialties. To identify flight nurses' competences, and to develop effective teaching methods and training programs (Braithwaite & Steele, 2020; Tsuchiya et al., 2021), numerous studies have been conducted (Reimer et al., 2013; Reimer & Moore, 2010; Senften & Engström, 2013). Stroller (1998), for example, interviewed six flight nurses with five or more years of experience. On this basis, the author identified four themes related to effective performance: (1) collaboration, (2) mutual respect and trust, (3) fitness standards, and (4) synergy. Also based on interviews with six experienced flight nurses, Pugh's (2002) study adopted a slightly different focus to identify three themes influencing flight nurses' decision-making processes: (1) ways of knowing the patient, (2) the context of knowing, and (3) reflective practices (for similar studies conducted in Japan, see, e.g., Funaki & Fukaya, 2015; Sakuta et al., 2020). Finally, based on interviews with doctors and nurses, Ebbs and Timmons (2008, p. 57) draw on the sociological concepts of "negotiated order" and "subordination" to analyze the practice of cooperation between flight doctors and flight nurses in a military setting. The authors' chief aim is to explain the relationship between the two groups in terms of power.

Issues concerning the flight nurses' competences discussed by these earlier studies rely solely on interviews. In contrast, our study investigates flight nurses' competences as embedded and displayed in actual prehospital activities-in-interactions alongside meetings among the coauthors of this paper, which include ethnomethodologists and experienced flight nurses, during which we held discussions of recorded data and informal interviews.

Studies of collaboration in healthcare settings

Studies on interprofessional collaboration in healthcare have focused mainly on the extent to which horizontal communication has been realized in practice

(Schot et al., 2020). From what can be gathered from Schot et al. (2020) and Braithwaite et al. (2016), the question of the extent to which individuals rely on the knowledge and skills they gain through socialization in each discipline to effectively carry out interprofessional collaboration has not received much attention.

Among studies on interprofessional collaboration in medical settings, ethnomethodological and conversation analytical studies are distinctive in that they focus on the social organization of collaboration by paying attention to situated actions.

In studying the organization of requesting immediate action in a hospital operating room, Mondada (2014) demonstrates ways in which such requests are organized as part of the activities in this setting. She argues that "immediate requests merge within the ongoing activity; they structure it, they exhibit responsibilities and entitlements to request, but they also rely on it, they exploit its trajectory, they are occasioned by it, and they can merge with it" (p. 300). González-Martínez and Drew (2021) present a study of the organization of telephone conversations by which the recovery room nurse informs the Surgery Care Unit that a patient in the recovery room is ready to return to the unit after awakening following surgery. The study demonstrates how the nurse, through a brief informing, recruits a colleague nurse to transfer the patient to the unit, rather than the nurse accomplishing two distinct actions, i.e., informing and recruiting.

These studies focus on how specific sequences of actions (such as requests for immediate actions and appropriate actions, informing and recruitment) take place smoothly because things are known to members and the development of activities is adequately made accountable to members. However, the focus of their studies is not on describing what is exactly known to members in the setting, with which activities are adequately made accountable. For example, González-Martínez and Drew argue that the simplicity with which the nurse from the Surgery Care Unit is recruited is possible because participants draw on a routine organization of tasks and an established division of labor, but what is exactly known to members about the division of labor itself is not the focus of the study.

One set of studies looks at cases where things are not adequately made accountable to members. Bezemer et al. (2011a,b) examine the organization of talk and body movement when a nurse is not able to immediately respond to a doctor's request for a particular tool during a surgery, e.g., scissors. This trouble emerges due to the nurse's lack of information about different doctors with different backgrounds using both different tools for different purposes and different names for the same tools. Thus, this study highlights that there are things known to competent members working in an operating room that are crucial for members to be able to accomplish their tasks.

Certain things that are taken for granted by members in the setting, i.e., things known to the members prior to the actual actions, constitute members' competences for performing tasks. Our paper also pays attention to what is known to members in the setting prior to the actual actions and how they get elaborated by the actual development of the course of actions to constitute what is known and how it is known to members at this moment, i.e., an occasioned corpus of knowledge (Zimmerman & Pollner, 1970).

Lastly, Lunkka et al. (2022) study a person who works as a "hospitalist," a new role at university hospitals. A "hospitalist" is defined as "a specialist physician who works in a surgical ward but is not a surgeon, primarily to ensure that patients receive holistic medical care, and thus enhance the quality of care and patient orientation within the ward" (Lunkka et al., 2022, p. 7). Based on a categorization analysis of work development meetings, the authors identified that hospitalists find their own unique positions while respecting the authority and functions of existing physicians and nurses in their units. Although this study (Lunkka et al., 2022) did not examine actual work involving the hospitalist in the ward, their findings suggest that the person acting as a hospitalist tried to find tasks that could be uniquely taken up by this new role, while paying close attention to tasks that are normally carried out by other specialists, such as surgeons and nurses.

One of the things Lunkka et al. (2022) seem to highlight is that when there is a change in an organizational formation for carrying out a set of tasks, the participants carefully observe which tasks are to be carried out by whom and when, and coordinate with others. In other words, they try to work out a reconfigured "boundary of spheres of operations" (Anderson et al., 1990, p. 242). In the setting we investigated, for both the flight doctor and the flight nurse, flying by emergency helicopter to accomplish prehospital care is a reconfigured boundary of spheres of operations. For both of them, when they receive patients transferred by the emergency crew, things are not as routinized as in the hospital. Thus, there is a sense in which each professional needs to work out what needs to be done at each moment, in each individual's capacity, still under the division of labor that is known to them in the setting (Anderson et al., 1990).

Study setting

Our study focuses on the activities of doctors and nurses who work in the Emergency Medical Unit of University Hospital A, which receives requests for emergency medical treatment that require a flight doctor and a flight nurse to fly to the rendezvous point to which the patient is brought by ambulance. Emergency helicopters usually have a pilot, an air mechanic, a flight doctor, and a flight nurse on board. After providing a full range of life-saving medical care to the injured and sick in the ambulance, they normally transport the patient by helicopter to their hospital. The flight doctor and flight nurse continuously manage the condition of the wounded during this transportation.

While there are guidelines for prehospital care for nurses (see our discussion above), a variety of educational programs for flight nurses can be found at each base hospital in Japan. As part of flight nurses' training at Hospital A, the nurse puts on a wearable camera during boarding to record the details of their work. During on-the-job training, these recordings are used as part of the training materials to allow trainees to assess their own behaviors and reflect on their work (Tsuchiya et al., 2021). The present study is also based on video recordings made in this way.

Since only one camera is used, suspended from the flight nurse's neck, whatever is in front of the nurse is shown in the video recording. For this reason, the nurse is not shown in the video data; and what is happening outside of the camera angle, including behind the nurse, cannot be seen either. Only the nurse's voice can be heard clearly.

We obtained official permission from the hospital to conduct the research using six such video recordings, together with documents related to each incident. We held research meetings on a monthly or bimonthly basis from January 2019 to January 2022 with two experienced flight nurses who were certified instructors working at the same hospital and who coauthored this chapter, a researcher in nursing, a psychologist, and three ethnomethodologists. In the meetings, we discussed the video data, prehospital care practices, educational programs for flight nurses, and the different studies conducted by the participants of the research meetings. Thus, informal interviews also took place on prehospital care practices and the researchers were able to check their analyses with the two flight nurses. One of them worked as a flight nurse in the data we analyzed. The flight nurse also interviewed the flight doctor, who features in the studied data, about some details. Through these meetings, the ethnomethodologists and flight nurses collaboratively developed the analysis and coauthored this chapter. This can be said to be our way of compensating for our (ethnomethodologists') "vulgar competence" (Garfinkel, 2002, p. 175; Garfinkel & Wieder, 1992, p. 182; Ikeya, 2020, p. 33) while Garfinkel is known to have set a high standard for the achievement of hybridity in studies of work, in particular with his unique adequacy requirement: ideally, the researcher should have the same competence as members of the field (Garfinkel, 2002; Garfinkel & Wieder, 1992; Ikeya, 2020; Lynch, 1993; Pollner & Emerson, 2001; Wilson, 2003).

Our analysis will address a central problem for members conducting activities in the setting as a *topic* for analysis. It focuses on how actions are organized from the members' point of view of accomplishing the practical management of prehospital care. By selecting this as a topic, we aim to investigate a topic that is relevant from members' point of view, and by carefully studying and describing how members organize and coordinate their actions, we aim to achieve topical relevance for both members and researchers. This, we think, is one way to satisfy the hybridity of topical relevance Garfinkel advocated (Garfinkel, 2002; Ikeya, 2020). To this end, we pay close attention to the development of the organization of talk that is intertwined with the embodied actions, which should be a primary focus. In this way, our analysis will also concentrate on what is known to members in the setting, which constitutes the competences involved in the practical management of prehospital care. The close collaboration between the ethnomethodologists and the flight nurses and other prehospital professionals allowed us to gain members' insight/expertise in the analyzed setting.

We also conducted two full days of fieldwork at the hospital in January and at the beginning of April 2020. (We halted fieldwork at that point due to the COVID-19 pandemic.) In the fieldwork, we observed how the flight doctor and flight nurse prepare and go to a rendezvous point when a request for an emergency helicopter is received by the Communication Specialist Room located beside the Emergency Medical Unit, how patients who are transported by the ambulance get initial treatment in the Emergency Medical Unit of the hospital, and how they are treated.

When the Emergency Medical Unit receives a patient transported by ambulance, five to six doctors, including interns, and three to four nurses are involved in the initial treatment. Figure 1 illustrates a scene showing the moment when a patient is taken into an Initial Treatment Room at the Emergency Medical Unit. In contrast, in the prehospital care setting, the flight doctor and flight nurse work on their own, with occasional assistance from the ambulance crew team. Figure 2, filmed by a video camera worn by a flight nurse, presents a scene occurring inside an ambulance at a rendezvous point. A flight doctor is taking care of a patient with the help of an ambulance crew member.

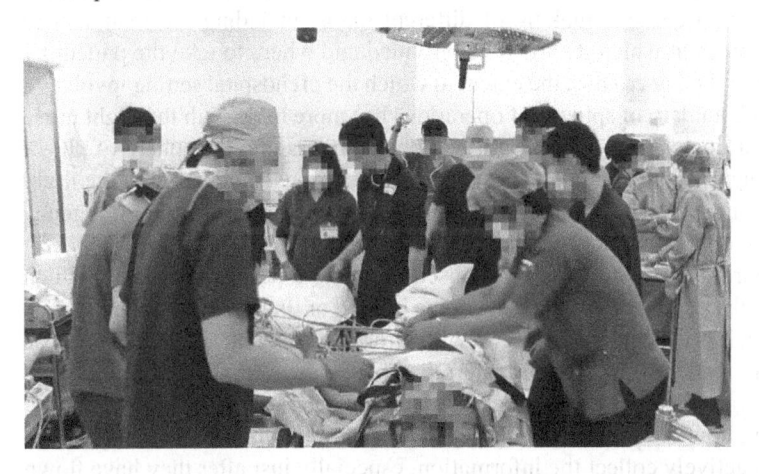

Figure 1 Initial outpatient treatment being administered in the Emergency Medical Care unit at the hospital.

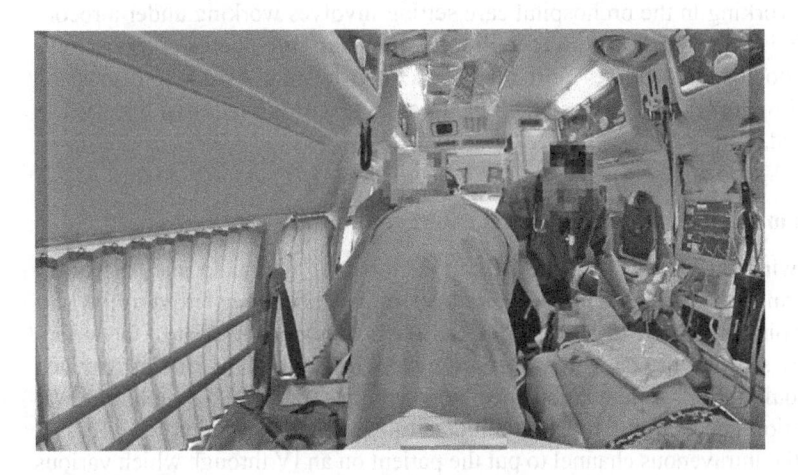

Figure 2 Emergency prehospital treatment in the ambulance.

As shown by Figures 1 and 2, the initial treatment provided to a patient in each setting occurs in extremely different environments. As mentioned earlier, textbooks and guidelines emphasize that flight nurses should be aware of the differences between prehospital care and the initial care at a hospital. For example, in the Emergency Medical Unit of the hospital, when they receive a patient in serious condition, a team of doctors normally conducts a physical assessment of the patient and then on that basis they decide among themselves what tests and treatment to provide. The nurses help the doctors to provide those tests and the treatment as well as documenting detailed information about the patient and their treatment. The nurses are normally not directly involved in the physical assessment or the decision-making with regard to examinations and treatment. In the prehospital care setting, in contrast, the flight nurse is directly involved in the entire process, from the physical assessment to decision-making of different kinds, including the treatment to provide, the order in which it should be provided and where to take the patient by helicopter or ambulance. Thus, the extent to which the prehospital setting involves a reconfigured boundary of spheres of operations has more to do with the flight nurse than the flight doctor, as it is the flight nurse who enters into the sphere of physically assessing the patient and making treatment decisions, together with the flight doctor. In contrast, when they treat a patient in serious condition in the Emergency Medical Unit, only doctors are in charge of these activities.

Furthermore, the flight nurse is supposed to create a patient document, which includes details of how the patient came to be injured or ill, while in the Emergency Medical Unit, it is the emergency crews who inform the doctors and nurses of these details for the patient they transferred. Thus, it is normally the flight nurse who gathers various types of information about the patient, including the accident situation, i.e., how the patient got injured or became ill. However, the flight doctor may also actively collect the information, especially just after they have flown to the rendezvous point, as the information is essential for conducting prehospital care, as we will see in the analysis in the next section.

Thus, working in the prehospital care setting involves working under a reconfigured division of labor with a reconfigured boundary of spheres of operations, as flight doctors and nurses normally work at a hospital (see our discussion above). However, how this is so and what competences are required have yet to be explored.

Practical management of prehospital emergency care

The following case is unusual for the flight doctor and flight nurse since they have been informed that more than one injured person has been transferred to the rendezvous point. When the flight doctor and flight nurse open the door of the ambulance, they see that the patient lying on the stretcher is moving around so much that he would fall off it if an ambulance crew member was not holding him down. This situation makes it difficult for the nurse to follow the normal procedure, i.e., securing the intravenous channel to put the patient on an IV through which various medicines can be administered.

Identifying priority patients

By the time the flight doctor and flight nurse arrive by helicopter, the ambulance crew members are usually found taking care of the patient. They would already have conducted a general assessment of the patient, including checking vital signs, noting the general appearance, and taking the patient's history. The doctor and nurse who have flown over from the hospital obtain more information about the patient from the ambulance crew members. At this point, the ambulance crew members hand the patient over to the flight doctor and flight nurse and may remain in the ambulance to assist them both, if they see it is necessary. In the case examined here, however, not only the ambulance crew members but also an air mechanic (which is quite rare) eventually join in to help the doctor and nurse, as the patient is quite unsettled and may fall if not restrained.

In the first part of Excerpt 1, the flight doctor (FD) and the flight nurse (FN) have arrived at the ambulance and are entering it (Figure 3):

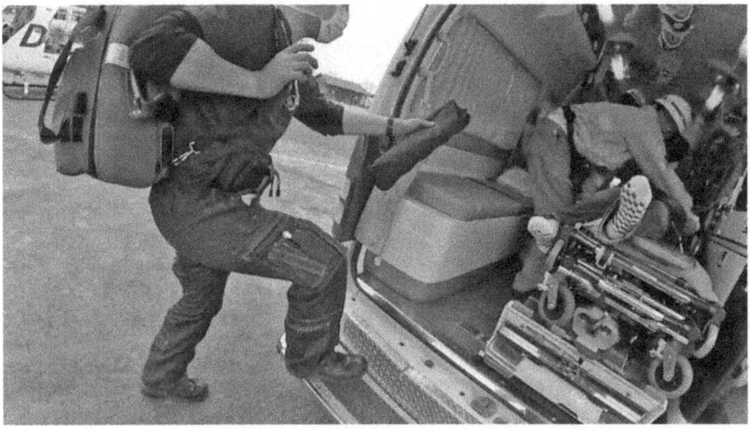

Figure 3 (00:12) Ambulance crew members holding the patient down on the stretcher as the flight doctor enters the ambulance with a bag of equipment.

Excerpt 1
FD: Flight Doctor; CC: Ambulance Crew Member

```
((00:11))
8    FD:    Etto juhsyoh ichimei keisyoh sannmei tte kiiteru nn desu kedomo=
            ITJ severe-injury one minor-injury three PT heard PT COP L
            Well, I heard there is one with severe injuries and three others
            with minor ones.
9    CC:    =Hai
            Yes
            Yes
10   FD:    Kono kata ga juhsyoh no kata de ii [nn desu ka?
            this person SP severe-injury L person PT right PT COP QP
            Is this person the one with severe injuries?
11   CC:                                       [Sou desu ne=
                                                Yes COP FP
                                                Yes,
```

```
12  CC:  =Soudesu
         Yes COP
         he is.
13  FD:  Keisyoh no sannin ha dou suru houkou ni nari masu ka?
         minor-injury L three SP what do direction O COP QP
         What has been decided on the three with minor injuries?
14       (1.0)
15  CC:  Keisyou no kata mo kochira ni ki masu
         minor-injury L person SP here PT come COP
         Those with minor injuries are also coming here.

16  FD:  Keisyou mo kuru, naruhodo
         minor-injury SP come ITJ
         Those with minor injuries are also coming, I see.!
17  P:   Ah::
         ITJ
         ((moaning))
         ((FN starts to prepare an IV bag))
18  CC:  Hora abare nai abare nai yo hora
         ITJ  behave-violently don't behave-violently don't FP ITJ
         Hey, don't move violently.
19  CC:  Abare nai yo
         Behave-violently don't FP
         Don't be violent.
20  CC:  Arimase n
         have FP
         I don't have it.
21  FD:  Wkari masu ka::?
         aware COP FP
         Are you aware of me?
22  P:   Ah:::
         ITJ
         (moaning)
23  CC:  Sugoi fuon ga sugoi desu
         extreme restlessness SP extreme COP
         He is extremely restless. ((Turning his face toward FN))
24  FN:  Sugoi doukou dou desu ka ne?
         extreme pupil how COP QP FP
         Extreme. How is his pupil?
25  CC:  Doukou tte yon yon jouten shite masu
         pupil P four four supraduction do COP
         His pupil is 4-4 and supraducted.
26  FN:  yon yon jouten
         four four supraduction
         4-4 and supraducted
27  CC:  (hai) taikou ha nibui desu
         yes light-reflex SP sluggish COP
         Yes, his light reflex is sluggish.
28  FD:  Kono kata ga tsukkonda kata desu ka?
         this person SP crashed person COP QP
         Is this the person who crashed?
29       (0.5)
30  CC:  Sou desu
         yes COP
         Yes.
31  FD:  ha::i
         ITJ
         OK.
((00:39))
```

Working out interprofessional collaboration 57

Based on the information obtained before they arrived at the rendezvous point (see our description above), FD asks members of the ambulance crew to first confirm whether the patient in the ambulance is the one with severe injuries (l. 8–10). After CC's confirmation (l. 11–12), he inquires whether a decision has already been made regarding the patients with minor injuries: "What has been decided on the three patients with minor injuries?" (l. 13). In response, CC replies that they will also be transported to the scene (l. 15). The flight doctor responds by repeating the crew member's sentence (l. 16), by which means this information is made known to the flight nurse. Moreover, by adding "I see" at the end, he highlights this fact for both himself and the flight nurse as this means an additional task must be carried out before they leave the rendezvous point, which we will deal with later. However, this topic is suspended by the patient's increased movements and the medical staff become occupied with him (l. 17-31).

While the flight doctor asks about the patients (l. 13), the flight nurse enters the ambulance with three bags of medicine, some equipment, and some packages of lactate ringer solution. Immediately after FN puts the bags down (00:18), he puts a package of lactate ringer solution on a hook in the ambulance (00:22) and extends the line of an IV drip that is attached to the solution (Figure 4). FN then asks about the patient's pupillary reflex (l. 24) and starts cutting small pieces of surgical tape from a roll, sticking each piece to the edge of a cupboard in the ambulance (00:34–00:39, Figure 5).

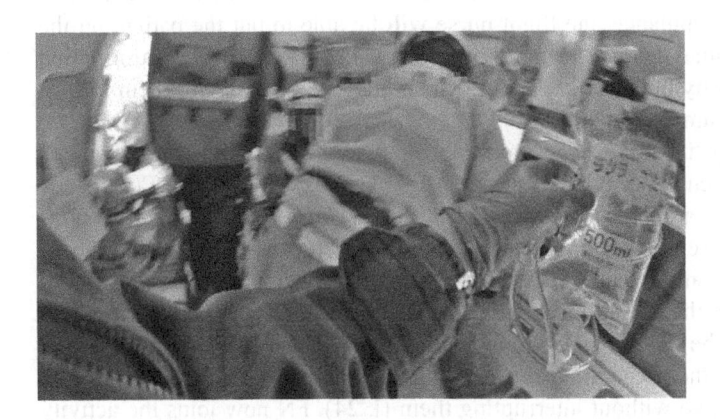

Figure 4 (00:22) The flight nurse hanging a pack of lactate ringer solution on a hook as he enters the ambulance with two bags of medicine and equipment.

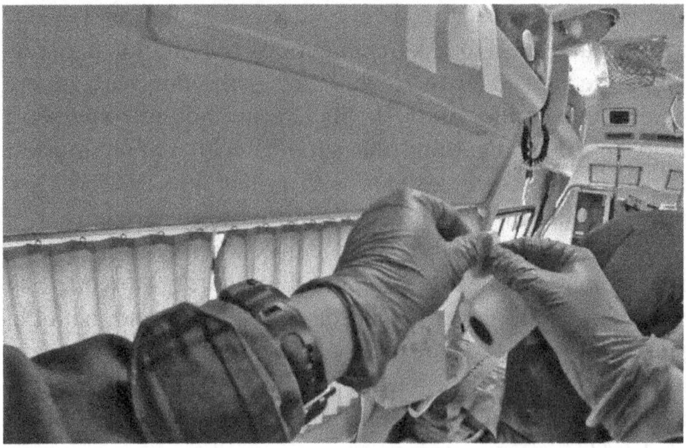

58 *Nozomi Ikeya et al.*

Figure 5 (00:39) The flight nurse cuts small pieces of surgical tape from a roll and sticks each piece to the edge of the cupboard.

This series of actions, from putting the package of solution on a hook to preparing short pieces of tape (to affix the line of the IV drip) (Figures 4 and 5), show that FN immediately starts preparing to secure an intravenous route to administer the solution. This preparation by FN takes place while FD tries to identify the priority patient to be treated. By preparing to secure an intravenous route as soon as he enters the ambulance, the flight nurse will be able to put the patient on the IV drip with minimal delay. This takes place while the doctor collects information to be able to identify the priority patient, which makes it possible for them to start administering treatment smoothly.

The first thing the flight nurse normally does as he enters the ambulance is prepare the intravenous drip by securing an intravenous route. In the Emergency Medical Unit, it is a doctor (often a resident doctor) who secures an intravenous route, and the nurse would normally just help the doctor by preparing the pieces of tape. Here we can see that FN and FD are working under a modified division of labor compared to the one at the hospital.

It should also be noted that FN overhears the talk between FD and CC while FN is engaged in the preparation for the IV drip. Thus, FN was able to enter the talk between the two without interrupting them (l. 24). FN now joins the activity of finding out about the patient by asking about the patient's pupillary reflex. This allows FN, together with FD, to prepare for the physical assessment of the patient, a task that will be conducted by both of them.

Later on (Excerpt 4, l. 84), an agreement is eventually reached to sedate the patient by intramuscular injection, as he is moving around frantically and may fall off the stretcher unless several people keep holding him in place. Immediately after this decision is made, the doctor returns to the earlier topic and asks about the three patients with minor injuries (Excerpt 2, l. 90):

Excerpt 2
FD: Flight Doctor; FN: Flight Nurse; CC: Ambulance Crew Member

```
((01:45))
90  FD:  Hoka no sannnin no johhoh tte nanka kiite masu ka?
         other L three L information PT any hear COP QP
         Do you have any information about the other three patients?
91  CC:  Nain desu moushiwakenai desu [ehto
         don't COP sorry COP ITJ
         Sorry we don't uhm.
92  FD:  [Nain desu ne
         don't COP FP
         You don't.
93  CC:  Zatto mita tokoro ha ritsui de taikishi te mashi ta
         quick look where PT standing-position PT wait PT COP PST
         From a quick look, they were waiting in a standing position.
94       ((D tries to get out from a front door.))
95  FD:  Maji ka [sore kocchi tsurete kuru [tteiu handan ha[
         really QP them here bring come L decision SP
         Really? They will be brought here?
((01:56))
```

The doctor asks whether the ambulance crew is aware of any specific symptoms or conditions ("any information") pertaining to the patients with minor injuries (l. 90). By asking about these patients' conditions, he seeks to identify what further tasks will be involved in taking care of them in addition to their first patient. CC initially responds by apologizing that they do not have any information (l. 91). However, immediately after the flight doctor's full repeat of what was said by CC (l. 92), the crew member adds: "from a quick glance, they were waiting in a standing position" (l. 93). FD responds by displaying that he disagrees with the decision made by the ambulance crew to bring "them" (the three patients with minor injuries) "here" (the rendezvous point) (l. 95). Generally, flight doctors and nurses are supposed to concentrate only on critically ill patients – normally the most critically ill patient, if there is more than one, since only one patient can be transported in a helicopter at a time. Thus, from the doctor's point of view, it is the ambulance crew who should deal with the three patients with minor injuries. However, CC's statement (l. 93) is understood to mean that the patients have already been brought to the rendezvous point and that they are in good enough condition to be able to stand and wait.

As has been demonstrated so far, identifying the priority patient to administer care to is the flight doctor and flight nurse's immediate task when they arrive at the ambulance and speak with the crew. They seek to obtain information from the ambulance crew, as it is they who have dealt with the patients from their original location to their arrival at the rendezvous point. It is important for the flight doctor and flight nurse to learn about the situation – including whether the patient in the ambulance is their priority patient, especially if other people were involved in the accident – to ensure that the *right* decision is made regarding priority. Thus, identifying how many patients there are and whom they should prioritize is critical for the flight doctor and nurse when they initiate their work at the rendezvous point, although this information is not initially extensive enough from the point of view of accomplishing the prehospital care. While the flight nurse may not ask questions directly, he or she can ask for information as necessary while listening to the exchanges between the emergency crew and the flight doctor. In this way, the flight nurse remains aware of which necessary tasks are already being handled by someone else while at the same time carrying out other tasks himself or herself.

Identifying and agreeing on priority tasks and task coordination

One important feature of prehospital care activities is that the patient is in serious condition and treatment-related decisions must be made quickly. For such decisions to be made, information on the patient's condition and injury mechanism must be collected from the emergency crew and a physical assessment must be conducted by observation – a task shared by the flight nurse and the flight doctor. Thus, once priority patients are identified as we have seen in Excerpt 1 and 2, treatment decisions are made by identifying and agreeing on priority tasks based on the patient's condition they jointly identify (Excerpt 3), agreeing on the coordination of priority tasks (Excerpt 4), and agreeing on timing for the accomplishment of remaining tasks (Excerpt 5). We examine how newly identified and shared information in the course of action is dealt with in relation to what is known to the doctor and nurse including the areas of expertise of the doctor, nurse, and members of the ambulance crew and the division of labor among them.

Identifying and agreeing on priority tasks based on the patient's condition

The patient has been in a severely disturbed state, moving his arms and legs around wildly, and four ambulance crew members are trying to respond to this situation. The flight doctor was informed before he arrived at the rendezvous point that the patient was involved in a car accident. At the beginning of Excerpt 3 (l. 32–33), CC is holding the patient down with his colleagues, while at the same time responding to FD's question (see Excerpt 1, l. 28) of how exactly this patient was involved in the car accident:

Excerpt 3
FD: Flight Doctor; FN: Flight Nurse; P: Patient; CA, CB, CC: Ambulance Crew Members

```
((00:39))
32  CC:   Eh, mokugeki johhou ni yoruto, torraku wo sake you to shite taikou no
          ITJ eyewitness information PT according, truck O evade PT PT try
          Well, according to an eyewitness, he crashed into an oncoming car
33        kuruma ni tsukkonda=
          oncoming L car O crashed
          when trying to avoid a truck
34  FN:   = Te toka dase masu ka ne kore chotto?
          arm PT pull COP QP FP this little
          Can you pull his arm up a little bit?
35  CA:   Muri(ssu)
          can't (FP)
          I can't.
36  CC:   Fuku bu no akiraka na gaisyou mirare nai nde
          abdominal region L observable L injury seem NEG FP
          There is no observable injury in the abdominal region.
```

```
37  CA:   ((Turning his face toward CB and CC)) [Ato hitori ni, sumimasenn
          hitori ote moratte ii?
          more person O ITJ person ride can ask QT
          another person, can we get another person over?
38  FN:                                           [Chi, chin, chinseika chinseika
                                                   se-  seda- sedation sedation
                                                   Sedation, sedation
39  CC:   Ushiro, ushiro osaete kudasai
          back back hold FP
          Back, back. Hold his back.
40        (.)
41  FN:   Chotto kono [te no(.)uhhnto ne.   [Kono te wo chotto Nobase masu kane?
          a bit this hand L   ITL FP         this hand OP a bit straighten FP QP
          A bit, could you straighten this arm a bit?
42  FD:                                     [Chotto nai (        )
                                             little NEG
                                             There is no (    )
43  CC:                                     [Hai
                                             ITJ
                                             Yes
44  FN:   Soujanaito tennteki tore nai nd=
          Otherwise IV put NEG L
          Otherwise, I cannot put an IV in him.
45  CA:   =a, hitori, ima, nori masu [node (.) chotto matte kudasai
          ITJ person now join FP L moment wait FP
          Oh, another person will join us, so please wait a moment.
46        ((The ambulance crew member is holding the patient's upper body down,
          but he keeps moving violently))
47  FN:                              [Oh::: sugoi ne
                                      ITJ extreme FP
                                      Wow, extreme
48  FN:   Sugoi ne (.) ohh mou daijoubu kore
          hard FP     ITJ PT all right this
          This is hard, are we all right, this
49  FN:   ((holding the patient's right hand))
50        (0.9)
51  P:    Uhhh
          ITJ
          ((moaning))
52        (1.1)
53  FN:   Te [wo ne
          hand OP FP
          His hand.
54  FD:   [Muri sou dattara: serushin kinn chu shichai masu kedo=
          difficult FP if diazepam muscle inject COP FP L
          If it's too difficult, I'll inject diazepam into his muscle.
55  FN:   =Ah::mou serushin [kin chu shi masu ka?
          ITJ now diazepam muscle inject COP FP QP
          Yeah, shall we then inject diazepam into his muscle now?
56  FD:   [sorede (.) ah (.) un
          then ITJ yeah
          Then, yeah.
((01:10))
```

FN is preparing to secure the intravenous channel with a rubber band in his left hand. He asks the ambulance crew member (CA) whether he could pull the patient's arm up (l. 34, Figure 6). CA, with his head slightly turned toward the nurse, says he cannot do this (l. 35) and then makes a request to colleagues to fetch another person to join them (l. 37).

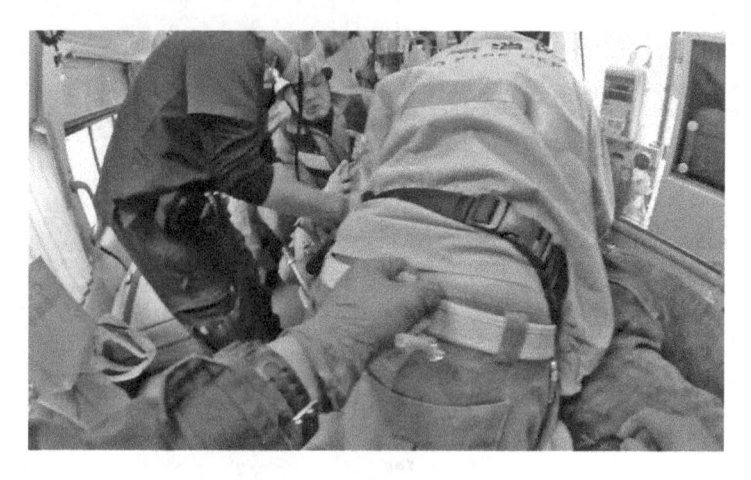

Figure 6 (00:45) The flight nurse asks the ambulance crew member (CA) "Can you pull his arm up a little bit?" (1.34).

While CA asks his colleagues to bring over another person, the flight nurse says the word "sedation" twice in succession (l. 38). At this point, it is not clear whether FN is making a suggestion to the others or talking to himself about the task that needs to be performed at *this* moment. However, it is certain that the suggestion is primarily addressed to FD and not to the ambulance crew members, as sedation is a treatment-related task for which the flight doctor and flight nurse are responsible. Immediately after the nurse's utterance, CC asks his colleague to hold the patient's back (l. 39), while the flight nurse again asks the ambulance crew if anybody can pull the patient's arm up while grabbing the patient's right hand (l. 41). Then, in line 44, FN indicates explicitly that not being able to do this is an obstacle to securing an intravenous route to put an intravenous drip into the patient's arm: "Otherwise, I cannot put an IV in him" (l. 44). Immediately after this, CA reports that one more member is coming soon.

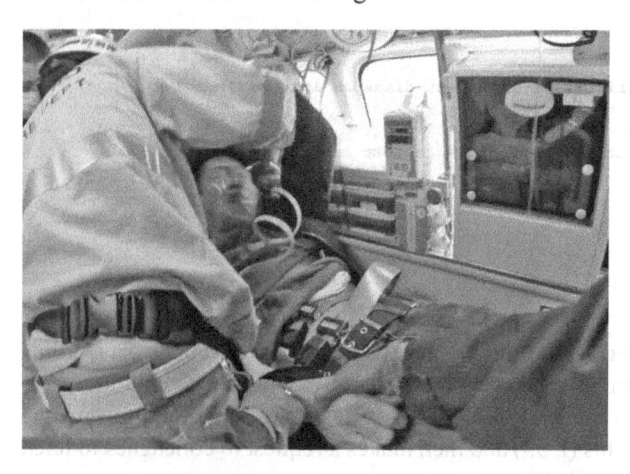

Figure 7 (00:58) The flight nurse tries to pull the patient's arm up "Wow extreme" (1.47).

From l. 46–52, it is evident that the patient is struggling violently while the team tries to restrain him. FD is holding the patient's right arm, still attempting to secure an intravenous channel, while CA is also holding the patient's right wrist. FN exclaims, "Wow, extreme" (l. 47, Figure 7). FN, by saying "This is hard. Are we all right, this" (l. 48), displays that they are at their limits in terms of controlling the situation. FD, watching them struggle, makes a suggestion: "If it's too difficult, I'll inject diazepam into his muscle" (l. 54). He suggests sedating the patient into a non-restless condition using an intramuscular injection of diazepam. In other words, the doctor suggests sedation and a concrete method of achieving it. This doctor's suggestion seems to have been made in response to the nurse's more general suggestion "sedation" (l. 38). Moreover, the first part of the suggestion can be reconstructed as meaning "'If it's too difficult' to sedate the patient through intravenous injection." Sedation through intravenous injection is generally preferred over intramuscular injection since the sedation takes longer with the latter method. Besides, intramuscular injection involves extra steps (after waiting for the patient to be sedated, they still need to secure an intravenous route to administer other medicine).

FN immediately gives his consent (l. 55) to the suggestion that was made by FD (l. 54): "shall we then inject diazepam into his muscle now?" By adding "now," the nurse displays that he agrees with the doctor's suggestion to do the sedation through intramuscular injection "now," instead of first securing the intravenous route and then administering an intravenous injection, which is normally the preferred way of injection. Thus, the nurse agrees with FD's judgment that securing an intravenous route would probably be difficult given the patient's relentless movements.

As we have noted, FN's earlier utterance "Sedation, sedation" (l. 38) itself does not appear to be addressed to anybody and it seems almost as if FN is talking to himself. However, when FD makes his suggestion "If it's too difficult, I'll inject diazepam into his muscle" (l. 54), FD's suggestion is heard as a response to FN's "Sedation, sedation" (l. 38), which now seems to have been heard by FD as both FN's judgment of the patient's condition with regard to their procedure and his consequent suggestion that sedation is needed. However, attention needs to be paid to the fact that FD's suggestion is made not just in response to FN's "Sedation, sedation" (l. 38), but also to the patient's movements and the struggles of the team of emergency crew members, FN, and FD himself since the moment FN said "Sedation, sedation" (l. 38). In this way, although FN's "Sedation, sedation" was not said clearly to be understood as a suggestion to the doctor, since it was said at this specific moment it was heard as a candidate judgment of the situation and a candidate solution, which prompted the doctor to eventually suggest a particular method for sedation, with a set of tasks to be coordinated, as an appropriate option.

Agreeing on the coordination of priority tasks

The following Excerpt 4 occurs shortly after Excerpt 3 (21 lines omitted), in which FD and FN have agreed on injecting diazepam to achieve sedation. At the beginning of Excerpt 4, FD asks FN to confirm that there are no findings in the patient's chest at this stage:

Excerpt 4

FD: Flight Doctor; FN: Flight Nurse; P: Patient; CA, CC, CD: Ambulance Crew Members

```
((01:21))
72  FD:   Mune [ha syoken nasa sou desu yone::=
          chest SP observation NEG seem COP FP
          There seems to be no findings in his chest, right?
73  FN:   [Totto ttotto
          ITJ ITJ
          Oops
74  FN:   =Mune ha syoken nasa [sou
          chest SP observation NEG seem
          There seems to be no findings in his chest.
75  FD:                       [Un(.) dakara chinsei kakete tte kara
                              yes  thus  sedation  start  PT L
          Right, so after sedating him
76  FD:   Yukkuri mou ikkai soukan demo ii desu yone
          slowly more one-time intubation PT OK COP QP
          one more time, we intubate slowly. Is that OK?
77        (1.0)
78  P:    (Uh)
          ITJ
          Uh
79  FN:   Tada chotto [kono fuon joukyou ja tennteki toru nomo muzukashii ssune
!         But even this restlessness situation SP IV inject PT difficult FP
          But it's difficult to even get him on IV because of his restlessness.
80  CC:   (        ) Shimasu ((moving towards the space between CD and CA))
                              I'll
          I'll (      )
81  FD:   Neh [(.) dakara serushin utte(kara)
          ITJ so diazepam inject (L)
          Well (.) so (after) injecting the diazepam,
82  FN:   [Yappa serushin ucchai masyou hai=
          Yes diazepam inject let's ITJ
          Yes, let's inject the diazepam.
83  FD:   Un yukuri yari masyou
          Yes slowly do FP
          Yeah, let's do them slowly.
84  FN:   Ryoukai
          OK
          OK.
((01:39))
```

In response to FD's request for confirmation that there are no significant findings in the chest (l. 72), FN confirms this to the doctor by repeating FD's statement (l. 74). Then FD asks the nurse for his agreement on intubating the patient after sedation: "Right, so after sedating him, one more time, we intubate slowly. Is that OK?" (l. 75–76). Here, the doctor appears to be suggesting (although this is not clearly stated in words) that because they are going to intubate the patient after sedation, they will need to secure an intravenous route to administer a sedative (which is necessary for intubation) and conduct a chest inspection "one more time" before the intubation. However, as it will take some time for the patient to become sedated with the intramuscular injection, those tasks cannot be done yet. They need to wait until the patient reaches a non-restless condition. This is why FD says "we intubate slowly" (l. 76). As was discussed in the former section, sedation through intramuscular injection requires the doctor and the nurse to perform an extra step: securing an intravenous route to administer a sedative for intubation. By asking FN to agree to a series of tasks that will follow the sedation, FD also reminds FN of the series of tasks that will follow, which also means that the intramuscular injection takes precedence over the routine flow of prehospital care – securing an intravenous route to get a patient on an IV drip and performing a physical assessment including a chest inspection. FD also asks FN to agree to the sedation through intramuscular injection even though it will take more time to get the patient sedated this way than with intravenous injection. This is why the doctor says "we intubate slowly. Is that OK?" (l. 76).

In response, FN says that even if they were to try to secure an intravenous route now, it would be impossible because the patient is moving too much ("But it's difficult to even get him on IV because of his restlessness" (l. 79)). In this way, FN agrees to FD's suggestion to perform sedation through intramuscular injection instead of intravenous injection. Having heard FN's agreement, FD again tries to confirm what needs to be done after injecting a sedative (the diazepam). FN interrupts FD, saying, "Yes, let's inject the diazepam" (l. 82). Thus, FN urges FD to move on to the primary task that they have just identified and agreed upon (sedation through intramuscular injection).

As has been observed, the doctor is cautious in deciding to administer a sedative through intramuscular injection. According to the nurse who was involved in the case, this is partly because it delays the whole process, since it takes longer for the patient to be sedated (in comparison with the intravenous injection), and other tasks that constitute the routine flow of prehospital care (including securing an intravenous route and performing a physical assessment) cannot be started right away. For this reason, according to the nurses we collaborated with, some doctors try to avoid administering a sedative through intramuscular injection.

Returning to the topic of FN's "Sedation, sedation" (l. 38), it is a statement of his judgment based on his observation of the patient and the team's struggles with him. By presenting his judgment, i.e., one candidate priority task in front of FD (and emergency crew members), FN helped them to quickly identify and focus on the priority task. FD, being presented with FN's statement, eventually picked it up as a suggestion and responded to it with the option of performing a specific procedure, i.e., sedation through intramuscular injection, that would make their process deviate from the routine procedures. Thus, FD repeatedly asked FN to agree not only to the selection of a specific method of injection but also to a set of tasks that would follow to make sure that their task coordination would be managed smoothly. When we asked the FN, who is also a coauthor of this chapter, he said that his "Sedation, sedation" (l. 38) was like talking to himself and that looking back, he could have explicitly suggested it to the doctor. If this is the case, it can be said that FN saw that sedation would be necessary and stated this so that FD could think about it. In any case, the suggestion to the doctor was made in a very subtle manner, and the doctor promptly picked up the idea of sedation and even suggested a way to perform it.

Statements concerning medical judgments are made not so much in the form of overt suggestions to flight doctors, but rather as candidate actions for the flight doctor to think about. This is probably also related to the fact that, for the flight nurse, being involved in making treatment decisions is somewhat like working in the doctors' spheres of operations at the Emergency Medical Unit. It should be noted that even the experienced flight nurse in our study finds it more appropriate to make a subtle suggestion about treatment to the doctor. As far as we have observed in other recorded video data, and as a study of a flight nurse's communication suggests (Takahashi et al., 2018), newly trained flight nurses are less likely to make such suggestions. It is probable that newly trained flight nurses find it difficult to get involved in this reconfigured boundary of spheres of operations.

Some flight doctors pick items presented by flight nurses as their priority tasks, treating them as suggestions made to them. They also tend to get the nurse to agree to the task coordination that will follow, rather than giving instructions on tasks after presenting decisions they have made. Other flight doctors may prefer to decide upon the priority tasks on their own. This is closely related to the division of labor under which they normally deal with a patient in serious condition in the Emergency Medical Unit, where doctors make most of the decisions among themselves without consulting nurses. In such cases, the flight nurses adapt to the division of labor under which the doctor is operating, which is probably close to the one in the Emergency Medical Unit. This seems to show that the flight nurse is required to always be attentive to the division of labor under which the doctor operates. Yet, the flight nurse must still carry out the necessary tasks in this prehospital setting, albeit under a division of labor close to the one they operate under in the Emergency Medical Unit.

Agreeing on timing for the accomplishment of remaining tasks

Seeing that the patient has not yet been stabilized despite the intramuscular injection of diazepam, the nurse decides that it will still be a while before the next procedure can be performed – that is, checking the chest before the tracheal intubation. FN urges FD to go and attend to the other three patients waiting outside the vehicle because the nurse observes that there are already enough people to hold down and watch the first patient (Excerpt 5, l. 161).

Excerpt 5
FD: Flight Doctor; FN: Flight Nurse; CD: Ambulance Crew Member

```
((03:20))
160         ((FN walks towards CD))
161 FN:     Soshitara sensei osaseteru dake dakara sanmei mite ki masu?
            then doctor hold-down just so three see go COP
            OK doctor, now we are just holding him down, you'll go and see
            the three patients, won't you?
162 FD:     Chotto jaa itteki masu [ne
            a-little then going COP FP
            All right, I am going then.
163 FN:                            [Un
                                    OK
                                    OK.
164 FD:     Kusuri kiita ra oshiete kudasai
            medicine work when know please
            Let me know when the medicine starts working.
((03:39))
```

FD agrees with FN's suggestion (l. 162), although it means leaving the critically ill patient inside the ambulance. So he tells FN, "Let me know when the medicine starts working" (l. 164). From the point of view of performing the tracheal intubation, followed by the chest examination (the series of procedures they have planned), FD needs to know the *right* timing for starting the next procedure. It should be noted that FD's request is made under the presumption that the patient in the ambulance is still their priority over the patients waiting outside. Meanwhile, FN considers it appropriate for the doctor – who can make medical decisions based on his knowledge, competences, and qualifications – to go and see the patients waiting outside. He also knows that holding the patient down inside the ambulance while waiting for the sedative to kick in does not necessarily require the doctor's help. In this way, the nurse tries to manage different tasks with respect to expertise and specialization. Managing different tasks by coordinating different areas of expertise is an integral part of the division of labor in operation.

In this way, the nurse considers whether they have more than enough skills and manpower to do what they are doing for the time being in terms of the priority patient and, if so, what else they should do at *this* moment and what skills are needed for that. In fact, this requires them to think ahead when they move on to another phase, identify what tasks need to be conducted, and determine how different kinds of expertise must be coordinated. This is how the practical management of prehospital care is conducted with sensitivity to time constraints.

It should be noted that in and through the interactions between FD and the emergency crew members we observed earlier, FN viewed dealing with the three patients waiting outside the ambulance as their responsibility even though these individuals were apparently not critically ill. Without being told by anybody to do this, FN found time for the patients to be taken care of by the doctor. It should also be noted that FN explicitly suggests to FD that he could go and see the patients outside ("OK doctor, now we are just holding him down, you'll go and see the three patients, won't you?" (l.161)), which is a departure from his earlier approach with "Sedation, sedation" (see Excerpt 3, l. 38). This may be partly related to the time constraints, in that this is the only time the patients can be dealt with since FD and FN will be occupied with the most ill patient in a short time. It may also be partly related to the fact that FN saw he could comfortably make this type of judgment, as it has to do with managing the process of prehospital care so that the entire process, of which the flight nurse is supposed to be in charge, goes smoothly and quickly.

Conclusion

Through an examination of prehospital care activities, this chapter aimed to present various competences involved in accomplishing the activities within the limitations of the number of individuals involved and time. Their competences are embodied as part of the flight doctor and flight nurse's ways of dealing with these problems to ensure that appropriate care can be delivered to the patient.

The first competence concerns their methods of collecting information from the emergency crew. Patient-related information is gathered by the doctor and nurse throughout the process. This task is primarily defined as the responsibility of the flight nurse, who is also the main person in charge of reporting the patient's details to a team of doctors and nurses at the hospital to which the patient is taken, as well as creating a patient record (Japan Society for Aeromedical Services, 2017). Patient-related information is important first to identify who they should be dealing with as the priority patient (see Excerpt 1). Furthermore, the nurses also try to find out how the patient was injured, i.e., the injury mechanism, if it is from an accident, or the patient's medical history. They also ask for the patient's vital signs, e.g., consciousness level or pupillary reflex, which the emergency crew members will have taken (see Excerpts 1 and 3). These items of information are important for the flight doctor and flight nurse to know, as they want to determine what they should be specifically concerned with in carrying out the physical assessment and following procedures. Information about the patient's family is also important as they need to inform the family of the hospital to which they will transfer the patient if the family is not with the patient already. Emergency crew members are also aware of the kinds of information the flight doctor and flight nurse want to know; thus, they are prepared to provide it when asked by the doctor and nurse (see Excerpts 1–4).

The second competence concerns the flight nurses' management of the whole process of prehospital care to ensure that the process gets completed as smoothly and quickly as possible. To this end, the flight doctor and flight nurse try to achieve "multitasking" whenever possible. As we have seen, each of them was trying to be engaged with each task whenever possible, but at the same time, each was monitoring the development of the other's task. For example, while the flight doctor was trying to identify the priority patient, the flight nurse was starting to prepare to put the patient on an IV drip by hanging a package of lactate ringer solution on a hook and cutting small pieces of surgical tape from a roll (see Excerpt 1). The flight nurse was apparently listening to the conversation between the flight doctor and the emergency crew, as can be seen in the way the flight nurse joined the conversation by asking a question about the patient's pupillary reflex (see Excerpt 1), which had not yet been touched upon. Another example of multitasking was shown in Excerpt 5, where the flight nurse suggested that the flight doctor go out of the ambulance and see the patients waiting outside it. While this meant that the doctor had to leave the priority patient, the nurse saw there were enough people to look after this patient until he reached a non-restless condition. The nurse saw that until the patient was ready for them to start the next treatment, the doctor could do another task (attending to the three minor injured patients) that needed to be carried out before they could leave the rendezvous point. By working out multitasking in these ways whenever possible, the flight doctor and flight nurse coordinated the tasks throughout the prehospital care process in a way that allowed multiple tasks to be accomplished in a short period. This sphere of management, which involves coordinating different tasks to ensure that the whole process of prehospital care is accomplished as quickly and smoothly as possible, is something new to emergency nurses, as it is doctors who manage the entire process of treatment in the Emergency Care Unit.

The third competence concerns performing physical assessments and making treatment decisions. The flight doctor and flight nurse verbally share their judgments of the situation at every appropriate opportunity. Based on these judgments, step by step, they reach an agreement on the priority task and how they will coordinate different sets of tasks. For example, the flight nurse verbally shared his judgment that the patient would need to be sedated and prompted the flight doctor to eventually suggest sedating the patient through intramuscular injection, which is considered to be more appropriate than intravenous injection when a patient is restless (see Excerpt 3). Also, the doctor's shared judgment that there did not seem to be any problems with the patient's chest prompted the nurse to inspect the chest, and the nurse's confirmation of the doctor's judgment prompted them to agree on a sequence of tasks that would follow the sedation before they intubated the patient (see Excerpt 4).

These ways of working in prehospital care are certainly different from the ways doctors and nurses work in the Emergency Medical Unit, where a team of doctors perform the physical assessment and decide among themselves what tasks are to be carried out, and the nurses assist them in accomplishing these tasks. In other words, from the perspective of both doctors and nurses, this sphere of operations belongs to doctors treating a patient in serious condition in the Emergency Medical Unit, and some flight doctors may still see it this way, even in the prehospital care setting. This means that the flight nurse needs to pay attention to the reconfigured boundary of spheres of operations the flight doctors see themselves operating within, especially with respect to the one in which physical assessments of the patient are conducted and treatment decisions are made. This was shown, in our case, when the flight nurse was vague in suggesting sedation to be administered before moving on to other tasks, while he was explicit in suggesting what the doctor should do next when the judgment did not directly involve treatment decision-making. This seems to confirm certain difficulties involved, especially with newly trained nurses participating in this sphere of physically assessing the patient and making treatment decisions (Takahashi, et al., 2018).

This may be related to what the hospitalist (Lunkka et al., 2022) is also trying to do in taking up tasks as he or she works with others in actual situations. This can create some difficulties when there are differences and a more adequate decision may need to be made from the point of view of an experienced flight nurse working in the prehospital setting. This issue is also closely related to one of the central concerns of research when it comes to interprofessional collaboration in healthcare settings. This study has sought to demonstrate the social organization of interprofessional collaboration by examining how flight doctors and flight nurses work from the point of view of actually managing work in one particular kind of healthcare setting. Our results show how members' ways of communicating among themselves are interwoven with what is known to members about the setting, including the division of labor and members' competences. Hence, we have managed to describe not only competences concerning the conducting of various tasks in the prehospital setting, but also what the flight doctor and the flight nurse see as relevant ways of coordinating their actions in relation to the division of labor that is relevant in the setting. Our analysis reveals that the flight nurse needs to be more sensitive to the division of labor that is relevant to the flight doctor he or she is interacting with, as the doctor may still see the division of labor applied in the Emergency Medical Unit as more relevant. As our analysis has shown, the flight nurse acts differently depending on which spheres of operations they are operating in, i.e., physically assessing the patient and making treatment decisions. These findings are closely related to what has been discussed in research on interprofessional collaboration in healthcare, with notions such as vertical communication and power relationships.

The methodological considerations we took in conducting this study were to adopt Garfinkel's solution for achieving "hybridity," the topical relevance of a study to both researchers and members under study. Ethnomethodologists and flight nurses aimed to achieve hybridity by jointly examining the members' investigative topic, the practical accomplishment of prehospital care, in which the investigative topic of the members and the researchers was integrated. With the ethnomethodologists and flight nurses working together closely, the analysis was developed into descriptions of how the members accomplish the prehospital care to be presented as a coauthored chapter. This can be said to be one way of dealing with the unique adequacy requirement.

The development of activities was examined by the researchers, with special attention to how actions were organized moment by moment, through talk and body movement, in relation to things available to members in the prehospital setting. As a result, the competences we have presented here are unique in the sense that they are presented as closely interwoven with the actual management of activities. This may be particularly important for the training of flight nurses (and, potentially, for use in the training of flight doctors), who are obliged to work in isolation from their colleagues due to the limited space on board the helicopter. A presentation of the competences needed, with an explanation of how they are related to particular situated actions in the setting, may well compensate for their limited opportunities for socialization.

Acknowledgments

We are very appreciative of the insightful comments we received from Sara Keel as well as two anonymous reviews and Andrew Carlin, which helped us to think through what we wanted to say, although the responsibility for any errors is ours alone. We also thank Japan Foundation for Emergency Medicine for the research grant that supported our research team in 2019. The authors are furthermore grateful to the late Takayuki Sakagami, Morikatsu Tsuchiya, and Masato Anzai for their comments in our research meetings.

Abbreviations for translating Japanese are listed below:

COP   Copula
FP   Final particle

ITJ   Interjection
L   Linking particle
N   Nominalizer
O   Object particle
PST   Past tense marker
PT   Particle
QP   Question particle
QT   Quotation marker
SP   Subject marking particle

References

Anderson, R. J., Sharrock, W., & Hughes, J. A. (1990). The division of labour. *Réseaux. Communication - Technologie - Société, 8*(2), 237–252. https://doi.org/10.3406/reso.1990.3560

Bezemer, J., Cope, A., Kress, G., & Kneebone, R. (2011a). "Do you have another Johan?" Negotiating meaning in the operating theatre. *Applied Linguistics Review, 2*, 313–334. https://doi.org/10.1515/9783110239331.313

Bezemer, J., Murtagh, G., Cope, A., Kress, G., & Kneebone, R. (2011b). "Scissors, please": The practical accomplishment of surgical work in the operating theater. *Symbolic Interaction, 34*(3), 398–414. https://doi.org/10.1525/si.2011.34.3.398

Braithwaite, I., & Steele, A. (2020). "Flight nurses," or "nurses who fly"? An international perspective on the role of flight nurses. *Air Medical Journal, 39*(3), 196–202. https://doi.org/10.1016/j.amj.2019.11.005

Braithwaite, J., Clay-Williams, R., Vecellio, E., Marks, D., Hooper, T., Westbrook, M., Westbrook, J., Blakely, B., & Ludlow, K. (2016). The basis of clinical tribalism, hierarchy and stereotyping: A laboratory-controlled teamwork experiment. *BMJ Open, 6*(7), e012467. https://doi.org/10.1136/bmjopen-2016-012467

Ebbs, N., & Timmons, S. (2008). Inter-professional working in the RAF Critical Care Air Support Team (CCAST). *Intensive and Critical Care Nursing, 24*(1), 51–58. https://doi.org/10.1016/j.iccn.2007.06.003

Funaki, J., & Fukaya, C. (2015). Furaitonasu no kango jissen no kouzou [Structure of nursing practice of flight nurses]. *Nihon Kyukyu Kango Gakkai Zasshi* [*Journal of Japanese Association for Emergency Nursing*], *17*(2), 1–11. https://doi.org/10.18902/jaen.17.2_1

Garfinkel, H. (1986). *Ethnomethodological studies of work*. Routledge.

Garfinkel, H. (2002). *Ethnomethodology's program: Working out Durkheim's aphorism*. Rowman & Littlefield.

Garfinkel, H., & Wieder, D. L. (1992). Two incommensurable, asymmetrically alternate technologies of social analysis. In G. Watson & R. M. Seiler (Eds.), *Text in context: Contributions to Ethnomethodology* (pp. 175–206). Sage.

González-Martínez, E., & Drew, P. (2021). Informings as recruitment in nurses' intrahospital telephone calls. *Journal of Pragmatics, 186*, 48–59. https://doi.org/10.1016/j.pragma.2021.09.013

Ikeya, N. (2020). Hybridity of hybrid studies of work: Examination of informing practitioners in practice. *Ethnographic Studies, 17*, 22–44. https://doi.org/10.5281/zenodo.4050533

Japan Society for Aeromedical Services. (Ed.). (2017). *Furaito nasu handbook: Kyukyugenba Deno Katsudo to Hanso no Tameni* [*Handbook for flight nurses: For activities and transfer in emergency*]. Herusu Shuppan.

Japanese Association for Emergency Nursing. (Ed.). (2018). *Gaishou shoki kango gaidorain JNTEC* [*Japan nursing for trauma evaluation and care* (4th. ed.)]. Herusu Shuppan.

Lunkka, N., Jansson, N., Mainela, T., Suhonen, M., Meriläinen, M., Puhakka, V., & Wiik, H. (2022). Professional boundaries in action: Using reflective spaces for boundary work to incorporate a new healthcare role. *Human Relations*, *75*(7), 1270–1297. https://doi.org/10.1177/00187267211010363

Lynch, M. (1993). *Scientific practice and ordinary action: Ethnomethodology and social studies of science*. Cambridge University Press.

Mondada, L. (2014). Requesting immediate action in the surgical operating room: Time, embodied resources and praxeological embeddedness. In E. Couper-Kuhlen & P. Drew (Eds.), *Requests in interaction* (pp. 271–304). John Benjamins.

Pollner, M., & Emerson, R. M. (2001). Ethnomethodology and ethnography. In P. Atkinson, A. Coffey, S. Delamont, J. Lofland, & L. Lofland (Eds.), *Handbook of ethnography* (pp. 118–135). Sage.

Pugh, D. (2002). A phenomenologic study of flight nurses' clinical decision-making in emergency situations. *Air Medical Journal*, *21*(2), 28–36. https://doi.org/10.1016/S1067-991X(02)70083-7

Reimer, A., Clochesy, J., & Moore, S. (2013). Early examination of the middle-range theory of flight nursing expertise. *Applied Nursing Research*, *26*(4), 276–279. http://doi.org/10.1016/j.apnr.2013.07.006

Reimer, A., & Moore, S. (2010). Flight nursing expertise: Towards a middle-range theory. *Journal of Advanced Nursing*, *66*(5), 1183–1192. https://doi.org/10.1111/j.1365-2648.2010.05269.x

Sakuta, H., Ogushi, A., & Sakaguchi, M. (2020). Furaitonasu no shokumu suikou no kouzou [Structure of nursing practice of flight nurses]. *Nihon Kangoka Gakkaishi* [*Journal of Japan Academy of Nursing Science*], *40*, 252–259. https://doi.org/10.5630/jans.40.252

Schot, E., Tummers, L., & Noordegraaf, M. (2020). Working on working together. A systematic review on how healthcare professionals contribute to interprofessional collaboration. *Journal of Interprofessional Care*, *34*(3), 332–342. https://doi.org/10.1080/13561820.2019.1636007

Senften, J., & Engström, Å. (2013). Critical care nurses' experiences of helicopter transfers. *Nursing in Critical Care*, *20*(1), 25–33. https://doi.org/10.1111/nicc.12063

Takahashi, S., Tsuchiya, M., & Sakagami, T. (2018). Furaitonasu no keikenkaisu ni okeru hatsuwakodo no tokucho [Characteristics of utterances by flight nurses of different number of flights]. *Nihon Kangokagaku GakkaiGakujutsushukaienshu* [*Proceedings of the Academic Conference, Japan Academy of Nursing Science*], *39*, O57-01, 435.

Tsuchiya, M., Ito, K., Takahashi, S., Sakagami, T., & Manabe, K. (2021). Uearabulu camera no doga no kaiseki niyoru purehosupitaru kea niokeru kangoshi no jukurensei hyoka no kokoromi: furaitonasu niokeru jukurensha to shoshinsha no hikaku. [Assessment of nurses' proficiency in pre-hospital care using activity based on wearable camera video: comparison between expert and novice rlight nurses]. *Nihon Kango Kagakkaishi* [*Journal of Japan Academy of Nursing Science*], *41*, 71–78. https://doi.org/10.5630/jans.41.71

Wilson, T. P. (2003). Garfinkel's radical program. *Research on Language and Social Interaction*, *36*(4), 487–494. https://doi.org/10.1207/S15327973RLSI3604_8

Zimmerman, D. H., & Pollner, M. (1970). The everyday world as a phenomenon. In H. B. Pepinsky (Ed.), *People and information* (pp. 33–65). Pergamon. https://doi.org/10.1016/B978-0-08-015624-8.50006-6

3 Senior staff member walks ahead, nursing intern follows

Mobility practices in hospital corridors

Esther González-Martínez

Introduction

Clinic personnel spend a considerable part of their time traveling through the hospital, achieving the configurations of people, places, items, and information required to conduct their activities (Bardram & Bossen, 2005). Going in and out of the rooms and walking through the corridors, they engage in interaction and common activities with coworkers and build situation awareness (González-Martínez et al., 2017a, b; Long et al., 2007). Through local mobility, clinicians in training and newcomers are instructed in their profession and get to know the functioning of the care units, for instance while shadowing a senior member during their first days or weeks in the wards (Messmer et al., 2004). When studying the staff's independent local mobility (Luff & Heath, 1998; Psathas, 1976) in a hospital outpatient clinic,[1] we became interested in the way nursing interns walk through the corridors with senior staff members. In this chapter, we focus on a specific mobile interactional configuration (Kendon, 1973): the senior member walks ahead and the intern follows. We present how this spatial, orientational, and practical arrangement of co-present bodies is produced by the participants, in situ and in real time, through deftly combined multimodal practices that question the condition of interns as not-yet-fully-competent members. In line with Sacks's (1992) emphasis on identifying the internal grounds of sequential structures, we will account for the intern's walking-behind by referring to the organization of the activities at hand, in contrast to an external system such as deference rules based on professional status (Shils, 1968).

In "The Techniques of the Body," Mauss (1973 [1935]) argues that individuals walk in ways that are socially transmitted and acquired, specific to social groups, contexts, and moments in time. To study ways of walking, Mauss recommends starting with detailed observations on the ground. The mobility and spatial turn in ethnography (Ingold & Vergunst, 2008) and social interaction research (McIlvenny et al., 2009) was in fact fueled by a long-standing tradition of ethnomethodological studies on the "endogenously achieved details of structure" of locomotive action (Garfinkel, 2002, p. 164); see Garfinkel and Livingston (2003), Livingston (1987), and Psathas (1976). Ryave and Schenkein (1974) consider walking as "the concerted accomplishment of members of the community involved [...]... in its production and recognition" (p. 265). Watson (1995) argues that the practical organization of walking is in line with a moral order: a natural, normal way of moving on which participants' inferences and actions are grounded. Relieu (1999) shows that the respective organizations of the walking activity and the participants' talk are reflexively connected. First and foremost, walking substantiates the ethnomethodological claims that "there is order in the most ordinary activities of everyday life in their full concreteness" (Garfinkel, 1996, p. 7) and that well beyond presenting properties of order, social facts are and exist as phenomena of order (Garfinkel, 1988). This applies to walking activities, as well as the organizational tasks, identities, and relationships emerging from them. Such phenomena of order are achieved in methodical, concerted, practical ways, moment-by-moment, on the spot, and in the midst of unavoidable contingencies (Garfinkel, 2002) by skillful members who are at odds with the "cultural dope" (Garfinkel, 1984[1967], p. 68), who acts following preestablished, standardized expectations and is characteristic of the social reproduction paradigm. Methodologically, the real-time practical work involved in endogenously producing these phenomena of order is available when going "inside-with the stream" (Garfinkel, 2002, p. 164) and through descriptions that could be misread as instructions for reproducing them (Garfinkel, 1996); such is the sociological perspective guiding the study presented in this chapter.

Setting, data, and methods

The origin of our study is a video-based research project on mobile and contingent work interactions in an acute-care hospital in the French-speaking part of Switzerland; see González et al. (2017a) for a detailed presentation. The research team concentrated on the local mobility practices of the staff of an outpatient clinic that provided scheduled and walk-in care services in general and orthopedic medicine. The clinic occupied the ground floor of a wing of the hospital and comprised a total of 22 rooms served by two long, parallel double-loaded corridors connected in the middle and at the ends by shorter corridors (see Figure 1). The main centers of activity were the day hospital room, used mainly for administering treatments to chronic patients, and the urgent-care room for non-life-threatening emergencies. Besides these, there were several other consultation, examination, and treatment rooms, a reception office, and several other spaces such as a waiting room, restrooms, and stock rooms. The clinic's staff was formed of a secretary-receptionist, a head physician, a senior resident, several non-appointed regular fellows and junior residents, a head nurse, nurses (working permanently at the clinic or on a rotating basis), nursing aides (permanent or rotating), and nursing interns; 14 staff members worked at the clinic on an average working day. Some staff members had assigned workstations but the actual spatial distribution of the staff frequently changed depending on the moment-by-moment needs of the clinic's functioning. All the staff moved around in the clinic extensively throughout the day.

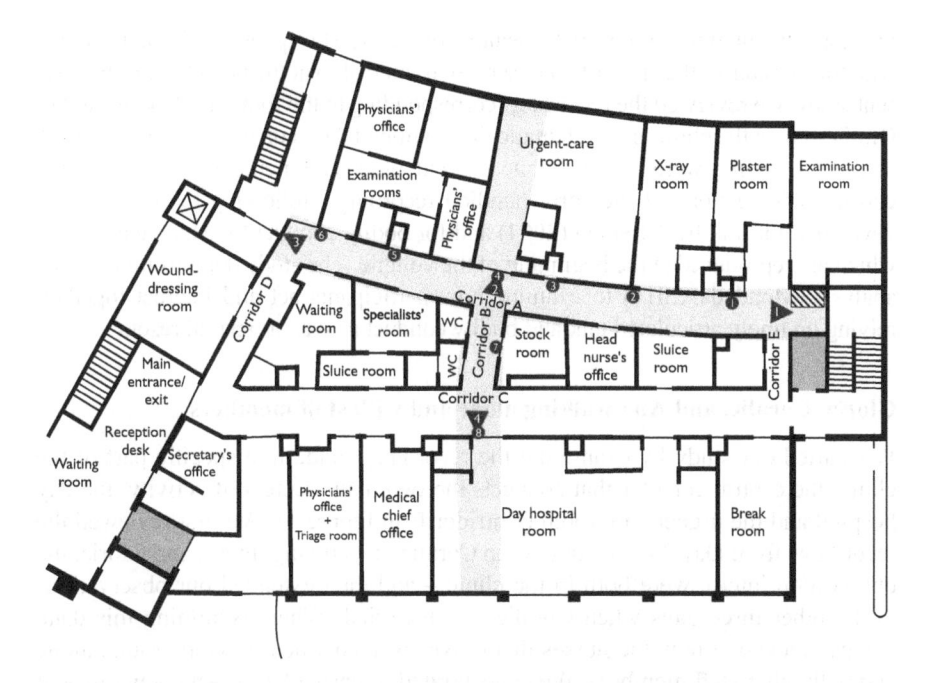

Figure 1 Clinic premises and recording set-up. The triangles represent the video cameras, the dots the wireless microphones, and the striped rectangle the rectangle/mixing/editing station. The area covered by the video cameras is represented in gray. Corridor A is 27.40 meters long, Corridor B (the section between A and C) 4.16 meters long, and Corridor C 31.50 meters long.

The research project entailed 66 days of fieldwork including seven consecutive days of video recordings, 12 hours per day, in the corridors of the clinic. We used four video cameras suspended from the ceilings and eight wireless microphones suspended from wall fixtures, all recording simultaneously. In this way, we collected 331 hours of video recordings, which the research team coded in full, identifying a total of 7,506 corridor occupations. The hospital's board of directors accepted the research project and the clinic staff consented to participate in it and have their activities video recorded. All footage of individuals other than the hospital staff and the research team (37 people in total) was discarded. The research protocol provided for the reproduction, for the purpose of scientific publications, of still images of the participants taken from the video recordings. We replaced the personal information, such as legal names, of recorded individuals or people referred to in the recordings with fictitious information.

During the recording period, the nursing intern was Coralie. She was doing an eight-week internship at the clinic as part of her bachelor's studies to become a nurse. She was on her 12th day at the clinic when she was recorded for the first time, on the second day of the recordings, and makes an appearance in the recordings of four full days. On the sixth day of the recordings, there was also Gloria, a young person interested in pursuing studies in the healthcare sector, who spent one day at the clinic with the nursing staff as part of an observation internship at the hospital. For the present study, we reviewed the recordings corresponding to the four days Coralie and/or Gloria were at the clinic and systematically examined their corridor occupations (418 in total) when they were walking alone and with other staff members. We transcribed considerable sections of the corresponding recordings, following the conventions developed for talk by Jefferson (2004) and for bodily conduct by Mondada (2019), which are reproduced at the beginning of the volume. The study deploys multimodal analysis (Mondada, 2014) to examine how participants act and interact together, relying on finely articulated talk and bodily conduct as well as spatial resources.

Gloria, Coralie, and Ana walking alone and with staff members

We started our study by examining the recordings made in a specific part of the clinic: the central corridor that connects the two main centers of activity, the day hospital and the urgent-care room (Corridor B in Figure 1). We first reviewed the recordings from Day 25 – the day when Coralie, the nursing intern, and Gloria, the observation intern, were both in the clinic – and then extended our observations to the other three days when Coralie was recorded. When examining this data, we also looked at how the nurses themselves walked when moving around alone and with other staff members. We concentrated in particular on Ana, a permanent nurse who had been at the clinic for the past several years and was working there the day Gloria visited it. The same day, there were two other nurses at the clinic: Alexandria, who worked on a rotating basis, and Hazel, who was a permanent nurse but was still recovering from foot surgery – for these reasons, we focused on Ana. The description that follows presents some characteristic features of the behaviors of Gloria, Coralie, and Ana when walking alone and with other staff members, based on systematic examination of the recordings.

Gloria never walks alone the morning of the day that she visits the clinic. At the beginning of the day, she always walks with Cybele, the clinic's rotating nursing aide, who is in charge of showing her around. At first, they walk side-by-side and talk (Figure 2, Image 2.1) while Cybele starts explaining the clinic's functioning to her.[2] However, very soon, Gloria starts walking behind Cybele, although staying close, often in silence, as they move from one room to the next (2.2). When Cybele starts her regular chores, Gloria follows her around the clinic. On several occasions, she waits in the corridor for the nursing aide while she is inside one of the rooms. Gloria always occupies the last position when walking in a group of several senior members, which sometimes means moving immediately behind a person other than Cybele (2.3). Gloria walks alone only in the afternoon, in particular for a short time after lunch. At these times, she walks carrying a glass of water in her right hand, goes to the restroom, and strolls through the corridors, sometimes rather slowly. While walking, she checks her personal cellphone and adjusts her uniform and the street clothes she is wearing underneath it (2.4). She also adjusts her hair, playing with it, and rubs her hands with the disinfection product, as she exits the restroom, in very conspicuous way. While moving through the corridors, she also engages in contact with the material environment; for instance, she slides her hand along the handrail (2.5) and playfully hangs onto the restroom door handle. She makes one single move from the day hospital to the urgent-care room and back, apparently to bring a pair of scissors, which is the only time she transports clinic equipment (2.6).

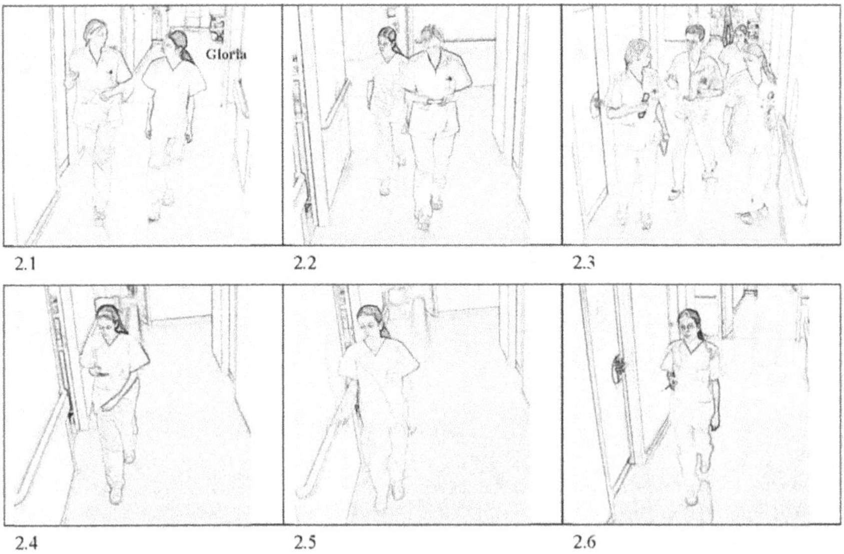

Figure 2 Gloria, the observation intern, walking alone and with senior nursing staff. View of camera 4 except for 2.2, 2.4, and 2.5, which correspond to the view of camera 2.

In contrast to Gloria, Coralie, the nursing intern, often walks alone, in most cases for quick back-and-forth trips to/from the reception and to/from the stock room. She often walks very rapidly, following straight trajectories, transporting documents and clinic equipment, sometimes several items at once (Figure 3, Image 3.1). As she walks, she produces systematic and rapid lateral visual checks of the adjacent rooms and corridors, thus monitoring the clinic premises as she passes by each area (3.1). While walking, she often engages in physical contact with her own body – she touches her face, ear, hair, and neck – but far less conspicuously than Gloria (3.2). The recordings from Day 25 show only two instances of Coralie walking with someone in the central corridor: Cybele, the rotating aide. Coralie walks side-by-side with her and they talk with each other (3.3). On Day 26, Coralie walks on many occasions with two nurses: Mae, a permanent nurse in the clinic, and Alexandria, a rotating nurse. When she is with Mae, who is the nurse educator supervising her internship, she always walks behind her, sometimes at a considerable distance and often without talking (3.4). When she is with Alexandria, she usually walks behind her (3.5). Coralie almost always occupies the last position when walking in a group of several senior members, even if this means taking a distance from the nurse she has been working with, such as Mae (3.6). Over the four days she was recorded, when Coralie walks with a nurse, she usually walks behind her, sometimes at a considerable distance

78 *Esther González-Martínez*

and often without talking. If a nurse talks to her, she tends to do it while walking ahead.

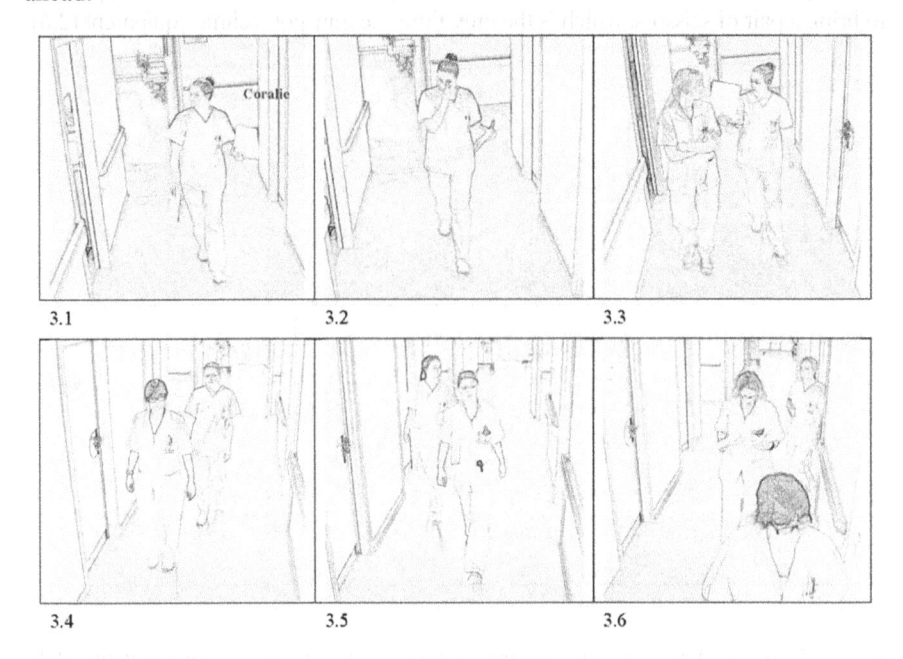

Figure 3 Coralie, the nursing intern, walking alone and with senior nursing staff. View of camera 2 except for 3.4, 3.5, and 3.6, which correspond to the view of camera 4.

Like Coralie, Ana, the senior nurse, often walks alone, most of the time for trips following straight trajectories to/from the reception and to/from the stock room. That said, she has a slower, more relaxed gait (Figure 4, Image 4.1) than the nursing intern. For instance, she often walks with one hand in the pocket of her pants and makes her visual checks of adjacent rooms and corridors more slowly. Moreover, she very often smiles and laughs while moving around.

She sometimes carries documents and clinic equipment, but less often than Coralie. In contrast, she often handles the triage nurse's cellphone and keys while walking (4.2). Ana does not often walk with coworkers: she does this only 13 times over the four days she was recorded. In one occupation, she is followed at a great distance, and without talking, by Coralie. In another, she walks second in a group of four in which Gloria occupies the last position, behind Cybele. She sometimes walks side-by-side with other senior nursing staff members, but more often, she walks behind or ahead of them. In most cases, she keeps talking to them, even from a great distance (4.3). In one case, in which she seems to be in a hurry, she walks ahead of a fellow nurse but says to her "I am listening to you" thus giving her an assurance of recipiency and marking "togetherness." She may walk with the same coworker behind (4.4), side-by-side (4.5), or in front (4.6), varying the positions even during a single trip.

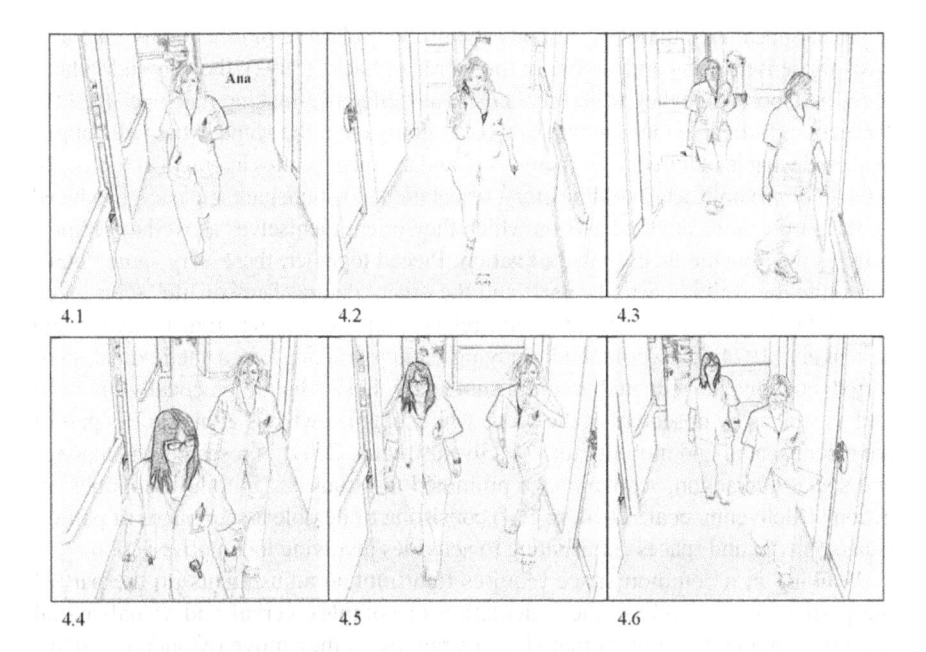

Figure 4 Ana, the senior nurse, walking alone and with senior nursing staff. View of camera 2 except for 4.2 and 4.3, which correspond to the view of camera 4.

A common point between Gloria and Coralie is that when one of them walks with a senior nursing staff member, it is overwhelmingly behind. Moreover, this serial order tends to remain stable during the course of the trip. Even if there is talk, the staff member speaks to the intern while walking ahead of her. In contrast, Ana, the senior nurse, may walk in front of, behind, or beside senior nursing staff, sometimes even changing positions in the course of the same trip. The staff members are careful not to occupy the entire width of the corridor so that there is some free space for other people to pass by. Nevertheless, the corridors of the clinic are very rarely obstructed, as the staff is eager to organize things so that patients and their relatives can stay in the rooms and to ensure that objects like wheelchairs and carts are put away immediately. Moreover, no physical obstacle prevents a senior nursing staff member from walking behind an intern. The argument that the senior member may walk ahead of the intern because they know where to go does not really hold for Coralie, the nursing intern, who has already spent two weeks in the clinic at the times of the recordings and often makes trips alone. In the following section, we will focus on considering the interns' walking behaviors with regard to the ethnomethodological literature on independent travel.

Studying walking alone and with others

In sociology, Goffman (1966 [1963], 1972 [1971]) is credited for spotlighting how individuals walk and interact when in public and semi-public places. He argues that they are attentive to gaze, facial expressions, movements, and manifold aspects of physical appearance that they embody themselves, observe in others, and take as a basis for sensemaking and action. In the words of Sacks (1992), the way individuals move and look while they walk functions as an "inference-making machine" (p. 115) for them to form an understanding of what is going on in the scene, what will happen next, and what is required from themselves and the other parties in practical terms. An array of observable details of trajectory, orientation, position, gait, and pace, produced by the participants, are the basis on which they orient themselves as well as reciprocally as they pursue their course of action. Pieced together, these very same details constitute the walking activity itself and the other "natural facts of life" (Garfinkel, 1984 [1967], p. 35), like identities and relationships, emerging from it. Ryave and Schenkein (1974) thus propound studying "doing walking" as a methodical, concerted, ongoing, and situated accomplishment by those who are practically involved in it as well as by observers of the scene who recognize what is going on. As part of the recent spatial and mobility turn (McIlvenny et al., 2009) in research on language and social interaction, scholars have promoted the study of "mobile formations-in-action" (McIlvenny et al., 2014, p. 104) consisting of flexible assemblages of participants, objects, and spaces contributing to activities involving locomotive action.

Walking in a common space requires tight mutual adjustments on the part of the participants as well as the articulation of complex verbal and visual-spatial resources in an environment that changes rapidly as they move (Mondada, 2014). Participants are confronted with the "navigational problem" of walking (Ryave & Schenkein, 1974, p. 266), meaning establishing the right-of-way (Liberman, 2013), avoiding collision (Goffman, 1963 [1963], 1972 [1971]), and finding their way around dealing with other people, objects, and practical contingencies. They build mobile courses of action that are predictable and understandable, for all practical purposes, at a glance (Sudnow, 1972).

Respecifying the notion of "individual," Goffman (1972 [1971]) reflects on pedestrian traffic as involving vehicular units formed of one or more members. He writes: "A vehicular unit is a shell of some kind controlled (usually from within) by a human pilot or navigator" (p. 6). He defines a "with" as "a party of more than one whose members are perceived to be 'together'" (p. 19). Ryave and Schenkein (1974) invite us to identify the methodical practices involved in producing and recognizing "walking-alone" and "walking-together" (p. 267). They refer to assemblages of specific times, places, participants, activities, and occasions that make "aloneness" and "togetherness" observable and also point to aspects related to the direction, trajectory, orientation, proximity, pace, degrees of body contact, and involvement in talk of the pedestrians contributing to the production of distinct mobile formations. Thus, two people walking, one closely behind the other, may be observably "walking together" or just moving in a "walking behind" configuration depending on features like the synchronicity of movements and gaze (Schmitt, 2012). De Stefani (2013) shows that supermarket customers are recognizable by their recurrent "stop-and-go" walking (p. 147), as they pick products from the shelves, and become observable as customer couples when engaging in "object-focused interaction" (p. 147). In an art museum, visitors produce embodied proposal-acceptance sequences when moving together, in a pair, from one exhibit to the next (vom Lehn, 2013).

Pedestrians crossing an intersection organize their mutual passage by walking in groups led by "front runners" (Livingston, 1987, p. 22) who inspect the opposing group, identify the individuals in a similar arrangement, open paths ahead, and take the openings provided to them. During a guided visit, the guide is observably "not just 'walking ahead' but also 'leading' the group, whose members are 'following' him" (Mondada, 2021, p. 106). Smith (2017) identifies interactional practices like "adjusting trajectories" and "recruiting and dismissing resources" (p. 12) deployed by duos of pedestrians crossing an intersection space together and a distribution of labor – one takes the lead, the other follows – between the parties.

A series of publications on guided visits (Broth & Mondada, 2013; De Stefani & Mondada, 2014; Mondada, 2014) have shown that the organization of talk and the organization of walk are finely interrelated. "[W]alk is organized, as talk, within initiating and responding as well as aligning or disaligning moves" (Mondada, 2014, p. 397). A speaker may mark the imminent completion of a turn at talk when they start walking away. Moving away may also mark the imminent transition from one sequence to another and from one activity to the next. Mondada (2021) emphasizes the identity work produced through these moves, which are ways of displaying and embodying membership categories, like "guide" and "guided person," that are associated with distinct ways of looking, walking, and talking, and features like differential degrees of expertise among participants.

Analysis

When an intern moves with a member of the senior nursing staff, the senior member often walks in first position and the intern follows behind. Our analysis concentrates on four practices involved in producing this serial order: (1) keeping the way clear, (2) adopting the mill position, (3) yielding the right-of-way, and (4) minding the distance. These practices are the product of both participants even if we named them taking the perspective of the intern. Their names refer to what is at stake rather than their results as these are sometimes inconclusive: the intern may for instance not yield the right-of-way but the senior member forges ahead and manages to go first. Each practice relies on complex arrays of moves like stopping or walking, taking steps in specific directions, modifying the orientation of the body and gaze, and altering the walking pace. The practices are often at work, simultaneously or in close temporal contiguity, in a single instance of a "walking-with-someone-following-them" configuration, as we will show in the following analytical subsections.

Keeping the way clear, adopting the "mill position," and yielding the right-of-way

A perspicuous moment to study the interactional work involved in establishing and maintaining a "walking-with-someone-following-them" configuration is when, after a stop, the intern and the senior member resume walking. At that point, the participants work to keep the way clear for the leading party to start walking again unobstructed when the time comes. This often involves the intern adopting a "mill position," which we named in reference to the board game mill, with respect to the senior member.[3] The intern moves approximately one meter and a half away,

82 *Esther González-Martínez*

which is a distance that is easily compressible but allows her room to maneuver, orients toward the senior member, and the scene in which the latter is involved, and stands in a place from which she can easily be seen by the senior member but in which she does not block her view. When the senior member resumes walking, both participants maneuver so that she has the right-of-way and can take the front position. The intern follows behind the senior member, often slightly to her side, in a mobile version of the mill position.

Excerpt 1 documents the moves of Coralie (Cor in the transcripts), the nursing intern, and Mae, the nurse educator supervising her internship. Coralie has been following Mae throughout the morning, moving between the urgent-care room (UCR) and the day hospital room (DHR), where the pair has been taking care of patients, as well as other parts of the clinic. Before the beginning of Excerpt 1, Mae walks from the DHR to the UCR's corridor entrance, where she opens the wall closet on her left and takes out several items. A minute later, Coralie goes out of the DHR herself and walks toward the UCR (line 1).[4]

Excerpt 1: 1368_26A_032454

```
1               €(0.2) $(7.0)$
     mae        €moves towards closet, adopts a static position--->
     cor               $goes out of DHR, walks towards UCR$
2               $(1.0)#  (2.5)$ $(2.0)€
     cor        $goes into UCR, walks more slowly towards Mae$
     cor                    $takes one stepR to the side, orients towards
                Mae, takes one stepL back, adopts a static position--->
     mae               --->€
     fig            #5.1
3               *€(1.0)#  (2.0)€ +(0.4)+$#  (1.0)$# $(0.7)# (0.7)€*
     cor        *looks towards Mae/DHR/Mae---------------------*
     mae        €takes one stepL back, closes closet with right foot and
                right hand----€reorients and walks towards UCR's entrance€
     mae                    +looks at Cor+
     cor                       --->$takes one stepL to the side$
     cor                                    $turns left, walks
                towards UCR's entrance--->
     fig            #5.2          #5.3      #5.4     #5.5
4               €(1.4)$#  (2.0)€ (1.9)$ (1.6)
     mae        €goes out of UCR, walks towards SR€goes into SR--->>
     cor        --->$goes out of UCR, walks towards SR$goes into SR--->>
     fig            #5.6
```

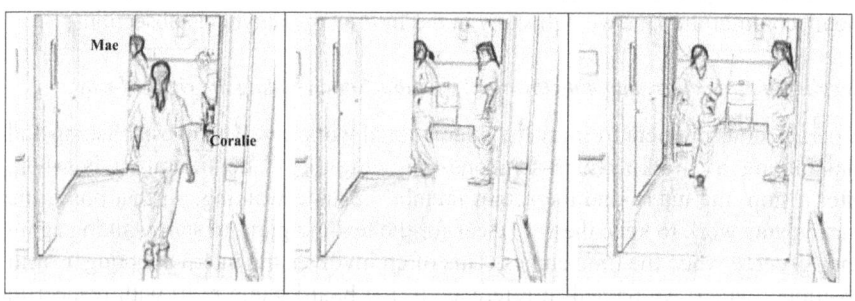

5.1   5.2   5.3

| 5.4 | 5.5 | 5.6 |

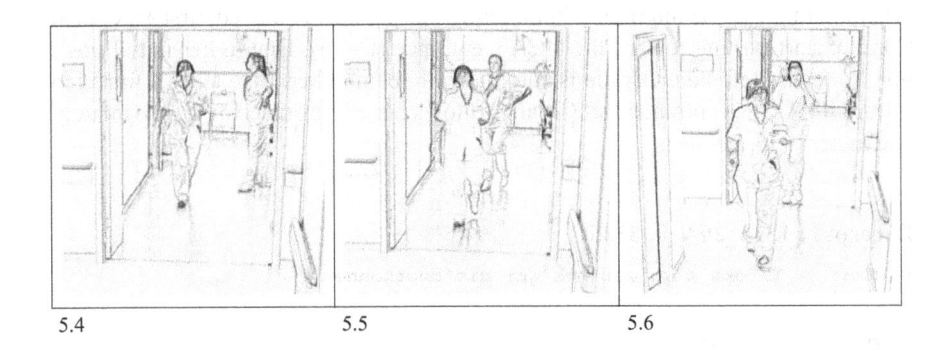

As Coralie gets near Mae, she slows her walking pace (2, 5.1). When she is approximately one meter from Mae, she takes one step to her right, pivots her body on her right foot, and brings her left foot back, parallel to the right one. This way, she adopts a static position behind Mae, to her left side, approximately one meter and a half away (2, 5.2). Coralie's position leaves Mae room to maneuver freely where she is and anticipates her walking moves. Indeed, Coralie keeps the way clear for Mae to withdraw from the closet, turn, and exit the UCR by the same path she used to enter it. She also leaves clear the space immediately behind Mae, through which she could have instead walked to enter the central section of the urgent-care room. Moreover, Coralie being positioned diagonally behind Mae permits the intern to observe what the nurse is doing. This is instrumental for the intern's practical training but also for her adjustments to the nurse's moves. Mae can also easily see Coralie from the corner of her eye. From their respective positions, the pair can easily hear each other and talk together. This diagonal mill position is instrumental in keeping the way clear for the senior member as well as preparing for and sustaining a "walking-behind" configuration.

Mae indeed steps back, closes the closet, turns left, and starts walking toward the UCR's entrance (3). As she takes her first step forward, she turns her head slightly to her left and looks toward Coralie, who has been watching her (2, 5.3). The mutual gaze functions as a signal for them to set sail, Coralie following her. Crucially for the reinstatement of the "walking-behind" configuration, Coralie first turns very slowly, taking just a small step to her left (2, 5.4). It is only when Mae is already three steps ahead of her that Coralie sets off in the same direction herself, behind Mae (2, 5.5). She thus yields the right-of-way to Mae. As the pair moves forward, toward the stock room (SR), Coralie adopts a mobile version of the mill position, walking at a close distance behind Mae and slightly shifted to her left (4, 5.6); she can thus see the scene ahead of Mae and adjust to it as the duo moves forward (Smith, 2017).

At the beginning of Excerpt 2, Mae, the nurse, is talking with Caspar (Cas in the transcripts), the chief nurse, at the end of the corridor of the urgent-care room (UCR). Caspar is facing Mae and Coralie, the nursing intern, is with her, standing to her left. Mae and Caspar produce a closing sequence corresponding to a formulation of the situation that has been discussed (1–2), and Caspar turns left, as if

84 *Esther González-Martínez*

orienting to the nurse/intern duo imminently moving away. Indeed, first Mae, then Coralie, start turning toward the UCR's entrance (12–13). Due to her initial position, to Mae's left side, Coralie is automatically behind her. Mae takes a first step toward the UCR's entrance and Coralie follows her at a distance of approximately one meter (3, 6.1).

Excerpt 2: 1316_26A_035725

```
1   Mae:   ¥>˚oké˚< (c'est eux qui disfonctionnent)
             okay it is them who mess up
    cas    ¥turns left--->
2   Cas:   €(>ouais<)¥
             yeah
    mae    €walks towards UCR's entrance--->
    cas           --->¥
3          $(0.5)# (0.8)
    cor    $walks towards UCR's entrance--->
    fig            #6.1
4   Cas:   t'oublie pas ta ↑canne
             you do not forget your cane
5          (0.3)€
    mae           --->€
6   Mae:   €>j'ai ↑pris.< ( )
             I have taken
           €turns around left towards Cas, takes one stepL to the side
           --->
7          (0.5)$
    cor           --->$
8   Cas:   $ah tu as pris.=#
             oh you have taken
    cor    $shifts to her left--->
    fig                #6.2
9   Mae:   =j'ai embarquée€ justement parce que$ j'ai- (0.3) j'me
             I have loaded precisely because I have I
    mae              --->€adopts a static position--->1.13
    cor                                 --->$reorients towards
           Mae, takes a stepR back, adopts a static position--->1.14
10         suis dit j'vais de nouveau# ou[blier        ]=
             have told myself I am going again to forget
    fig                      #6.3
11  Cas:                              [(donc) eh oui: ]=
             so of course
12  Mae:   =et puis ce soir j'ai l'chariot machin, (.) .h donc je
             and then this evening I have the cart whatsit so I
13         l'ai-j'l'ai pris et€ p'is je (lui ai dit de la mettre
             have it I have taken it and then I have told them to put it
                                 --->€turns around right , walks towards
           UCR's entrance--->
14         de nouveau) dans ma bagnole.$#
             again in my ride
    cor                                 --->$
    fig                                  #6.4
15  Cas:   $<par↓fait>€ (0.5)# nickel$
             perfect impeccable
    cor    $takes one stepL to the side, walks towards UCR's entrance$
    mae              --->€goes out of UCR, walks towards DHR--->>
    fig                #6.5
```

```
16         $(3.5)#  (6.3)
    cor    $goes out of UCR, walks towards DHR--->>
    fig         #6.6
```

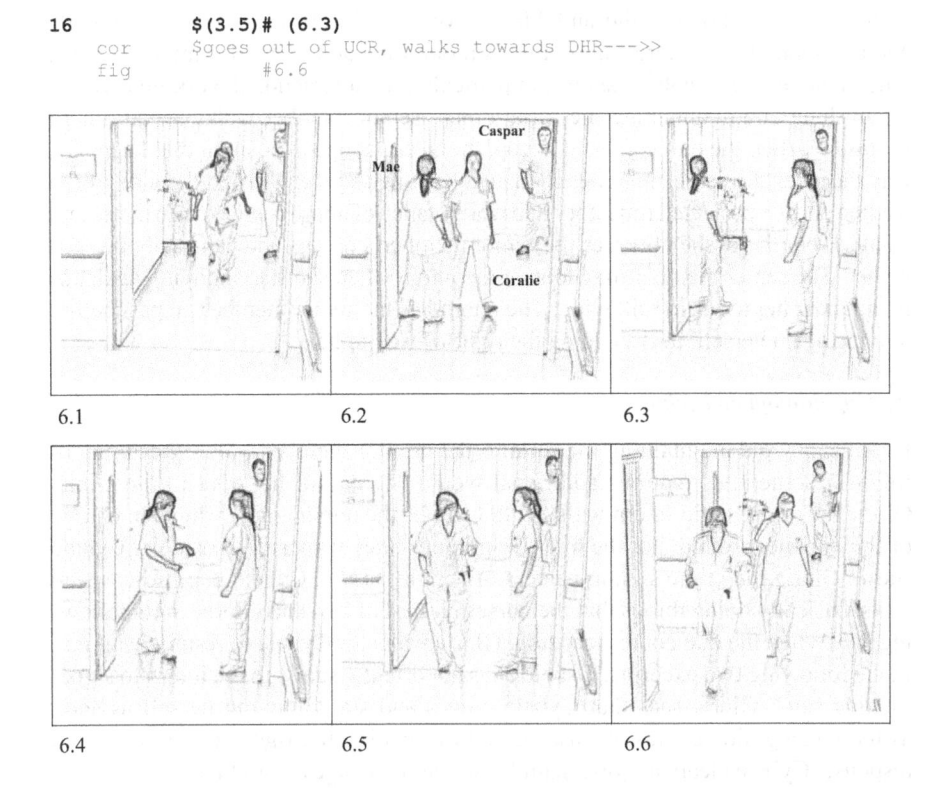

6.1   6.2   6.3

6.4   6.5   6.6

As Mae, followed by Coralie, is heading toward the UCR's exit, Caspar speaks to Mae again, enjoining her not to forget a cane that she plans to take with her in the evening (4). As she replies (6), Mae makes a sharp U-turn to her left, reorienting toward Caspar. Coralie, who is walking behind, avoids stumbling into Mae by shifting to her left (8, 6.2). Mae also helps prevent a collision by taking a step to her left side and moving close to the wall. Coralie passes Mae by, takes one additional step forward, then turns toward her, steps back, and adopts a static position at a distance of approximately one meter and a half (9, 6.3). Coralie has thus moved out of Mae's way and adopted a mill position from which she can easily monitor Mae's moves and adjust to them. Mae can see Caspar, and could even walk toward him, without the intern standing between them. Moreover, Mae could also resume walking toward the day hospital room unobstructed. In the meantime, the nurse and the intern keep the access to the UCR clear as one stands against the left wall and the other to the right. Mae starts moving again as she is about to finish explaining her dealings with the cane to Caspar (13): she turns right and starts walking toward the UCR entrance. As she turns, she can see Coralie, who is looking at her (14, 6.4). Coralie waits for Mae to pass her by to start moving herself, at first very slowly, just moving her left foot to the side (15, 6.5). The intern thus yields the right-of-way to the nurse, who takes the lead. Even though she was positioned closer to the exit than Mae, she goes out of the UCR second, walking behind her, shifted to the left, in a mobile mill position (16, 6.6).

86   *Esther González-Martínez*

In these excerpts, Coralie and Mae move very fluidly in a "walking-behind" configuration. This requires close mutual monitoring and tight adjustments to each other's moves. The analysis shows, in particular, the interactional work involved in establishing and maintaining the serial order "senior member walks ahead, intern follows." When the duo comes to a stop, the intern adopts a position that keeps the way clear for the senior member to maneuver. She stays slightly to the side of the leading party's projected trajectory and at a distance of approximately one meter and a half. From there, she observes the senior member's doings and can easily be seen by her. The senior member may look at the intern when she starts moving again, as if enjoining her to begin following. The intern lets the senior member go past before moving again herself, thus yielding the right-of-way to her.

Pushing through and going first

Establishing and maintaining the serial order "senior member walks ahead, intern follows" sometimes requires additional work. The day of her visit to the clinic, Gloria the observation intern walks with Cybele, the nursing aide who is in charge of showing her around. For the first five minutes, they walk side-by-side as Cybele shows Gloria the clinic's main centers of activity. Then, Cybele begins her usual tasks, basically doing things that the nurses request of her, and Gloria starts following her. When the duo comes to a stop, Gloria waits for Cybele to resume walking. In the following two excerpts, Cybele does not orient visually to the intern to signal "setting sail." Gloria sees that Cybele moves and starts moving herself as soon as the nursing aide comes abreast instead of yielding the right-of-way to her. In response, Cybele clears her own path herself and manages to go first.

Before Excerpt 3 begins, a nurse (Alexandria, Ale in the transcripts) has called on Cybele (Cyb in the transcripts), the nursing aide, from the central section of the day hospital room (DHR). Cybele draws the curtain that isolates the patients from the DHR's entrance section and Gloria (Glo in the transcripts), the observation intern, stays on the other side, waiting for Cybele to come back. At the beginning of the excerpt, Gloria is oriented toward the opening in the curtain used by Cybele to get through. Gloria is two steps away from Cybele and looking downwards (1). Cybele is talking to the people inside the DHR (2), behind the curtain.

Excerpt 3: 1182_25A_021106

```
1            $*(0.3)
   glo       $stands in a static position inside DHR's entrance
             section--->1.7
   glo       *looks down---->1.6
2  (Cyb:)    ( ) mais: voilà.
             but that is it
3            €(0.8)€
   cyb       €walks into the central section of DHR€
4  Cyb:      €oula
             oops
             €adopts a static position--->
5            (0.6)€
   cyb          --->€
```

```
6  (Ale:)  €(donc tu vas)* le chercher# ( )
           so you are going to pick it up
    cyb    €approaches curtain-->1.8
    glo            --->*looks towards curtain--->
    fig                                    #7.1
7          ®(0.2)* (1.5)$ (0.2)
    cyb    ®puts right hand on curtain, draws curtain--->1.9
    glo    --->*looks towards Cyb--->
    glo            --->$takes one stepL back--->
8  Cyb:    ben j'vais$ a↓ller:: >l'cher↑cher<$€#
           bah I am going to go pick it up
    glo            --->$takes one stepR back, adopts a static position$
    cyb                                         --->€
    fig                                         #7.2
9          €(0.4)® &+(0.8)*#
    cyb    €goes out of the central section of DHR, walks towards DHR's
           entrance--->
    cyb    --->®
    cyb        &orients upper body to the right--->
    cyb        +looks right--->
    glo        --->↓*
    fig        #7.3
10         *$(0.6)€+&# ®+(0.8)®$# $(0.5)# (0.5)* (1.3)
    glo    *looks down------------------------*
    glo    $walks towards DHR's entrance$
    cyb        --->€goes out of DHR, walks towards reception--->>
    cyb            ®moves her right arm in front of Glo®
    cyb            +looks ahead--->>
    glo                    $goes out of DHR, walks towards
           reception--->>
    glo                                *looks ahead--->>
    fig        #7.4        #7.5    #7.6
```

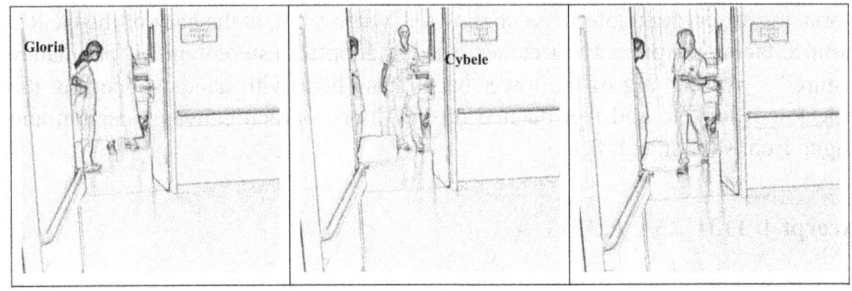

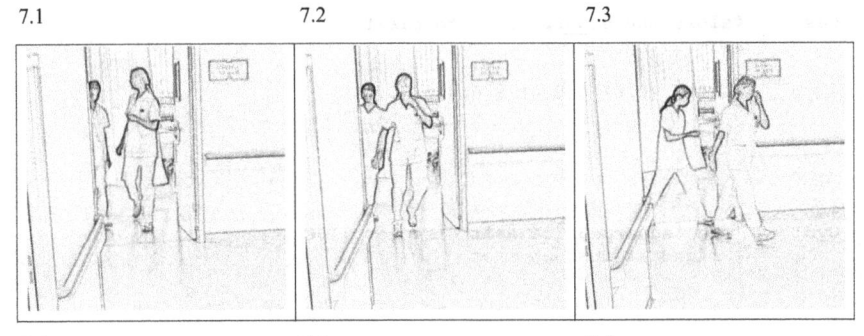

| 7.1 | 7.2 | 7.3 |

| 7.4 | 7.5 | 7.6 |

Cybele approaches the curtain as Alexandria tells her to go pick something up (6) (the aide will return later to the DHR with a folder). Gloria raises her head and looks toward the curtain (6, 7.1). As Cybele starts drawing the curtain open, Gloria looks at her, straightens up, and starts moving back: she takes first one small step (7), then a second one as Cybele confirms to Alexandria that she will go (8); Gloria then adopts a static position. When Cybele goes out of the central section of the DHR (9) and starts walking toward the entrance, Gloria is approximately one meter and a half away from her, to her right, in a mill position that leaves the way clear for Cybele to proceed (8, 7.2). She is oriented toward Cybele, monitoring her moves. Cybele can freely see ahead of her and still realize that Gloria is nearby.

Cybele takes a first step in front of her, toward the DHR's entrance, then orients to her right, looking beyond Gloria as if checking for something that will be at the back of the entrance section (9, 7.3). Contrary to Excerpt 1, here, the senior member does not seem to exchange a "setting sail" gaze with the junior one (who is nevertheless looking at her). Gloria starts moving when Cybele comes abreast of her. At this point, the bodies of the aide and the intern are very close as a result of Cybele orienting to her right. When Gloria starts moving ahead, she finds just enough space to place her right foot perpendicular to the left one, legs crossed (10, 7.4). Cybele deftly slips her right arm between herself and Gloria and moves it in front of the intern. She thus takes a leading position (10, 7.5). Cybele is the first one to step out of the DHR, into Corridor C, and turn right toward the reception. By the time Gloria herself steps into Corridor C, she is clearly following her, slightly shifted to the left, in a mobile version of the mill position (10, 7.6).

At the beginning of Excerpt 4, Caspar, the clinic's head nurse, is taking care of a patient in the urgent-care room (UCR), assisted by Cybele, the nursing aide. Gloria, the observation intern, is standing to Cybele's left, at the back of the UCR's entrance facing the patient's stretcher. She has adopted a stereotypical "pregnancy posture" – overarching of the lower back, arms bent with hands supporting the back, knees locked, and feet planted on the floor – which conveys inaction and fatigue from standing (1, 8.1).

Excerpt 4: 1131_25A_021617_A

```
1             (3.0)#
   fig              #8.1
2  Cas:     ¢alors une écharpe s'il te plaît.
            so a sling please
   cas      ¢walks with trolley in front of Glo--->
3             (1.6)¢ (0.6) €(0.6) $(0.4)# (0.4)
   cas      --->¢
   cyb                       €turns left, walks around Glo, towards
            closet--->
   glo                              $turns around towards Cyb/closet--->
   fig                                    #8.2
4  Cyb:     °une ↑écharpe$ (ça doit être ça::)°$€
            a sling it must be that
   glo             --->$takes one stepR back$
   cyb                                        --->€
```

```
5            $(0.2) ®(0.3) €(4.1)
    glo      $takes one stepL back, walks three steps towards
             UCR's entrance, reorients towards Cyb--->
    cyb              ®opens closet, looks inside--->
                         €adopts a static position--->
6            ¥(1.0)$ €(1.3)€®# (2.0) ∞(0.8) +(1.0)®€ (1.8)$
    ale      ¥goes out of DHR, walks towards UCR--->1.8
    glo      --->$adopts a static position---------------$
    cyb                 €takes one stepL back€
    cyb                 --->®closes closet holding a grip bar in
             right hand-------------------------®
    ale                              ∞looks towards UCR/Cyb--->1.8
    cyb                                  +looks towards Ale--->1.9
    cyb                                      --->€reorients,
             walks towards UCR's entrance--->1.9
    fig                      #8.3
7   Cyb:     #$tu sais où ↑c'est les écharpes?
             you know where it is the slings
    glo      $reorients towards Cyb, walks towards UCR's entrance--->1.10
    fig      #8.4
8            ®(0.4)® °(1.0)¥∞#
    cyb      ®moves grip bar from right to left hand®
    glo              °joins hands--->1.11
    ale              --->¥
    ale              --->∞
    fig                      #8.5
9   Ale:     ¥ça doit être ↑là non?€+
             it must be there no
    ale      ¥turns around towards SR, walks towards SR--->1.12
    cyb                      --->€
    cyb                      --->+
10           €(0.6)$ (0.8)
    cyb      €goes out of UCR, walks towards SR--->
    glo      --->$goes out of UCR, walks towards SR--->
11  Ale:     mais a↓près- h°
             but once
    glo                  --->°
12           (0.3)¥ (0.2)# (0.8) €(1.6) $(3.7)
    ale      --->¥goes into SR--->>
    cyb                      €goes into SR--->>
    glo                          $goes into SR--->>
    fig              #8.6
```

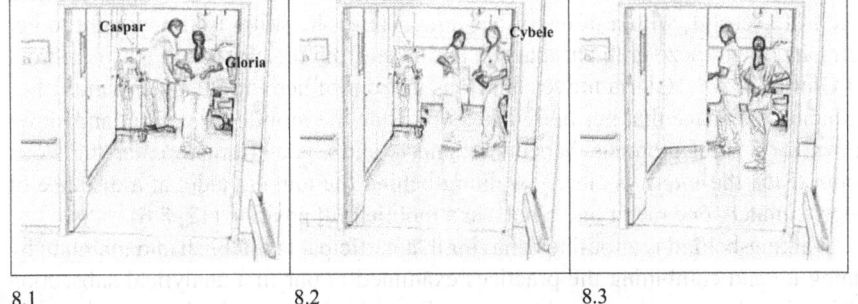

8.1 8.2 8.3

8.4   8.5   8.6

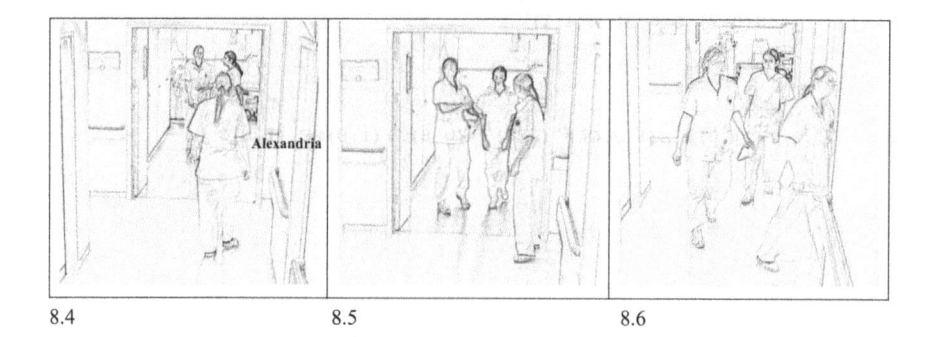

Caspar asks Cybele for a sling as he passes in front of Gloria with the dressing cart (2). Cybele then turns to her left and moves toward the wall closet on the left side of the UCR's corridor (3). She thus encounters Gloria along the way and needs to walk in a semi-circle around the intern to approach the closet (3, 8.2). Meanwhile, Gloria has also started turning around, looking to stay oriented toward Cybele (3). Cybele passes by Gloria and extends her right hand toward the closet. At this point, the intern is to her right, just in front of the handles of the closet, which makes it difficult to access it. Gloria clears the way when she takes two steps back (4–5), behind Cybele. From there, she moves away again, toward the UCR's entrance, turns, reorients toward the aide, and adopts a static position (6, 8.3). Gloria has thus afforded space to Cybele, who can maneuver freely in front of the closet and easily return toward Caspar with the sling or go out of the UCR to look for it elsewhere. From her mill position, Gloria can look at what Cybele is doing and can easily be seen by the aide from the corner of her eye or by means of a slight turn of her head. Cybele indeed finds her way clear when she closes the closet (6), looks at Alexandria (Ale in the transcript), a nurse that is approaching her, walks toward her, and asks where the slings are kept (7, 8.4). Like in Excerpt 4, here, Cybele does not seem to exchange a "setting sail" gaze with Gloria (who is nevertheless looking at her); she is concentrating on Alexandria. Like in Excerpt 4, Gloria starts moving as soon as Cybele comes abreast of her (7). She lets Cybele go first but walks just behind her. Cybele manages to create some space between her and the intern, like in Excerpt 4, with a move of her arms. Here, she shifts from her right to her left hand the trapeze grab bar that she has taken from the closet and puts it in front of Gloria (8, 8.5). Gloria moves her arms in front of her and joins her hands, thus reducing the space that her body takes up inside the mobile formation, and slows down for a brief moment. When Alexandria and Cybele turn to enter the stock room (SR), the intern is clearly walking behind the nursing aide, at a distance of approximately one meter and a half, in a mobile mill position (12, 8.6).

Walking-behind is a routine behavior that participants establish and maintain by lining up and combining the practices examined in our first analytical subsection ("Keeping the way clear......"), repeatedly and with great fluidity as the most normal and natural thing to do. When they come to a stop, the intern clears the way for the senior member to maneuver and stands in a mill position. When the latter resumes walking, the intern yields the right-of-way and follows her. This is conspicuously the case with the moves of the nurse/nursing intern duo. The analysis of this second subsection ("Pushing through......"), focused on the nursing aide/observation intern duo, adds nuance to the portrait. It shows, first, that the spatial, orientational, and practical arrangement of the participants does not always go without a hitch, and, second, that the serial order "senior member walks ahead, intern follows" ought to be followed and that the senior member can deploy subtle but forceful moves to uphold it. In Excerpts 3 and 4, the intern anticipates the resumption of the senior member's walking and steps back, freeing the way for the leading party to proceed when the time comes. Nevertheless, the senior member sets off without visually acknowledging the intern's presence: there is no "setting sail" gaze as her attention is focused somewhere else. The intern jumps on board as soon as the senior member comes abreast, as if concerned not to be left on the shore. The senior member enforces the serial order: she pushes her way through with an arm movement and takes the first position.

Minding the distance

The intern closely follows the senior member but takes care to stay out of her way. This requires, to start with, continuously handling proximity in physical terms, as the pair progresses, comes to a stop, and then sets off again. For instance, the aide steps back, providing maneuvering space to the senior member; she lets her go first or the senior member pushes her way through; the pair mutually adjust their walking pace; if the leading party shifts slightly to one side, for instance to drop off an object in a room adjacent to the corridor as they go by, the intern slows down and stays behind. Minding the distance is a practice that is particularly relevant for the participants, and perspicuous for the analyst, in cases when the leading party abruptly reverses direction and the participants take measures to avoid a collision and reinstate the serial order "senior member walks ahead, intern follows."

In Excerpt 5, Cybele, the nursing aide, goes out of the urgent-care room (UCR) and heads toward the wound-dressing room (WDR). She is followed by Gloria, the observation intern, who walks approximately one meter and a half behind Cybele, who is shifted slightly to the aide's right (3, 9.1).

Excerpt 5: 1131_25A_021617_B

```
1            €(2.2) $(1.2)
    cyb      €walks towards UCR's entrance--->
    glo              $walks towards UCR's entrance--->
2   Cas:     o:ké ça marche mer˚ci˚
             okay that works thank you
3            (1.5)€ (0.9)#
    cyb      --->€ goes out of UCR, walks towards WDR--->
    fig                  #9.1
4   Cas:     euh: cy↑bele$
             um Cybele
    glo                 --->$
```

```
5               $(0.2)€
    glo         $goes out of UCR, walks towards WDR--->
    cyb         --->€
6   Cyb:        €OUAIS?$#
                yeah
                €stops, turns around left, walks towards UCR--->
    glo         --->$
    fig                  #9.2
7   Cas:        $tu pourrais# me chercher le problème# ophtal↑mo?#
                you could get me the ophtalmo problem
    glo         $turns around right, stops, walks more slowly towards UCR--->
    fig                       #9.3                    #9.4          #9.5
8               (0.6)€
    cyb         --->€
9   Cas:        €<comme ça dino peut voir (s'il) faut:
                this way Dino can see (if we must)
    cyb         €goes into UCR, walks towards UCR's central section--->
10              (1.3)$
    glo         --->$
11  Cas:        $qu'on l'envoie# directement en [ophtalmo ou pas,    ]=
                send them/it straight to ophtalmo or not
    glo         $adopts a static position in front of UCR's entrance--->
    fig                       #9.6
12  Cyb:                                           [le problème ophtalmo:]=
                the ophtalmo problem
13  Cas:        =(y'a: une) urgence
                there is an emergency
14              (0.4)
15  Cyb:        d'accord,
                all right
16              (0.3)
```

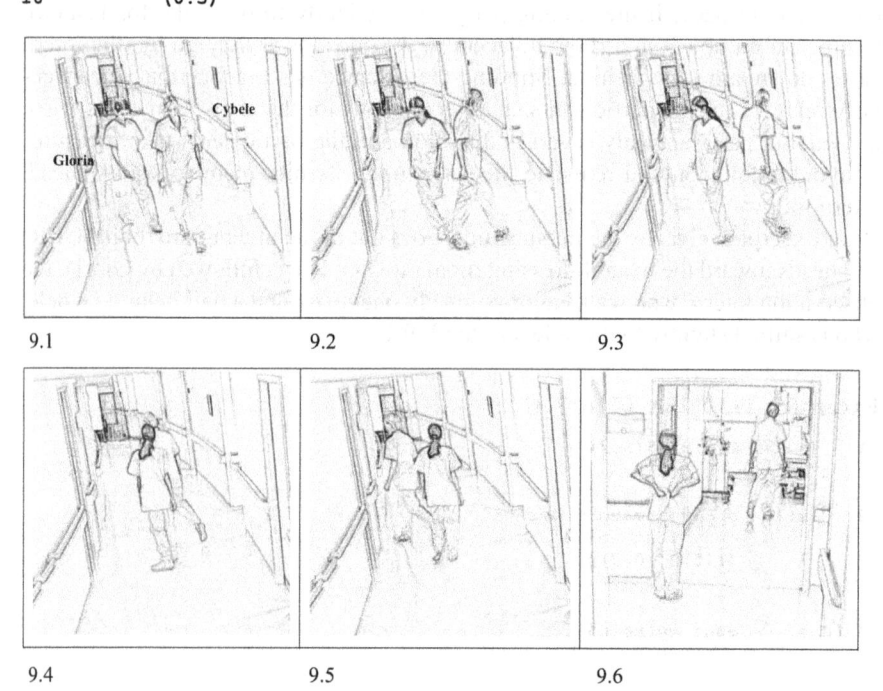

9.1   9.2   9.3

9.4   9.5   9.6

Caspar, the chief nurse, summons Cybele from inside the urgent-care room (4). Cybele produces a go-ahead response (6) that displays recipiency of the summons and availability for interaction and the upcoming activity that the summons foreshadows (Schegloff, 2007). As she answers, Cybele plants her right foot next to her left one, which abruptly halts her forward movement, and orients her body to her left, toward the UCR (6). From there, she makes a sharp U-turn to her left, pivoting on her right foot. Behind her, Gloria, who has kept moving forward, encounters Cybele's right foot (6, 9.2) in her way. She too makes a U-turn in the opposite direction from Cybele, to her right, by which she follows the aide's reversing direction but avoids stumbling into her (7, 9.3). She then stops and lets Cybele circumvent her and pass her by (7, 9.4). When Cybele is approximately one meter and a half ahead, the intern starts moving forward again but very slowly, taking only short steps, and pausing between each one (7, 9.5). Cybele then enters the UCR (9) and Gloria waits for her outside, facing the entrance, in the stereotypical "pregnancy posture" (11, 9.6). She may have heard that Caspar had asked Cybele to go pick up a patient (7) and thus anticipates that the nursing aide may stay in the UCR only for a brief moment, during which she does not need to follow her and can wait outside.

In Excerpt 5, the observation intern, Gloria, is focused on the senior member, Cybele, walking ahead when the latter suddenly reverses direction. Gloria adjusts to this with great nimbleness, quick and light-footed, reproducing symmetrically, and almost simultaneously, the same U-turn. Having avoided a collision, she then slows down and lets Cybele forge ahead. In contrast, in the following excerpt, proximity during another U-turn is handled with some minor hiccups. At the beginning of Excerpt 6, Ana, a nurse, walks into Corridor A from the plaster room (PR) to the physicians' office (PO) next to the urgent-care room's entrance (UCR). She is followed by Coralie, the nursing intern, at a distance of approximately two meters. The intern is shifted to the nurse's right, in a mobile mill position.

Excerpt 6: 1209_25B_034741

```
1           €$(4.2)
    ana     €walks towards PO--->
    cor     $walks towards PO, walks more slowly by the UCR's entrance--->
2           &(0.3) +(0.5) ¥(0.4) *(0.2)€#
    ana     &leans on the PO's door frame--->
    ana            +looks inside PO--->
    haz                   ¥goes out of SR, walks towards DHR--->1.6
    cor                          *looks towards Haz--->
    ana                                 --->€
    fig                                        #10.1
3           ∞€(0.2)&+ (0.2)* (0.4)$# (0.5)+ (0.2)# (0.2)∞
    haz     ∞looks towards Cor/Ana----------------------∞
    ana     €turns around left, walks towards UCR--->
    ana     --->&
    ana            --->+looks towards Cor--->
    cor                   --->*looks towards Ana--->
    cor                          --->$turns around right, walks towards
                   UCR--->
```

94 *Esther González-Martínez*

```
     ana                            --->+looks towards Haz--->>
     fig                                 #10.2          #10.3
4    Haz:    ∞ça ↑va?∞#
             going okay
             ∞looks ahead∞
     fig                  #10.4
5            (0.2)*
     cor     --->*
6    Ana:    €*tu t'es d'jà# arrêtée$ hazel du ↑coup$¥ [ou pas.    ]$
             you have already stopped Hazel in fact or not
             €adopts a static position in front of UCR's entrance--->>
     cor     *looks towards Haz, towards Ana, towards Haz--->>
     cor                     --->$adopts a static position in front of
                     UCR's entrance$
     haz                                        --->¥turns around
                     left towards Ana, adopts a static position--->>
     fig                  #10.5
7    Haz:                                       $[j'me $suis]
             I have
     cor                                              $takes one step∟back$
8            arrêtée$ juste cinq minutes avant là#=
             stopped just five minutes before there
     fig                                       #10.6
9    Ana:    =$<j'irai juste au moins cinq minutes °moi: a[près:]°
             I will go just at least five minutes myself after
     cor     $adopts a static position--->>
```

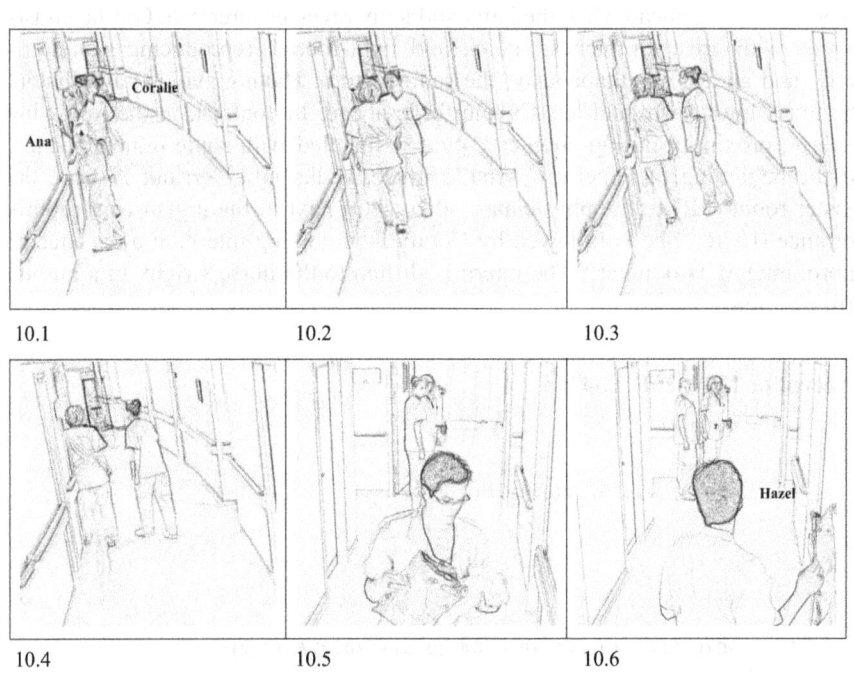

10.1

10.2

10.3

10.4

10.5

10.6

At the beginning of the excerpt, Ana leans on the door frame of the PO and looks inside (2, 10.1). Coralie, who has slowed down when approaching the UCR's entrance, has her attention caught by Hazel (Haz in the transcripts), a nurse, who has gone out of the stock room (SR) (2). When Ana turns around and starts walking toward the UCR (3), she almost stumbles into Coralie, who is walking nonchalantly behind her and looking at Hazel. Coralie then turns her attention toward Ana and the two find themselves into a nose-to-nose position (3, 10.2). Coralie prevents the stumbling by making a U-turn to her right (3, 10.3), thus clearing the way for Ana, who passes her by, approaches the UCR's entrance, and turns toward Hazel. Following eye contact between the two nurses, Hazel asks Ana if everything is going okay (4), a common in-passing check between staff members (González-Martínez et al., 2017a). Here, in contrast to Cybele and Gloria in Excerpt 5, Ana and Coralie walk toward the UCR almost side-by-side, with the intern standing to the nurse's right (4, 10.4). Indeed, Coralie starts moving in the direction of the UCR in parallel to Ana without waiting for the nurse to overtake her and go first. As a result, when Ana stops by the UCR's entrance, her head turned to her right to answer Hazel, Coralie obstructs her view because she is standing to her right (6, 10.5). Ana is then forced to stretch her neck forward to have a view of Hazel. At this point, Coralie takes one step back, thus clearing Ana's line of vision and action, and taking a position behind her, shifted slightly to the right (8, 10.6).

In this third analytical subsection ("Minding the distance"), we have looked at the interactional work involved in handling proximity when the leading party reverses course. The contrasting excerpts show that, at least in the examined data, the intern's deftness at this may not be a matter of individual experience in following senior staff members (after all, similar activities are common in everyone's early years of social life) but rather of contingent appropriate attention and the situated achieved intelligibility of the course of action. In Excerpt 5, it is the observation intern who replicates the senior member's U-turn as it happens, whereas the nursing intern, in Excerpt 6, who had her attention focused elsewhere, finds herself in the way. Moreover, the observation intern contributes to reinstating the serial order "senior member walks ahead" as soon as she completes her own turn, whereas the nursing intern first walks side-by-side then retreats. The truth is that the observation intern, in Excerpt 5, is guided to stay behind by what she hears, the head nurse's request to the aide, and what she sees, the aide's expeditiously aiming for the urgent-care room. In contrast, the nursing intern, in Excerpt 6, attends to a check to an unspecified recipient and is with a nurse who stops on the spot and engages in interaction with a colleague, in which it turns out that the intern is to take an observer role.

On the whole, the excerpts considered in the chapter's analytical section hint at what might be the practical reason for the intern staying behind the senior staff member: the senior member is the one who is at the wheel of the ongoing activity, who deals up front with anything happening on the path, and who will get involved first and foremost in action at the destination point. It is the nurse who is looking for an object in the closet and later in the stock room (Excerpt 1), and who is addressed by the head nurse (Excerpt 2). It is the aide who agrees to pick up the folder in the reception (Excerpt 3) and is recruited (González-Martínez & Drew, 2021) by the head nurse to get him a sling (Excerpt 4) and to bring a patient to the UCR (Excerpt 5). It is the nurse who is looking for someone or something in the

PO and deals with the check of her fellow nurse inquiring in return on the latter's doings (Excerpt 6).

Discussion and conclusion

In his lectures of fall 1967 and 1968, Sacks (1992) comments on Albert's (1964) article on precedence rules among the Burundi. Albert claims that the order in which individuals take the floor in the studied setting is determined strictly by their social status inside their society. In contrast, Sacks identifies an internal system accounting for the sequential organization of ordinary conversation. A basic principle is that interlocutors need to listen and pay attention to each other as they orient themselves reciprocally. Sacks also argues that social mechanisms, like politeness rules, are often derived from the rules of the internal system of organization. For instance, the rule "do not interrupt" is built up around the internal requirement of listening to know when and how one should speak.

The intern's walking behind the senior staff member could be accounted for by referring to an external system of organization: for instance, deference rules based on professional hierarchy (Shils, 1968), which will classify the intern's not giving way to the senior member as rude and insisting on walking by her side as pretentious. In contrast, we suggest considering the "senior member walks ahead, intern follows" configuration as a resource for projecting and building distinct opportunities for participation in ongoing and forthcoming activities. Walking ahead allows the senior member to establish the destination, trajectory, and pace of the vehicular unit, to confront contingencies first and to initiate the projected activity as soon as the destination is reached. By walking behind, the intern affords the senior member space to maneuver, shift, or reverse course. The intern is thus interactionally included in ongoing and forthcoming activities in a specific spatial and interactional configuration (behind senior staff members) that orients her possible contributions. She pays attention to what the senior member is doing, remains unobstructive in the background, lets her handle things, and stays ready to respond to her requirements. In reality, the senior member "takes the intern with her" and the intern walks with the senior member. They are a "with" (Goffman, 1972 [1971], p. 19) but they are not "doing walking together" (Ryave & Schenkein, 1974, p. 267). They produce a distinct mobile formation: "intern follows senior member," with its own structure of positions, first and second, and its own participation framework for talk and body behavior.

This chapter identifies four relevant practices when it comes to moving around in a "walking-with-someone-following-them" interactional configuration: (1) keeping the way clear, (2) adopting the mill position, (3) yielding the right-of-way, and (4) minding the distance. We show how these practices work when they are deployed with ease but also what happens when they are not and the senior member must for instance push through to go first (Excerpts 3 and 4). Our analysis underscores the interactional work involved in maintaining the studied mobile configuration and the active role played by both participants, which is made up of close mutual attention and reciprocal adjustment. We thus show how the participants jointly and methodically achieve the "seen but unnoticed" (Garfinkel, 1984 [1967], p. 36) features of an everyday-life scene – participant B walks following participant A – and how a phenomenon of social order, which is a matter of concrete serial order, is accomplished through embodied action. In particular, the chapter contributes "to develop[ing] a descriptive vocabulary of elementary practices" (Lerner & Raymond, 2017, p. 312) that is useful for studying walking as a methodical accomplishment (Ryave & Schenkein, 1974) and, specifically, for analytically describing the mobile interactional configuration: walking with someone following them. It distinctively furthers ethnomethodological studies on walking practices by focusing on professionals traveling in a semi-public work environment. Moreover, it offers glimpses of the organization of "in-passing activities" like recruitment moves and checks (González-Martinez et al., 2017a; González-Martinez, 2023).

The nursing interns can be considered mobile novices (Rauniomaa et al., 2018) in that part of their on-the-job experience is to move around in the clinic as a means of getting acquainted with its functioning and the activities of the staff members; this is deftly captured by the English expression "walk the wards." Our study touches on a component of the fabric of the intern's instruction-on-the move (Rauniomaa et al., 2018): following (literally) senior members as they conduct their daily activities, paying close attention to their doings but staying in the background, which is this chapter's main contribution to the present volume's topic. The participants' orientation to an on-the-job training situation could account for the studied mobile configuration that, first of all, prompts interns "to read embodied, real-time action" (Hindmarsh & Pilnick, 2002, p. 161) and "to display intercorporeal knowing" (Hindmarsh & Pilnick, 2007, p. 1414) starting by unobtrusively following senior staff. Moreover, the trips provide opportunities to assist with mobile nursing activities like, in the studied excerpts, picking up patients in the waiting rooms, leading them to the examination rooms, and gathering the documents and medical devices necessary for treatment. Besides, the studied walking configuration also demonstrates specific ways of carrying oneself professionally – following implicit rules such as "do not run even if in a rush" or "limit physical contact" – of practicing restraint in professional relationships and of dealing with the requirements of hospital work in terms of multi-tasking, interruptions, and time pressures. The functionalist approach – through training, the intern is introduced to a future professional role – is nevertheless tempered with the interactionist approach: what is at stake is to "pass" as an intern, which requires occupying a spatial position (behind the senior members) in line with a hierarchical system (Melia, 1987). The classic discrepancy between professional ideology and bureaucratic roles (Simpson, 1979) could furthermore be showing in the limited agency afforded to the "walking-behind" intern compared to the ideals of team integration and training self-reliant professionals. After all, internships are designed to "[provide] a real-world experience while maintaining the student-learner role" (Udlis, 2008, p. 21) with the attached perpetual challenge of overcoming the model of the student as a "passive receptacle" of knowledge (Psathas, 1968, p. 191).

This being said, we would like to be cautious when discussing any more general implications of our study. We have shed some light on just one aspect of the ordinary work involved in a nursing internship, which we have, furthermore, very broadly defined. The goal of our study – to present some practices related to the production of a mobile interactional configuration – differs from the aim of identifying what makes one course of action what it is and produces the participants' correlative identities. By itself, the studied interactional configuration generates the identities "holders of first and second positions in a serial walking order" and is central to the enactment of the identifies "junior and senior participants in the realization of a course of action." It also contributes to the interactional achievement of the identities "nursing staff member" and "nursing intern" but only together with far more consequential practices: being in a hospital setting, wearing a specific type of uniform and badge, doing distinctive nursing activities, etc. In other words, the studied interactional configuration does not make the participants "nursing staff members" and "nursing interns" (Garfinkel et al., 1981, p. 133). The specificity of a nursing internship is not walking following a senior member of the nursing staff. "Walking-with-someone-following-them" is not a constituent of the nursing occupation that could account for its distinctiveness. Quite the contrary, the studied interactional configuration can arguably be at play in a diversity of ordinary and institutional settings in which a senior member "takes with them" a junior member for the latter to see "how we do things here." We can legitimately, and conveniently, refer to the studied participants as nursing aide, nurse, and intern because these are the terms the participants use to refer to themselves. Nevertheless, the difference between the identities generated by the studied mobile configuration and the participants' professional identities is to be analytically reckoned with (Watson, 1997; Mondada, 2021).

Acknowledgments

This chapter was prepared in the framework of the research projects *Mobile and Contingent Work Interactions in the Hospital Care Unit* (SNSF grant no. 134875) and *Requesting in Hospital Nurses' Unscheduled Interprofessional Interaction* (SNSF grant no. 185152). Over the years, the author has presented preliminary analyses of the data at several scientific gatherings, including the Swiss Sociological Association Conference, University of Zurich, June 22, 2017; the International Pragmatics Association Conference, Winterthur, July 2, 2021 (paper with Sylvia Trieu); and the Conversation Analysis Symposium, Università degli studi di Modena e Reggio Emilia, May 20, 2022; she thanks the participants for their comments. She is especially grateful to the volume's editor for encouraging her to publish the results of the study, to the anonymous reviewer for their insightful comments, and to Elisabeth Lyman for the editing work.

Notes

1 Studying the mobility of persons and objects in relation to collaboration in professional settings, Luff and Heath (1998) draw a distinction between micro-mobility in

an "at hand" domain, local mobility in a common workspace, and remote mobility between several settings. When studying mobility, Psathas (1976) focuses on the traveling in space of the entire body and on independent travel, in contrast to being transported.
2 The images are taken from video data collected by the author and principal investigator of the research projects from which this study originates.
3 The game is also called nine men's norris, merrills, ninepenny marl, and cowboy checkers, among other names, in English; see https://en.wikipedia.org/wiki/Nine_men%27s_morris
4 Underneath the original French talk (in bold), the transcripts provide an English translation (in italics) that is in line with its organization yet as natural as possible. We describe the embodied actions (in gray) but do not specify their trajectory to single out a preparatory phase, an apex, and a withdrawal phase, as Mondada (2019) does. In the following analytical section, the numbers in parentheses refer to the lines of the excerpt and the images in the corresponding figure; "(2, 5.2)," for instance, equates to "(line 2, Image 5.2)."

References

Albert, E. M. (1964). "Rhetoric," "logic," and "poetics" in Burundi: Culture patterning of speech behavior. *American Anthropologist, 66*(6–2), 35–54. https://doi.org/10.1525/aa.1964.66.suppl_3.02a00020

Bardram, J. E., & Bosen, C. (2005). Mobility work: The spatial dimension of collaboration at a hospital. *Computer Supported Cooperative Work, 14*(2), 131–160. https://doi.org/10.1007/s10606-005-0989-y

Broth, M., & Mondada, L. (2013). Walking away: The embodied achievement of activity closings in mobile interaction. *Journal of Pragmatics, 47*(1), 41–58. https://doi.org/10.1016/j.pragma.2012.11.016

De Stefani, E. (2013). The collaborative organisation of next actions in a semiotically rich environment: Shopping as a couple. In P. Haddington, L. Mondada, & M. Nevile (Eds.), *Interaction and mobility: Language and body in motion* (pp. 123–151). Walter de Gruyter. https://doi.org/10.1515/9783110291278.123

De Stefani, E., & Mondada, L. (2014). Reorganizing mobile formations: When "guided" participants initiate reorientations in guided tours. *Space and Culture, 17*(2), 157–175. https://doi.org/10.1177/1206331213508504

Garfinkel, H. (1984). *Studies in ethnomethodology*. Polity Press.

Garfinkel, H. (1988). Evidence for locally produced, naturally accountable phenomena of order, logic, reason, meaning, method, etc. in and as of the essential quiddity of immortal ordinary society, (I of IV): *An announcement of studies. Sociological Theory, 6*(1), 103–109. https://doi.org/10.2307/201918

Garfinkel, H. (1996). Ethnomethodology's program. *Social Psychology Quarterly, 59*(1), 5–21. https://doi.org/10.2307/2787116

Garfinkel, H. (2002). *Ethnomethodology's program: Working out Durkheim's aphorism*. Rowman and Littlefield Publishers.

Garfinkel, H., & Livingston, E. (2003). Phenomenal field properties of order in formatted queues and their neglected standing in the current situation of inquiry. *Visual Studies, 18*(1), 21–28. https://doi.org/10.1080/1472586032000010029

Garfinkel, H., Lynch, M., & Livingston, E. (1981). The work of a discovering science construed with materials from the optically discovered pulsar. *Philosophy of the Social Sciences, 11*(2), 131–158. https://doi.org/10.1177/004839318101100202

Goffman, E. (1966 [1963]). *Behavior in public places: Notes on the social organization of gatherings*. The Free Press.
Goffman, E. (1972 [1971]). *Relations in public: Microstudies of the public order*. Harper Colophon Books.
González-Martínez, E. (2023). Faire du coude avec un énoncé 'il y a x': Inciter à l'action et recruter une personne responsable d'agir en milieu hospitalier. *Langage et Société*, *179*(2), 111–139.
González-Martínez, E., Bangerter, A., & Lê Van, K. (2017a). Passing-by "Ça va?" checks in clinic corridors. *Semiotica*, 215, 1–42. https://doi.org/10.1515/sem-2015-0107
González-Martínez, E., Bangerter, A., & Lê Van, K. (2017b). Building situation awareness on the move: Staff monitoring behavior in clinic corridors. *Qualitative Health Research*, *27*(4), 2244–2257. https://doi.org/10.1177/1049732317728485
Hindmarsh, I., & Pilnick, A. (2002). The tacit order of teamwork: Collaboration and embodied conduct in anesthesia. *Sociological Quarterly*, *43*(2), 139–164. https://doi.org/10.1111/j.1533-8525.2002.tb00044.x
Hindmarsh, J., & Pilnick, A. (2007). Knowing bodies at work: Embodiment and ephemeral teamwork in anaesthesia. *Organization Studies*, *28*(9), 1395–1416. https://doi.org/10.1177/0170840607068258
Ingold, T., & Vergunst, J. L. (Eds.). (2008). *Ways of walking: Ethnography and practice on foot*. Ashgate Publishing.
Jefferson, G. (2004). Glossary of transcript symbols with an introduction. In G. H. Lerner (Ed.), *Conversation analysis: Studies from the first generation* (pp. 13–31). John Benjamins. https://doi.org/10.1075/pbns.125.02jef
Kendon, A. (1973). The role of visible behavior in the organization of social interaction. In M. von Cranach & I. Vine (Eds.), *Social communication and movement: Studies of interaction and expression in man and chimpanzee* (pp. 29–74). Academic Press.
Lerner, G. H., & Raymond, G. (2017). On the practical re-intentionalization of body behavior: Action pivots in the progressive realization of embodied conduct. In G. Raymond, G. Lerner, & J. Heritage (Eds.), *Enabling human conduct: Studies of talk-in-interaction in honor of Emanuel A. Schegloff* (pp. 299–314). John Benjamins. https://doi.org/10.1075/pbns.273.15ler
Liberman, K. (2013). The local orderliness of crossing Kincaid. In K. Liberman (Ed.), *More studies in ethnomethodology* (pp. 11–30). State University of New York Press.
Livingston, E. (1987). *Making sense of ethnomethodology*. Routledge and Kegan Paul.
Long, D., Iedema, R., & Lee, B. B. (2007). Corridor conversations: Clinical communication in casual spaces. In R. Iedema (Ed.), *The discourse of hospital communication: Tracing complexities in contemporary health care organizations* (pp. 182–200). Palgrave Macmillan. https://doi.org/10.1057/9780230595477_9
Luff, P., & Heath, C. (199814–18 November). Mobility in collaboration. In *Proceedings of the 1998 ACM conference on computer-supported cooperative work*, Seattle, United States (pp. 305–314). Association for Computing Machinery Press. https://doi.org/10.1145/289444.289505
Mauss, M. (1973 [1935]). Techniques of the body. *Economy and Society*, *2*(1), 70–88. https://doi.org/10.1080/03085147300000003
McIlvenny, P., Broth, M., & Haddington, P. (2009). Communicating place, space and mobility. *Journal of Pragmatics*, *41*(10), 1879–1886. https://doi.org/10.1016/j.pragma.2008.09.014
McIlvenny, P., Broth, M., & Haddington, P. (2014). Moving together: Mobile formations in interaction. *Space and Culture*, *17*(2), 104–106. https://doi.org/10.1177/1206331213508679

Melia, K. M. (1987). *Learning and working. The occupational socialization of nurses.* Routledge.
Messmer, P. R., Jones, S. G., & Taylor, B. A. (2004). Enhancing knowledge and self-confidence of novice nurses: The "Shadow-A-Nurse" ICU program. *Nursing Education Perspectives, 25*(3), 131–136.
Mondada, L. (2014). Bodies in action: Multimodal analysis of walking and talking. *Language and Dialogue, 4*(3), 357–403. https://doi.org/10.1075/ld.4.3.02mon
Mondada, L. (2019). *Conventions for multimodal transcription.* https://www.lorenzamondada.net/multimodal-transcription
Mondada, L. (2021). Membership categorization and the sequential multimodal organization of action: Walking, perceiving, and talking in material-spatial ecologies. In R. J. Smith, R. Fitzgerald, & W. Housley (Eds.), *On Sacks: Methodology, materials and inspirations* (pp. 101–117). Routledge.
Psathas, G. (1968). *The student nurse in the diploma school of nursing.* Springer.
Psathas, G. (1976). Mobility, orientation and navigation: Conceptual and theoretical considerations. *New Outlook for the Blind, 70*(9), 385–391. https://doi.org/10.1177/0145482X7607000904
Rauniomaa, M., Haddington, P., Melander, H., Gazin, A.-D., Broth, M., Cromdal, J., ... McIlvenny, P. (2018). Parsing tasks for the mobile novice in real time: Orientation to the learner's actions and to spatial and temporal constraints in instructing-on-the-move. *Journal of Pragmatics, 128*, 30–52. https://doi.org/10.1016/j.pragma.2018.01.005
Relieu, M. (1999). Parler en marchant: Pour une écologie dynamique des échanges de paroles. *Langage et Société, 89*(1), 37–67.
Ryave, A. L., & Schenkein, J. N. (1974). Notes on the art of walking. In R. Turner (Ed.), *Ethnomethodology: Selected readings* (pp. 265–274). Penguin Books.
Sacks, H. (1992). *Lectures on conversation. I-II.* Blackwell.
Schegloff, E. A. (2007). *Sequence organization in interaction: A primer in conversation analysis.* Cambridge University Press.
Schmitt, R. (2012). Gehen als situierte Praktik: "Gemeinsam Gehen" und "hinter jemandem herlaufen". *Gesprächsforschung - Online-Zeitschrift zur verbalen Interaktion, 13*, 1–44.
Shils, E. (1968). Deference. In J. A. Jackson (Ed.), *Social stratification* (pp. 104–132). Cambridge University Press.
Simpson, I. H. (1979). *From student to nurse: A longitudinal study of socialization.* Cambridge University Press.
Smith, R. J. (2017). Left to their own devices? The practical organisation of space, interaction, and communication in and as the work of crossing a shared space intersection. *Sociologica, 11*(2), 1–31. https://doi.org/10.2383/88200
Sudnow, D. (1972). Temporal parameters of interpersonal observation. In D. Sudnow (Ed.), *Studies in social interaction* (pp. 259–279). The Free Press.
Udlis, K. A. (2008). Preceptorship in undergraduate nursing education: An integrative review. *Journal of Nursing Education, 47*(1), 20–29. https://doi.org/10.3928/01484834-20080101-09
vom Lehn, D. (2013). Withdrawing from exhibits: The interactional organisation of museum visits. In P. Haddington, L. Mondada, & M. Nevile (Eds.), *Interaction and mobility: Language and body in motion* (pp. 65–90). Walter de Gruyter. https://doi.org/10.1515/9783110291278.65
Watson, D. R. (1995). Angoisse dans la 42ème rue. In P. Paperman & R. Ogien (Eds.), *La couleur des pensées* (pp. 197–216). Editions de l'Ecole des hautes études en sciences sociales.
Watson, D. R. (1997). Some general reflections on "categorization" and "sequence" in the analysis of conversation. In S. Hester & P. Eglin (Eds.), *Culture in action: Studies in membership categorization analysis* (pp. 49–75). University Press of America.

4 Asking questions in the operating room

Lorenza Mondada

Introduction

Asking questions is a privileged and simple practice to learn – as shown by children asking questions to parents, pupils to teachers, and novices to experts. In professional settings in which being socialized and trained into skilled tasks is achieved through apprenticeship, participation, and companionship, questions are asked and made possible in the midst of the professional activity. This raises the issue of when and which kind of questions are asked, as well as which competences asking them relies on. Instruction on how to ask questions is part of the socialization of novices and an important prerequisite for them to actually ask questions and learn from the answers.

Whilst there is a wide range of studies on questions in the interactional literature, these essentially focus on the linguistic format of questions, as well as on the interpretability of various turn formats in posing a question. Much less attention has been given to the material ecology and the praxeological context in which questions are asked, which crucially make the question relevant and to which questions adjust. In this chapter, I adopt an ethnomethodological and conversation analytic (EMCA) perspective to address the contingencies and situatedness characterizing the sequential environments in which participants treat questions as adequate or not – including not only the sequentiality of talk but also the sequential organization of the surgical operation. The setting studied is surgery, which is a medical professional field in which operating on patients is also the occasion to teach the procedure to medical students. In the data studied, this double nature of the operating theater is enhanced by the fact that the operation, conducted by senior surgeons and their team, is being broadcasted on closed-circuit television (CCTV) to an amphitheater where an audience of trainees and experts watches it in real time. This technological configuration enables trainees to ask questions via an audio connection with the chief surgeon, and experts to support them in moderating the connection with him.

In this context, a recurrent issue for all participants – surgeons, trainees, and experts – is when it is relevant to ask questions. Specific moments in the operation are treated by these parties as relevant for asking questions. The chapter offers a systematic study of these moments, and the ways different participants orient to them. It shows how participants identify these moments, how questions are treated

DOI: 10.4324/9781003312345-6

as situated actions and as revealing the competent, socialized, skilled professional vision participants demonstrate of the surgical procedure. In other words, asking questions in the operating room is an action that can be referred to, invited to, and achieved by different parties. They instructably display that questions rely on relevant ways of seeing the unfolding moves in the operating procedure, as well as on the identification of relevant interactional moments in which asking a question is adequate. The chapter thus reveals how asking questions is orchestrated, instructed, and made possible within a plurality of participation frameworks, across locations and within multiple courses of action, orienting to the socialization of the trainees into understanding the unfolding of the professional activity in real time.

Background: The embeddedness of work and training in surgery as multiactivity

Contrary to formal education in classrooms, diverse professional settings integrate *in situ* the training of novices, students, and trainees within the work activity and as work unfolds. Trainees work with professionals and learn by witnessing and participating in the activity. In EMCA, such situations have been studied by Goodwin (2017), analyzing how junior members of an archeology team identify relevant colors and textures of the soil under the guidance of senior archeologists, how a student works with a geochemist on a fiber and learns how to categorize the blackness of black, and how students in geology learn to see the environing landscape of rocks.

Surgery is another exemplary setting in which professional activities are intertwined with instructional activities. EMCA studies of surgery have shown how surgical operations involve experienced surgeons and junior members with different levels of training (Mondada, 2007; Zemel & Koschmann, 2014; Zemel et al., 2011), and how the organization of surgical work integrates the presence of trainees (Sanchez-Svensson et al., 2009). In neighboring fields like dentistry, students not only participate but work under expert supervision (Hindmarsh, 2010). Even when trainees are not directly contributing to the ongoing work, they might participate and witness it, learning from following the procedure in real time.

In the context studied here, the use of visualization technologies serves both surgical work and training, thanks to the broadcasting in large amphitheaters of images used by the surgeons themselves for operating with the help of endoscopic cameras (Mondada, 2003, 2007, 2011, 2014a). Similar uses of video have been observed in university courses in endodontics where the microscope is connected to a video broadcasted in an auditorium (Lindwall et al., 2014; Lindwall & Lymer, 2014). In all these cases, trainees do not participate in the work, but share some visual access to it: their bodies are not directly involved in the operating activity, but their vision has access to what the professionals see and visually rely on for operating. Thus, a central issue in these settings is the socialization of trainees to see what the professionals see, that is, to learn a form of "professional vision" (Goodwin, 1994) making sense of the progression of the operation, its situated contingencies (Sanchez-Svensson et al., 2009), and the details of the anatomy relevant for it (Zemel et al., 2011). The local use of video further enhances the visual accountability of the operating theater (Mondada, 2003, 2007, 2014a; Lindwall & Lymer, 2014), building the professional vision of the trainees being socialized in the use of these images.

Thus, what characterizes these settings is multiactivity (Haddington et al., 2014), intertwining professional work (the surgical operation), and instruction (the demonstration, formulation, and explanation of how to operate). Both activities remain distinct, but reflexively shape each other, since the demonstration is built on the operation and the operation is adjusted to the demonstration. Both are performed by the surgeon, although they might privilege one aspect or the other depending on the difficulty of the operation (Mondada, 2014b). Moreover, their multiactivity is supported by the presence of experts, also located in the amphitheater away from the operating theatre, contributing to the instruction, and sometimes to the operation (Mondada, 2007). In this setting, trainees can participate by asking questions, and the expert might support them, as well as assist the surgeon in dealing with it. Questions are invited by the surgeon and the expert: they are integrated in the work as *in situ* training; at the same time, they adjust to the ongoing work, which constrains their production, acceptability, legitimacy, and even audibility.

Although questions have been massively studied in EMCA, the material ecology and the praxeological context in which they are asked, making the question relevant and to which questions adjust, remain understudied. Questions have been studied for their sequence organization, as adjacency pairs (Schegloff & Sacks, 1973), as pre-sequences, and as practices in the service of possible diverse actions, building their multi-barreled and ambiguous interpretations (Schegloff, 2007). Questions have been analyzed for their formats and their sequential implicativeness (De Ruiter, 2012; Enfield et al., 2010) and epistemic issues have been discussed in relation to their format and interpretability (Heritage, 2012). Moreover, questions have been characterized as the finger-print of some institutional settings, as in news interviews (Clayman & Heritage, 2002) and other media settings in which they are the backbone of the work of journalists (Clayman, 2010). In asymmetric institutional interactions, questions are often asked by professionals and experts, whereby questions asked by lay members are distinctive and distinctively treated – such as patients' versus doctors' questions in medical settings (Ten Have, 1991; Frankel, 1990; Roberts, 2000), students' versus teachers' in the classroom (Mehan, 1979; Duran & Sert, 2021).

Trainees' questions in the operating room have been discussed by Lindwall and Lymer (2014) in relation to their formats and topics. They contrast questions relative to the identification and recognition of anatomical structures ("What is X?" and "Is that X?" versus "Is that X?" which provides a candidate answer), the recognizability of the embodied action of the dentist ("What is X doing now?"), the provision of candidate understandings about the ongoing action ("But now X isn't doing Y"), and finally generic concerns about the routine and normative character of procedures and techniques ("Doesn't one always have to do X?"). In their study, the trainees asking questions are students watching the procedure with a member of the teaching staff – whereas in the cases studied here, the trainees are surgeons in continuous education, who address their questions directly to the operating surgeon, although they are supported by a chairperson, who is an expert and colleague of the surgeon.

This chapter thus explores a setting in which the opportunity to ask questions is offered from within the ongoing work activity – rather than in a separated realm – although preserving the status of the trainees as observers – rather than as intervening in the work. This particular configuration confronts them with the *in-vivo* unfolding of the action, which supports their socialization but also is revealed to be quite challenging, as the difficulties trainees have in asking questions will show.

Data: Laparoscopic surgery as video training

In this chapter, I study the intertwining of operating on a patient and instructing advanced medical practitioners in surgery, on the basis of a video-recorded corpus of surgical laparoscopic operations broadcasted live to trainees (about 15 h, recorded in 1996–1997 in collaboration with the surgeons, in a university hospital in France). Although the recordings were made some time ago, they document video-mediated instructional practices that were pioneering at that time and have become increasingly popular since.

The surgical team studied here has been experimenting early on with a double use of video devices, for the sake of the operation and for the purposes of instruction and demonstration (Mondada, 2003, 2007, 2014a). On the one hand, the chief surgeon directs the endoscopic camera while he operates laparoscopically. Laparoscopy (also called "key-hole surgery") is a minimally invasive technique that consists in placing the instruments and an optic system inside the patient's body through small incisions and by means of *trocars* in which the instruments are inserted. The camera is handled either by the surgeon or an assistant; the surgeon operates while looking at a monitor where the endoscopic image is made available for the entire team.

On the other hand, the operation is transmitted live via CCTV to an audience of advanced trainees and a board of experts, who are located in a distant amphitheater. Remote learning is made possible thanks to the transmission of the endoscopic image in the amphitheater. Moreover, another image is also produced for instructional purposes by a traditional camera mounted on the light above the operating theater, making visible the surgeons' hands operating on the patient's body. The chief surgeon can request the technical staff member in the control room, who edits the images in real time, to transmit a specific view, the external view or the endoscopic view, or a combination of both. Furthermore, while watching the operation in real time, the trainees and the expert can also talk with the surgeon thanks to an audio connection, provided by a microphone equipping each seat in the amphitheater, which can be activated at any time by each participant pushing a button to unmute it.

In this context of multiactivity (Mondada, 2014b), the surgical team is involved in two concurrent courses of action: the operation *in situ*, and its demonstration for the distant trainees. The team is supported by experts, who sit with the trainees, and in this position can mediate between the amphitheater and the operating room.

These experts are senior surgeons, who often also engage in the next operation: they share the embodied perspective of the trainees and the professional vision of the surgeons. Although the team, the trainees, and the experts are in different locations, they all rely on what is made visibly accessible by the video cameras. However, their visual perspectives are different, based on different practices, vision, and relevancies. The endoscopic view is produced by the embodied action of the surgical team in the operating room, looked at by them on small monitors on both sides of the room. The same view, completed by an external view of the operated body, is watched by the trainees on a magnified screen in the amphitheater and by experts on small inset screens in the board where they sit facing the trainees.

Looking at an image in the midst of an activity for which it is indispensable or watching it as a spectator sitting in an amphitheater are very different visual-embodied activities, although they involve looking at the "same" image (Mondada, 2007). Moreover, the images produced for the operation versus the demonstration are different: the former require a focus on relevant details for the procedure, the latter require magnified, easily recognizable, well-exposed details. Both are achieved through camerawork, dissecting practices, and explanatory talk by the surgeon *in situ*, supported by the distant expert. While the surgeon often focuses more on the operation, the formulation of its distinctive steps, and the demonstration of the anatomy, the expert supports a complementary focus by pinpointing and expanding relevant details, and by supporting the questions of the trainees. As we shall see, the fact that the surgeon conducts the operation makes them not always available for engaging in instructional activities, while the expert as a distant observer is closer to the perspective of the trainees. The issue for trainees is not just asking questions, but becoming socialized in identifying relevant environments for doing so and more generally in *seeing* the operation and the anatomy in a professional way.

The analysis is organized in two parts: first, I show how opportunities to ask questions are created for trainees by surgeons and experts, supported by the video editing team (Extracts 1–7). While these opportunities might be seized (Extracts 6–7) or not (Extracts 1–5), they point to relevant moments within the procedure where asking questions is relevant and possible. Displaying these opportunities works as an instruction about where and when questions are legitimate. Second, on this basis, I show how questions are asked (Extracts 8–14), not only by trainees, but also by experts. I differentiate between the format used by experts (Extracts 8–11: prefaced by a simple summons, introducing questions that might instruct the trainees) and by trainees (Extracts 12–14: prefaced by an apology, introducing "real" questions), as well as between the way they are responded to (unproblematically and immediately versus with some hitches and difficulties). The analysis reveals how the relevance of asking questions is treated as constitutive of trainees' socialization, that is, as contributing to the development of their professional vision and understanding of the ongoing operation and its detailed organization, and how asking questions is actually instructed, enabled, and thus (collectively) achieved through the distinct contributions of a diversity of participants (surgeon, expert, video team) involved in the activity.

Asking questions in the operating room 107

Creating opportunities for trainees to ask questions

Within the complex, multiactivity, multisite, multi-participative setting characterizing the surgical operation, it is not easy for distant trainees to directly ask questions to the operating surgeon. As a matter of fact, their access to the surgical field is more often mediated either by the surgeon himself, or by the expert co-present with them in the amphitheater. In this section, I discuss instances in which both create opportunities for trainees to ask questions and show the instructional character of these practices.

Surgeons' management of opportunities to ask questions

Engaged in the multiactivity of operating and demonstrating the operation, the surgeon orients to particular moments within the procedure as being relevant for trainees to ask questions. These moments are significant within the procedure: the fact that the surgeon inserts a sequence enabling possible questions serves as an instruction for the trainees to see these moments (to learn to identify and recognize them) as such. This happens generally at some transition point, when a phase (e.g., the completed installation of trocars, an anatomic demonstration, the end of a delicate phase of the operation), sequence, or action is visibly accomplished and the next one can be expected. Mentioning or giving the opportunity to ask a question instructably pinpoints a moment as organizationally important within the surgical procedure, thereby also highlighting the order of the procedure itself.

Opportunities for questions are typically created at the beginning of the operation, when the trocars have been inserted in the body: this is the case of the following two extracts, where the surgeon, having positioned some trocars and instruments, pauses and indicates the opportunity for a question.

In the first extract, the surgeon has inserted four trocars and the laparoscopic camera (fig. 1): he now checks if there is "any question" (l. 1). Multimodal transcripts integrate relevant embodied surgical actions (SUR: surgeon), as well as changes visible on the broadcasted image (scr: screen).

Extract (1) (k1d1/12'30/Q-about-disp—e7)

```
→ 1   SUR   .hh okay. (0.7) any question about the
  2         disposition (0.4) of *the tro#car?
                                 *2H open on abdomen->
        fig                           #fig.1
  3         (2.2)*
                ->*
  4   SUR   o|kay. (1.2) the next step (.) is, (0.2) the-
        scr  |internal image PIP->>
  5         *(0.4) the instrumentation,*# (0.5) we put a
            *appr w retractor---------*inserts rectr in trocar->>
        fig                             #fig.2
```

6   retractor of the liver, (.) in the subcostal area

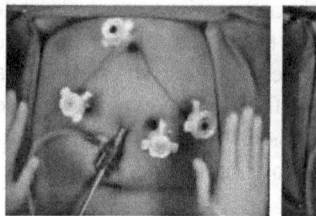

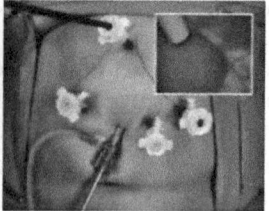

1: the question   2: projection of the next step

The check for possible questions (l. 1–2) is uttered (see →) while showing the patient's abdomen (fig. 1) with two open hands above it, where the trocars are visible. Not only the turn and the gesture, but also the image, are designed for the trainees. The way the visual access to the operation is orchestrated is clearly recipient-oriented: the camera used is the external one, showing the operating field from above, and the surgeon's gestures are made for that camera perspective. Neither the camera nor the gesture are functional for the surgery. Moreover, the surgeon does more than offer an opportunity to ask a question: he indicates, at the completion of the phase consisting in deciding where to put the trocars, that this is a relevant moment to retrospectively summarize the chosen location of the trocars (data not shown). In this way, the surgeon instructs the trainees about an important step of the procedure.

The surgeon's question is followed by an absence of response (l. 3). His "okay." (l. 4) retrospectively orients to the closure of that sequence and prospectively to the next action. The latter is explicitly announced ("the next step (.) is," l. 4), and manually initiated by inserting a retractor in the trocar (at the top of fig. 2). At this point, the transmitted image changes, making available the internal view within the abdomen in a picture-in-picture insert (fig. 2, PIP, on the upper right corner of the screen). This visually achieves the transition to the next step of the procedure, consisting in inserting the instruments to be used for the laparoscopic operation, as well as the transition to the view produced by the endoscopic camera, functional to the operation. So, by highlighting the position of a possible question, the surgeon also instructably highlights the sequential organization of the procedure and its articulation in "steps," drawing attention to the prerequisites for the "next" action.

Likewise, in the next extract, the surgeon checks if there is "no question" (l. 3) just after completing the insertion of the trocars and the instruments within them. Like Extract 1, he also utters his turn together with a showing gesture (fig. 3):

Asking questions in the operating room 109

Extract (2) (14'57/nice-case—e11)

```
   1  SUR  okay,
   2       (1.1)
→  3  SUR  Δno question about the #disΔposition of the trocar?
      scr  Δext.view + inset int.view-Δint. view-->
      fig                          #fig.3
   4       and about the::: mkt (0.4) the instrumentation?
```

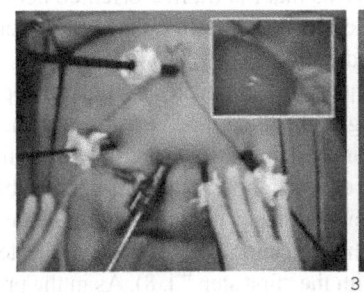

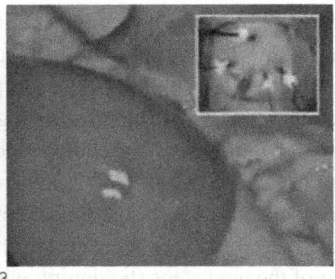

```
   5       Δ# (1.1)
      scr  ->Δint.v.+inset ext.v.->
      fig  #fig.4
   6  SUR  okay, we can start the di*ssection#
                                   *introduces retractor->
      fig                          #fig.5
```

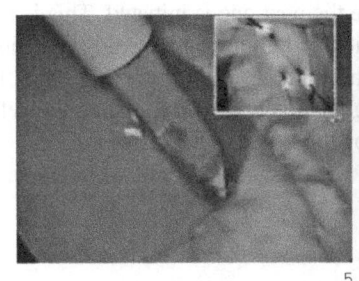

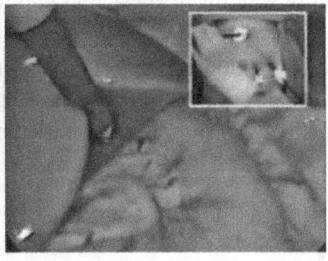

```
   7       (1.1)*
            -->*
   8  SUR  *first step, (0.4) is# the exposure (1.6) of
           *retracts progressively the liver--->>
      fig                        #fig.6
   9       the gastro (0.2) oesophagial (.) junction.
  10       (1.7)
  11  SUR  in order to do that, (0.4) we use the retractor
```

110   *Lorenza Mondada*

The surgeon's "okay," registers the completion of the previous action, the insertion of the last instrument in the relevant trocar (l. 1). He then checks (see →) if there are questions while showing the patient's body (l. 3–4). This is done for the external camera (fig. 3). We can notice that the team in charge of editing the broadcasted image, who sit in a control room outside the operating room, by changing the view at that point, orient to "okay" as closing the previous sequence and as projecting the relevance of an instruction. This reveals that the trainee-oriented action of offering the opportunity for a question is collectively achieved by the video team and the surgeon, in a perfectly timed tacit coordination.

The surgeon not only opens up a window for questions, but makes explicit the topical domain of potential questions (the positioning of the trocar and instrumentation, l. 3–4), retrospectively highlighting the choice characterizing the previous step. In this way, even in the absence of questions (l. 5), the orientation toward them instructably accomplishes a retrospective synthesis of the previous step. The transition to the next step is then explicitly formulated ("we can start the dissection" l. 6) and also indicated by the numbering of the next steps (beginning with the "first step," l. 8). As in the previous case, offering a space to ask a question occasions the explicit formulation of the sequential organization of the operation for the learning audience, instructing them how to see the unfolding procedure.

The first two extracts referred to the beginning of the operation and the prerequisites for engaging in it. Later, during the operation, opportunities to ask questions are created at the completion of significant steps, and before the next one is initiated. This is the case of Extracts 3 and 4, in which we join the action as the surgeon is already orienting toward the trainees, formulating his action or demonstrating the anatomy for them. In the next extract, the surgeon (SUR) is addressing the trainees by formulating the delicate action he is actually performing, supported by the expert (EXP, l. 5–6).

Extract (3) (k1d1/53'41/not-necessary—e10)

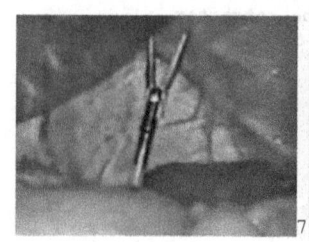

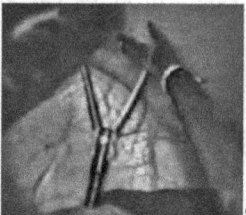

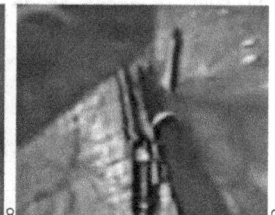

```
1         (6)#
    sur  >>tries to catch ligament w plier->
    fig   #fig.7
2   SUR  okay now i grasp (4.5)* the# triangular (1.3)
                              ->*helps w other plier->
    fig                           #fig.8
3        ligament#
    fig          #fig.9
```

```
    4          (1.4)
    5   EXP    do*n't forget this little (.) step, ©or you will have
               ->*
        cam                                          ©zoom back--->
    6          surprise© (.) [(with the articulator)] .hh he he]©
 →  7   SUR                  [no question?           ]
        cam    --->©zoom forth and adjustment---------------©
    8                                       [  (1.7)  ]
    9   SUR    you see (1.1) this is probably the z line, (2.0) two
   10          centimeter below (2.4) i make (.) the retro- (.)
   11          gastric channel,
```

The surgeon formulates the action he is performing (l. 2–3), thereby reflexively ensuring the intelligibility of the action that is visible on the screen (figs. 7–9). His descriptive turn is temporally adjusted to his manual attempts, and the completion of the turn is finely tuned with the success of the maneuver (fig. 9). At this completion point, this action is also commented on by the expert, highlighting its importance (l. 5–6). Thus, surgeon and expert identify the same relevant moment and collaborate to make this moment noticeable, intelligible, and learnable for the trainees. Having completed his manipulation of the ligament, the surgeon asks "no question?" (l. 7; see →), overlapping with the expert's final increment (l. 6). The camera also orients to the completion of this action, by moving back and offering a general view of the anatomical field, also orienting to its relevance for the trainees (versus a more detailed and focused view oriented to the operating team).

Thus, the sequential position of the surgeon's check, at the completion of an important action, instructs the recipients about the relevance of asking a question, and the target of a possible question, highlighting the relevance of that particular action. Here too, there is an absence of response from the trainees (indicated l. 8, overlapping with the expert's laughter, l. 6). Consequently, the surgeon initiates the next step (l. 9–11).

As observable in the previous and next extracts, the relevance of a surgical moment, and therefore of asking questions at that point, can be addressed both by the surgeon and the expert: this shows again that the operation is scrutinized in a recipient-oriented way not only for how surgery is accomplished, but also for opportunities to teach it. In the next fragment, the surgeon, at the end of an anatomical description, creates a space for a question, immediately supported by the expert:

Extract (4) (k1d2/7'25/they agree—e8)

```
    1   SUR    so:, *you see here the* upper part of the stomach,
                    *points w plier*
    2          (1.3)
    3          euh *fifteen* cc,
                   *points w plier*
    4          (0.8)
    5          and (.) the distal *part of the stomach.
                                  *grasps w plier and tends->
    6          (1.2)
    7          euh:°hh° zoom arrière.*
               ehm      zoom back
                                    -->*
```

112 *Lorenza Mondada*

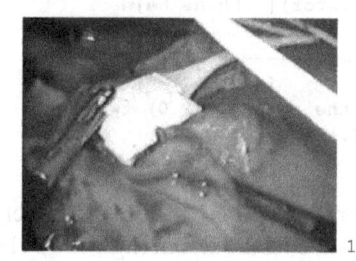

```
   8        +  (1.1)   +
      ast   +zooms back+
→  9  SUR   any question?# (0.4) about that?
      fig                #fig.10
```

[figure 10]

```
  10        (2.5)
→ 11  EXP   ever[ybody] agree that the balloon is in the stomach
  12  SUR       [okay]
  13  EXP   and not in the oesophagus?
  14        (4.0)
  15  EXP   o:kay. (.) they agree
  16        (0.7)
  17  SUR   °okay.°
  18        (0.8)
  19  SUR   NOW the problem is to avoid the: the slipping (0.9) of
  20        the::: (1.1) tsk (.) of the band, (0.5) and in order
  21        to avoid that we will put three stitches anteriorly
```

The surgeon demonstrates the anatomy of the stomach for the audience ("you see here" l. 1, 5), while also directing his team about operating tasks (l. 3), and the assistant (ast) holding the endoscopic camera (l. 7). The opportunity to ask a question (see →) is created after the assistant has been requested to zoom out (versus Extract 3 where the assistant was initiating it), to offer a broader view of the stomach for the trainees. Its sequential position as well as the turn format (with the demonstrative pronoun "that?" l. 9) indicate that the anatomical demonstration is completed. This opportunity is not taken by the trainees (l. 10).

At this point, as the surgeon moves on ("okay" l. 12), the expert inserts another question (l. 11–13), which topicalizes the current step of the procedure, where a "balloon" is inflated (as requested in line 3) under the nasogastric band (visible in fig. 10), and the importance of its location. Interestingly, while the surgeon was pointing to the relevance of a question about "that?" (l. 9), using a deictic expression, the expert unpacks the issue at hand, contrastively describing the possible positions of the balloon (l. 11, 13). So, the same sequential position is instructably used by the surgeon and the expert, albeit from different perspectives, one more indexical and the other more explicit. The absence of (audible) response is treated here as agreement (l. 15). The sequential position at which these possible questions are introduced is also retrospectively pinpointed by the fact that once the sequence is completed, the surgeon formulates a new step ("NOW the problem is" l. 19). In this way, highlighting opportunities for asking questions not only constitutes an instruction about the sequential environment in which questions are relevant, but also an instruction about the sequential intelligibility of the surgical steps.

As shown in the last fragments, both the surgeon and the expert orient to moments offering opportunities to ask questions, as well as to the absence of a response as (positively) interpretable:

Extract (5) (k2d1/41'30/any-questions—e9)

```
→ 1   SUR   are there any questions in the::
  2         (5)
→ 3   EXP   no que[stion?]
→ 4   SUR         [no?]   no question?=
  5   EXP   =and i can assure you that they are not sleeping
```

At this point, the surgeon is not engaged in operating, rather waiting for another action to be achieved. He checks if there are "any questions" (l. 1). After an observable absence of response (l. 2), the expert (l. 3) repeats the surgeon's turn in a reduced format, "no question?" (l. 3), followed by the surgeon's repeating of the question (l. 4). The checking by both shows their orientation toward the absence of a response: while the first one might orient to the optionality of a question, the second might point to the noticeability of the absence of the question (as an "instructional correction," Hindmarsh et al., 2014). The expert, who sits with the trainees in the amphitheater, and has direct access to them, further makes explicit the exclusion of a negative interpretation of this absence (l. 5).

In sum, in Extracts 1–5, the surgeon checks if there are questions, giving an opportunity to ask one. In all cases, a pause follows the surgeon's invitation, which manifests that a next turn by the trainees is expected and makes observable the absence of the projected question, treated as more or less problematic. The accountability of this absence can be elaborated on by the expert (who sits with the trainees), providing for its positive interpretation, as an agreement (Extract 4), or excluding a negative one (Extract 5), reporting on the attention and involvement of the trainees, showing that the absence is noticeable and accountable.

Formatted as checking if there are questions, these turns create the opportunity to ask them; moreover, even in the absence of a response, they instruct the trainees about particular moments within the surgical procedure in which questions could be relevant and about relevant topics for possible questions. Thereby, these moments are highlighted as completion points and transition phases, either after a surgical step (Extracts 1 and 2) or after a demonstration already oriented to trainees (Extracts 3 and 4), by the surgeon as well as by the expert, in a collaborative and complementary way. This reflexively pinpoints the recognizability of the global organization of the surgical procedure, its significant steps, and identifiable actions. In this sense, checking if there are any questions constitutes *per se* an instructive action.

Experts' management of opportunities to ask questions

As the last fragments show, the expert can join the surgeon in treating the same moments as opportunities for questions. The expert can also initiate the check for questions, like in the next excerpt:

114   *Lorenza Mondada*

Extract (6) (TC27038V/k1d1/9'25-Qfrom-buda)
```
  1            (1.5)
      sur   >>dissecting along a tissue->>
→ 2   EXP    are there any questions from budapest?
➔ 3   TRA    eh ya we have eh one questions. how can you deci:de
  4          eh: (.) that you perform that laparoscopically?
```

While the surgeon (sur) is silently progressing into an unproblematic dissection, the expert asks if there are "any questions" in Budapest (l. 2; see →), offering a trainee (TRA) distantly connected from there to ask one (l. 3–4; see ➔). On the basis of the available recording, we don't know if somebody in Budapest has contacted the expert in order to be preselected, which is not excluded; in any case, the expert's action enables them to successfully access the floor.

The action of the expert (l. 8) is followed by a trainee's question in the next case too, although some difficulties are encountered:

Extract (7) (k2d1-20'21/size-of-first-tr—e18)
```
  1   SUR   SO, (0.5) well h, .h let's start,
  2         (0.3)
  3   SUR   °écarteur de foie,°#
            liver retractor
      fig                         #fig.11
  4         (1.2)
  5   SUR   °parfait°
            perfect
  6         (0.6)
  7   SUR   [xxxx
→ 8   EXP   [okay no question about that?
  9   SUR   °non. >celui-ci celui-ci ce-< oui. (.) réducteur,
            no    this one this one th- yes       retractor
 10         et: (.) non i faut pas* de ré[ducteur# xxx°xx ici*
            and     no it's not needed any retractor xxxx here
                                  *shows R trocard---------*
      fig                                        #fig.12
```

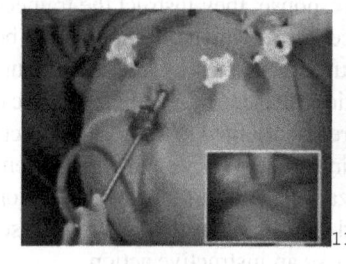

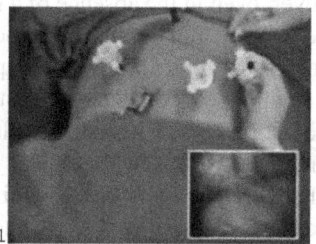

Asking questions in the operating room 115

```
→ 11  EXP                     [position? (.) pressure?
  12         *(0.8)
       sur  *takes retractor->
→ 13  EXP  [size of the *trocar? everything is clear?]
  14  SUR  [.hh so we're* going to put] away a little bit the*
                         ->*inserts retractor in upper trocar---*
  15       [fat
➔ 16  TRA  [what size is the first [trocar?
  17  SUR                          [xxx yan. (.) yan et nath?
                                    xxx Yan      Yan and Nath
  18       (0.2)
➔ 19  TRA  what si[ze is* the first tro*car?
  20  SUR         [xxxxxxx xxxxxxx
                          *points at R trocard*
  21  EXP  euh yves?
  22       (0.9)
  23  SUR  yes?
  24  EXP  a que€stion from the audience, what size is the
       eve       €bleeding->>
  25       first trocar? could *you (.) [euh remind us
  26  SUR                                [the first trocar?*
                               *approaches bleeding w gauze*
  27       *(0.7)
           *puts gauze on bleeding->>
  28       so *the first* trocar here is so a a TEN milimeter
            ->*,,,,,.....*points at optics->>
  29       trocar for my optical system
```

We join the scene as the surgeon has just finished introducing the trocars. By announcing "let's start," (l. 1) he initiates the next step, which consists in inserting the instruments in them. The first instrument is a liver retractor, requested from the team in French (l. 3), and apparently handed over by them (l. 4–5, not visible on the screen). Next, the surgeon requests another instrument (l. 7, 9–10), but does several repairs, pointing at a trocar on the right of the screen. In overlap with these repaired requests, and while on the screen any activity is not yet visible (fig. 11–12), the expert checks if there is a question (l. 8), using an indexical expression ("about that?" l. 8; see →) which refers to the position of the trocars. Thus, the expert orients to what is visibly (not) going on (treating it as a break in the operation), rather than what is audible (in French, addressed to the team) as preparing the next step. Furthermore, the expert expands his turn offering possible candidate topics for questions (l. 11). As the surgeon visibly manipulates the retractor (l. 12), requested before (l. 4), the expert provides for another expansion of his turn (l. 13). These revised questions pursue a question from the trainees (rather than a response from them, see Zemel et al., 2011). In overlap, the surgeon continues his action, inserting the trocar and formulating what he is doing (l. 14–15), thus also addressing the trainees. So, for a few seconds, two courses of action are unfolding in parallel, as the operation progresses while the expert addresses the trainees.

A participant asks a question (l. 16) and repairs it (l. 19; see →) as the surgeon continues to address his team in French (l. 17). While the question is repeated, the surgeon points to the same trocar on the right as before (l. 20, see fig. 12). Thus, the surgeon is observably continuously engaged with the same issue within the operation, oblivious of the other course of action, the communication with the trainees – which he might treat as having less priority and also as being less audible, within the noisy soundscape of the operating room. This prompts the expert to intervene, with a summons (l. 21, see also Extracts 8–11), responded to with some delay (l. 23), followed by the expert voicing the trainee's question (l. 24–25).

The expert organizes his turn by first announcing a question from the audience of trainees, clearly indicating that this is not *his* question, second, voicing their question, and third, adding "could you (.) euh remind us" (l. 25). With the latter increment, he displays an orientation to the fact that the question concerns a past event, the size of the very "first" trocar (l. 25), shown at the very beginning of the procedure, thus indicating that the question is slightly misplaced, or at least late. The surgeon delays the answer by repeating the question (Robinson & Kevoe, 2010); this repetition (l. 26) constitutes another repair-initiator treating the question as somehow problematic. The trainee remains silent, while the surgeon deals with another problem, some bleeding near the trocar on his left (eve: event, l. 24). Once that problem has been solved, the surgeon finally answers (l. 28–29). This shows another consequence of the misplacement of the question: the (past) detail targeted by the question and the present events are not only very different, but require different actions, one more urgent (fixing the bleeding), the other more postponable (answering the question, which as time passes, becomes less and less relevant, hence its surprising or problematic character, hinted by the repair initiation of the surgeon).

In this case, although the expert orients to a sequential position in which questions are recurrently made possible, he is a bit late with respect to the start of the next step by the surgeon (l. 2). He is even later when he expands his offer to ask questions simultaneously to the surgeon who is increasingly involved with his team and the instrumentation (l. 9–14). This produces a difficult context in which the trainee asks his question (l. 19), fully authorized by the expert, but unnoticed by the surgeon (l. 20). Thus, it requires some extra work by the expert mediating between the trainee and the surgeon (l. 21, 24–25; see further instances below), in order for the question to be addressed, suspending the operation (l. 28–29).

So, while roughly orienting to the same sequential environments as the surgeon, treated as making questions relevant, the expert might (partially) share the surgeon's view on the operation (see Extracts 4–5) but might also display a slightly divergent perspective (as in Extract 7). Both are senior members of the same professional community, but whereas the surgeon is fully engaged with the procedure, the expert only accesses the operating room through the mediation of the CCTV video, and an audio connection with the surgeon's microphone, which does not fully reproduce what is happening in the operating room. This asymmetry of access accounts for slight divergences, in which the surgeon orients first and foremost to the practical moments constituting the *in-vivo* progression of the operation, whereas the expert orients to the details that are relevant for socializing the trainees to specific difficulties of the procedure. Trainees too have an asymmetric access to the operation and this can produce some obstacles in them finding the right moment to pose their question. The expert, sharing the same location with the trainees, and having direct access to them, their reactions, and their attention (not broadcasted back to the surgeon), is thus able to address issues he considers relevant for them, while at the same time facilitating their production of questions.

Checking whether there are questions works as a pre-sequence, creating an opportunity to ask one. While the initial extracts (Extracts 1–5) showed that TRAs' questions can be observably absent, the last two extracts showed that the opportunity might be seized by them. In this latter case, the environment where questions are asked might be unproblematic (Extract 6) but might also generate some interactional troubles (like in Extract 7, where the question overlapped with the surgeon's talk and action, and can be finally addressed only thanks to the expert's mediation). We further develop these issues in the next section, targeting questions asked, both by trainees and experts.

Asking questions

The orientation of surgeons and experts toward relevant points at which to raise a question instructably defines particular moments within the procedure, not only manifesting the relevance of retrospective questions before a new step is initiated and highlighting the intelligibility of the sequential unfolding of the procedure, but also making the surgeon available for an exchange at that point. Thus, the orientation to and preparation of an adequate ground for questions is an essential part of the instructional dimension of the operating procedure.

In this section, we turn to questions asked, and distinguish those asked by the experts (Extracts 8–11) versus those of the trainees (Extracts 12–14), showing that they are formatted in very different ways, constitute different actions, and deal differently with the sequential environment in which they are produced. In turn, this addresses issues of expertise and competence: the position and format of the question exhibit the competence and authority of the person asking it (that is, express their epistemic stance, Heritage, 2012), as well as different engagements in the activity of operating-and-teaching/learning-the-operation. This further shows how the opportunity for questions during the operation shapes the ongoing event as an operation-and-demonstration, not only when asked by trainees, but also when prepared and managed by surgeons and experts. The socialization and instruction achieved by questions are not restricted to the trainees asking them, but are performed by the work of making space for questions and making possible questions instructably accountable within the operation.

Experts initiate questions (prefaced by a summons)

Experts regularly ask questions, addressing the surgeon with these as well as other types of actions (such as commentaries, critiques, jokes, etc.). They do so in very different ways than the trainees. In order to explore this contrast and before focusing on the trainees' questions, we turn to a recurrent format used by the experts and the praxeological and sequential environments in which they are produced.

The next extracts (8–11) show a small collection of questions asked by experts. All these questions are located within the ongoing procedure, as the surgeon is working, in silence, progressing in the operation in a routine way. Thus, when the expert asks a question, they do so on the basis of their witnessing, monitoring, and noticing the emergent *in-vivo* details of the ongoing procedure – by contrast with the environments in which surgeons invite the trainees to ask questions, which rather favor the completion of ongoing surgical steps. Moreover, the question of the expert orients to these environments as enabling multiactivity; despite the surgeon being engaged in dissecting, he is treated as being nonetheless available. In other words, the multiactivity regime identified here is a "parallel order" (Mondada, 2014b), in which the initiation of a new sequence, besides the current ongoing course of action, is not considered as creating any problem. This is treated similarly in the surgeon's response too:

Extract (8) (k2d1/30'30/liver-retractor)

```
    1   SUR   °zoom avant°
→   2   EXP   yves?
→   3   SUR   yes?
➔   4   EXP   don't you think the liver retractor could be (.)
    5         a little more to the left, so that it can help you?
    6   SUR   yes, yes, yes (.) [maybe
```

Extract (9) (k2d1/34'25/space)

```
    1   SUR   zoom avant, zoom avant, (.) pierre-alex essaye de
    2         nous montrer (.) oui:,
    3         (2.8)
→   4   EXP   yves?
→   5   SUR   yes
➔   6   EXP   you open the speen- euh the space between spleen and
    7         left cro[ss right?
    8   SUR           [yes, i have not so lot of choice
```

Extract (10) (30'27/balloon)

```
    1         (14)
→   2   EXP   euh pierre-alexan:d[re?
→   3   SUR                     [yes?
➔   4   EXP   is the balloon deflated now?
    5   SUR   yes
```

Asking questions in the operating room 119

Extract (11) (46'23/show us)
```
→  1   EXP   =eh pierre-alexandre?
→  2   SUR   yes?
➔  3   EXP   could you show us the FIRST short gastric vessel?
   4         [so that the audience [can (.) imagine?
   5   SUR   [yes                  [yes yes
   6         sure. je suis très collé à la rate. i create the
                  I am very glued to the spleen
   7         window (.) here, and the first short vessels is here.
```

In all these cases, the expert initiates the sequence with a summons, responded to positively by the surgeon (see →), without any delay. Next, the expert asks a question (see ➔), and the surgeon answers immediately. So, the sequence is unproblematically inserted in the ongoing course of the operation.

The sequence is prefaced by a summons, a practice that characterizes the opening of telephone calls (Schegloff, 1968) as well as situations of a continuing state of incipient talk (Schegloff & Sacks, 1973). The summons checks the availability of the addressee to talk topically and enables a "coordinated (re)entry" (Schegloff, 1968, p. 1092) into interaction. It has a "prefatory character" and is characterized by non-terminality (1968, p. 1091): a positive response establishes the obligation to continue speaking and listening.

The summons/answer sequence seems to be particularly efficient for the expert's interventions within the operation – in a context in which participants are engaged in multiple courses of action and, although being audio-visually connected, are not necessarily perceiving each other, and are not mutually available at the same time.

Moreover, experts use a particular and unique format for the summons, using the surgeon's first name, i.e., a basic sort of "recognitional" (Sacks & Schegloff, 2007, p. 15). The preference for recognitionals implemented here also obeys the preference for minimization, using not only the first name but its short form ("pierre-alex," Extract 9). This form also makes clear who is speaking, recognizable by his voice but also by the fact that he legitimately uses the first name (versus the full address term, possibly with the title, as in "Dr. Daccard"). Therefore, the alignment produced by these summonses is not just between co-participants, but between persons exhibiting and recognizing an informal relationship, and specific rights and obligations, relying on and making relevant the category of "close colleague" (cf. Risberg & Lymer, 2020) in contrast to other possible categories (such as "trainee").

The questions asked all refer to a current technique, tool, or anatomical detail visible on the screen, constituting the focus of the surgeon's work. They constitute relevant ongoing issues the expert has identified and makes explicit for the trainees. In turn, the questions highlight for the surgeon relevant aspects to be specifically instructed and paid attention to, thereby supporting his instructional work too. These questions can be uttered on behalf of the trainees, but also convey some criticism or advice addressed to the surgeon himself (like in Extract 8). In this way, the expert manifests what a professional vision (Goodwin, 1994) is able to recognize, and address, possibly competing with that of the surgeon. He also initiates a sequence in which these details will be confirmed, or elaborated on, creating an environment for further instruction of the trainees.

There is a clear distribution between sequential-praxeological environments during the surgical operation where the expert and the surgeon invite the trainees to ask questions (Extracts 1–7) and those where the expert self-selects and initiates his own questions (Extracts 8–11). The former environments are recurrently transition points, *at the completion* of steps, sequences, or actions; the latter are rather moments *within* phases or actions. In the former, the surgeon points retrospectively to central features of his work (e.g., the localization of trocars, the instrumentation, the anatomy, the technique used); in the latter, the expert points at emergent details of the ongoing procedure. These actions achieve different things too: they point to relevant moments for the trainees to ask recapitulative and confirming questions (Extracts 1–7) versus addressing questions emerging out of a specific moment within the procedure and situatedly pointing to details that are relevant and intelligible here and now, making the surgeon aware that they might constitute interesting issues for the trainees and generate relevant elaborations and instructions for them (Extracts 8–10).

Trainees initiate questions (prefaced by an apology)

Trainees regularly ask questions, either in response to the opportunity created by the surgeon or the expert (see previous Extracts 6–7) or by self-selecting and initiating a question/answer sequence. In the latter case, discussed in this section, they recurrently use a format for asking questions that strongly contrasts with the format used by the experts, characterized by a preface in the form of an apology ("excuse me" or "sorry"). Often, although these questions are relevantly placed with respect to the ongoing operation, they are not heard by the surgeon and encounter some trouble in being recognized and understood, and thus are not immediately answered. So, even when they are relevantly and competently located within the current activity in the first place, they often end up being delayed and even misplaced. In that case they are supported by the expert mediating between the trainee and the surgeon. This shows that the expert not only supports the instructing action of the surgeon but also gives him opportunities to develop his activity as an instructor. In this sense, the expert is crucial for orienting/treating/constituting the ongoing multiactivity (operating-and-demonstrating-the-operation) as a site of socialization/training/instruction.

We now turn to the sequential placement of the trainees' attempts, their format, and the way in which the difficulties they encounter are solved with the help of the experts.

Asking questions in the operating room 121

Extract (12) (26'58/from-espain—e21)

```
1   SUR  .h you c- okay (.) you can* pull out the:
             >>dissects---------------*
2            +(1.5) the naso-gastric tube
    ass  +rearranges plier->
3        (0.4)
→ 4 TRA  °sorr°[°°y°°      [xx]
5   SUR        [you see the [di]section?
→ 6 EXP  can you ge- eh please introdu:ce yourself when
7        you speak so eh pierre-alexandre can know (it)
8        (0.6)+
    ass      ->+tends tissue w plier again->>
→ 9 TRA  o:kay. eh: it's a question from ramos from espain
10       in madrid, (1.2) eh:: is there any reason eh::
11       *becau:se eh why do you u- you don't use a clip in
    sur  *burns some blood remains->
12       this vessel, (.) .h do you prefer: to use the
13       coagulation.
14       (0.8)
→ 15 TRA i think it's [t- more dangerous to have an hae- (.)
16  SUR              [(no i th-
17       haemorage
18  SUR  °oui on peut le retirer.°* no i think euh: (.) the
         yes we can take it out
                                 ->*dissects along a vein->>
19       coagulating hook here is is very nice (.) device,
```

The trainee's (TRA) turn (see →) is initiated (l. 4) just after the surgeon has requested his team to pull out the naso-gastric tube (l. 1–2): the consequences are visible on the screen, since the request occasions a rearrangement of the tools and the anatomy, making intelligible that some step has now been completed. Both the trainee and the surgeon himself orient to this point as such: the trainee by asking a question, prefaced by "°sorr°°y°°" and with a very low voice (l. 4), and the surgeon by asking for confirmation (l. 5) about the intelligibility of the current dissection, both in overlap. The question is thus well placed within the surgical procedure; but it is asked in an interactional environment where it is overlapped by the surgeon's turn, resulting in being difficult to hear.

Moreover, the expert initiates a repair of the trainee's turn (see →), asking him to introduce himself (l. 7–8). This also highlights for the surgeon that a question is underway. The trainee complies, and adopts a new format, with a louder voice: he uses a preface, formulating his ongoing action and giving his identity (l. 9). Then he gives the question proper (l. 10–13) expanded by a critical statement (his opinion, l. 15). During the question, the assistant uses the plier to tend the tissue again, making it possible for the surgeon to resume dissecting. The surgeon first burns some blood spots; at the completion of the question, he first addresses his team (l.

18) and then begins to dissect a tissue along a vein, while giving his answer. This way of engaging in multiactivity constitutes a response to the critical points of the question: by working with his hook along a vein, he rebuts the dangerousness (l. 15) of the tool's use hinted at in the question. Rather than only stating that it is a "nice" tool (l. 19), this is also demonstrated (cf. Sacks, 1992, II, p. 140, on the distinction between claiming versus demonstrating understanding).

This fragment shows how the ongoing surgical work is not only a condition that makes the answer (im)possible or the surgeon (un)available for it; it is also a praxeological context that can be mobilized to provide a relevant environment for the answer. In other words, the answer provided is not only verbal but is embodied in the ongoing action, which becomes an instructional demonstration.

Like the previous case, the next one shows a question that is placed at a moment of transition, thus relevantly positioned regarding the operation. Here too, it is overlapped by the surgeon, thus resulting in some interactional trouble, solved with the support of the expert helping the trainee to get an answer to his question:

Extract (13) (k2d1/11'32/deflexed-legs—e20)

```
   1  SUR  so all the fat is in the abdomen. (.) so we have some
   2       problems to rea:ch the patient, so i have to (.) eh .h
   3       ask euh a trot[toir, eh be*cause euh=*
                    staircase
                                    *climbs up*
   4  EXP1           [.hh           =you are too small
   5  SUR  yes i am a little small=
   6  EXP1                        =no he is too high h h h
   7  SUR  SO. (.) ehm there is a little more oxygen at this
   8       altitude, but i try to do my best. .h okay.
→  9  TRA  (°excuse-me°)
  10  SUR  external view, [so    i    put some # * [landmarks]
                                              *shows abdomen->
→ 11  EXP2             [yes, a que- a question [in the:
→ 12  ?                                         [a question]
         fig                                    #fig.13
```

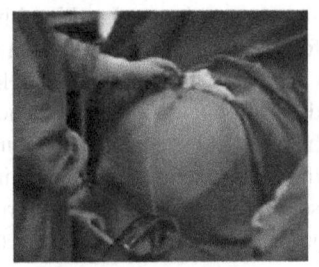

13

```
       13 SUR  you see here?
  → 14 EXP1 there is [a q- [ (.)     [pUsh (.) on, the button
       15 SUR           [the  [xiphois [a- (.) xiphoid appendix*
  → 16 EXP2                          [non. push on the: button mic
          sur                                                ->*
       17      (1.4)
  → 18 SUR  yes?
       19      (1)
  ➔ 20 TRA  eh .h (.) pardon me is the patient in a xxal (.)
       21      position, with the deflexed eh (.) legs?
       22      (0.5)
       23 TRA  [or the leg are standed
       24 EXP1 [yes
       25      (1.0)
       26 SUR  i i i i do''t did''t he- [hear the question
       27 EXP2                          [comment
                                         how
       28      comment eh sont posées les les jam:bes, est-ce
               how eh are placed the the legs          is
       29      qu'[il y a une flexion des jambes ou est-ce&
                  there a flexion of the legs or are
       30 EXP1    [elles sont droits? ou pas.
                   are they straight or not
       31 EXP2 &qu'elles sont droits? en extension? [ecartées?
                  they straight        extended       spread
       32 SUR                                        [yes, the the
       33      legs in fact are in extension here, but you can put
       34      them in flexion there is no problem.
```

The surgeon is not operating; at the beginning of the procedure, he explains that because the patient is big, he needs an extra step to be adequately positioned for the operation, and indeed he climbs onto it (l. 1–3). This occasions an extended joke (l. 4–8) to which expert1 contributes. Following the joke, the sequential moment is used by the trainee initiating a possible turn with "°excuse-me°" (l. 9) as well as by the surgeon himself by verbally and gesturally initiating the demonstration of the trocars' locations (l. 10, 13, 15, fig.13).

The simultaneity of these two actions is immediately seen by expert2 (l. 11), another participant (l. 12), and expert1 (l. 14), all referring to an incoming "question" or the difficulty of the trainee in accessing the floor (l. 14, 16). The expert supports the trainees in overcoming technology-mediated communication problems, which are not only related to the CCTV but also to the way trainees access the microphone: although the microphone can be unmuted by simply pushing a button on their desk, this constitutes an extra action to be performed when self-selecting, possibly occasioning further delay. Finally, the surgeon recognizes the trainee's attempt with "yes?" (l. 18): thereby, he not only affords the trainee an opportunity to ask a question, but, through its interrogative format, *obliges* the trainee to ask one (Schegloff, 1968: 1092). So, the question can be posed in the clear, while the operating activity is suspended. The question addresses the position of the patient's body (l. 20–23), which in a way relates (seriously) to an issue just addressed in the surgeon's joke. Instead of answering, the surgeon initiates a repair (l. 26), prompting the two experts to provide repairs in French (l. 27–29, 31), offering some candidate answers. Finally, the surgeon answers (l. 32–34).

As in the previous case, although the question is well-placed sequentially and praxeologically, it encounters some troubles: these are specifically related to the fact that the same precise moment is identified by various participants (the surgeon, the trainee) to initiate new actions at the same time, which result in overlaps. These difficulties are also more generally related to the multiactivity setting, and to difficult sound conditions, challenging the communication between two distant and audio-video connected locations.

The next fragment presents multiple similarities with the previous one, showing the recurrence of this interactional configuration, with the expert intervening as a mediator supporting trainees in their attempts to ask questions:

Extract (14) (d1k1/10'16/excuse-me—e22)

```
    1  SUR  okay. (.) the: (.) the (.) four(th) trocar is just BElow
    2       the xyphoïd appendix, (.) and first ah i app[reciate (.)
→   3  TRA                                              [°xxxxx°
    4       [the size the left euh liver it's     [xxxxxxxx&
    5  EXP1 [eh if you want to put (.) xx better[, yes
→   6  TRA                                          [excuse-me
    7  SUR  &xx[thosis the sickness of the left (.) eh liver is not
→   8  EXP1    [there is a question, il y a une question dans
    9       l'audience mais comme pierre-alex[andre  xxxx
›  10  EXP2                                  [PIERRE-ALEXANDRE
   11       PIERRE-ALEXANDRE (.) ther- there is a
   12       question for you, okay?
→  13  SUR  okay
→  14  TRA  excuse me do you employ the open technique for
   15       laparoscopy, or: do you employ the veress needle?
   16  SUR  if if euh we inform the patient that it's possible to:
   17       to convert in laparotomy? (.) that-
   18  EXP1 [xxx
   19  EXP2 [NON, est-ce que tu as util- est-ce que tu utilizes
             no   do you have us-       do you use
   20       l'OPEN laparoscopie [ou le needle optiqu[e, (.) enfin &
             the open laparoscopy or the optic needle       well
   21  SUR                      [non                 [okay okay
   22  EXP2 & ou le (needle) euh (.) [xxx
             or the needle  ehm
   23  SUR                           [i understand. (.) visiport or
   24       something like this, (.) no i euhm (.) i never use the
   25       open (.) euh laparoscopic access.
```

The trainee identifies a point of completion and transition for initiating the question, while the surgeon moves to the next point (l. 2–3). Like in the previous cases, there are significant overlaps between the surgeon and the distant interlocutors (l.

2–8) and the experts mediate in this difficult environment (l. 10–12). By instructing the trainee to use the microphone (l. 5) and using a louder voice (l. 10–11) they orient to this environment as noisy. Finally, in this case too, the question, even if uttered in the clear (l. 14–15), is repaired (like in the previous case, with a translation into French, l. 19–22). Finally, the surgeon answers (l. 23–25). So, here too, neither the sequential moment in which the question is initiated, nor the question itself is treated as problematic; rather, the multiactivity setting makes its audibility difficult.

The extracts studied in this section show that the identification of a sequential moment within the operation in which asking a question is relevant is not enough to secure a successful selection of the trainee and production of the question. First, this sequential moment is also identified by other participants for other actions – typically by the surgeon in addressing the audience (Extracts 7, 12–13), coordinating with his team (Extract 7), or initiating the next step of the operation (Extracts 7, 13–14). Second, this creates a sound environment in which not only overlaps make the trainee's questions difficult to hear/understand (Extracts 13–14), but access to the microphone is unevenly distributed (regularly, trainees encounter problems with the activation of the microphone, Extracts 13–14, whereas the expert seems to have a more direct and open access to it, Extracts 7–11). Third, the way trainees speak and format the beginning of their turn is tentative, apologetic, and in a lower voice (Extracts 12–14), which displays lower entitlement and makes them less easy to hear.

These conditions, assembled by interactional, praxeological, technological, and normative constraints, make trainees' questions in the operating room difficult to hear and to understand – in clear contrast with the way questions and other comments by the experts are heard. Recurrently, although relevantly placed, the trainees' (self-)selection and question are not responded to by the surgeon; the selection (Extract 12), the way to handle the technological devices (Extracts 13 and 14), and the question (Extracts 13 and 14) are all repaired by the experts, who mediate between the trainee and the surgeon, by making the selection clear (using the summons/answer sequence typical of experts; Extract 14), and also by repeating, rephrasing (with candidate answers), or translating the question (Extracts 13, 14).

Conclusions

This chapter offered an analysis of how *in situ* questions are instructed and achieved in the midst of a professional activity. It showed that asking questions is not only an issue for trainees, but also involves other participants. Drawing on early examples of distant learning thanks to the use of video technologies enabling trainees to watch surgical operations as they are performed in real time, the chapter showed that the possibility of asking questions is carefully designed, prepared, and instructed by surgeons and experts together. This creates a specific ecology, praxeological context, and sequential interactional environment in which questions are (to be) uttered, characterized by close contact with and access to the operating surgeon (versus the instructional configuration in which questions are raised during an endodontic operation studied by Lindwall and Lymer (2014), in which the separation of trainees and surgeons facilitates the pedagogical activity).

The focus on the interactional constraints of the local ecology enables a better understanding of the instructional features of questions, which are in no way limited to the information provided by the answers but are crucially related to the orchestration of and understanding by the trainees of the local circumstances making questions relevant as well as the local contingencies making questions possible and hearable. This crucially enables an approach to questions that fully considers their situatedness as a members' concern.

The analyses of this chapter showed how surgeons and experts mediating the interaction between the operating room and a remote amphitheater where the trainees are located creates opportunities for advanced trainees to ask questions: the surgeon checks if they have any questions (Extracts 1–5), and the expert supports him (Extracts 3–4) as well as creating opportunities himself (Extracts 6–7). These pre-sequences not only create opportunities for questions; more fundamentally, by highlighting the moments in which a question is relevant, they also instructably pinpoint the intelligibility of the procedure at that point, its local order, and relevant details. The pre-sequences instruct the trainees to see these moments in that way, socializing their professional vision, guiding their attention to the anatomical details, the instrumentation, and delicate maneuvers characterizing its step-by-step progression, and the decisions to be taken at key points.

The analyses have also focused on the questions asked, and in particular how two types of participants ask questions (Extracts 8–14). Whereas the experts preface their questions with a summons (Extracts 8–11), the trainees preface them with an apology, displaying different rights, obligations, and entitlements to ask a question (Extracts 12–14). Whereas the experts' questions are unproblematically uttered and immediately answered, the trainees' questions are produced with some difficulty, often overlapped by the surgeon addressing something else; consequently, they are supported and mediated by the experts. Whereas the experts ask questions-with-known-answers (Macbeth, 2003), in environments they competently recognize, and even project, trainees ask "real" questions, in environments they progressively identify as relevant. Different types of engagements, related to several asymmetries, are observable: when the surgeon creates the opportunity to ask a question, the trainees tend not to seize it (Extracts 1–5); when the trainees initiate a question, they run into various difficulties (Extracts 12–14). The experts access the floor and initiate actions with fewer problems (Extracts 8–11) and mediate in the latter case.

The trainees' questions are generally sequentially placed in a relevant position within the course of the operation and their content is treated as relevant. Their difficulties rather point to other contingencies – interactional and technological – showing the complexity of the instructional activity orchestrated by the CCTV device and the multiactivity connecting the operating room and the amphitheater. They arise from the fact that the same sequential and praxeological environments are identified and exploited not only by them, but also by the surgeon, to initiate new actions; consequently, trainees' and surgeons' turns often overlap and compete with each other. The trainees' difficulties are aggravated by a noisy environment and asymmetries of access to the floor. Moreover, these difficulties delay the production of the question proper, meaning it is produced *later* than when initially initiated, therefore resulting in being slightly *misplaced*. These problems are in part solved thanks to the mediation of the experts, who have both direct access to the trainees, sitting with them in the same room, and authorized access to the surgeon colleague (Heritage, 2012).

Work settings are often also instructional settings for trainees: however, the configurations in which instructional actions for and by trainees are embedded within the professional activity vary. Likewise, questions are an important pedagogical practice: however, the way questions are made possible in the classroom (Duran & Sert, 2021; St. John & Cromdal, 2015), in a safe space watching an operation (Lindwall & Lymer, 2014), or in the midst of the work activity (Risberg & Lymer, 2020) suppose very different relations and engagements with the ongoing professional course of action. The ecology studied in this chapter shows the advantages and the difficulties of a setting in which questions can be directly addressed to a senior surgeon while he is operating: the CCTV device enables a distance between the trainees and the operating room; the audio-video connection with the surgeon provides an immediacy and proximity with the *in-vivo* details of the surgical procedure here and now. The complex distribution of actions between surgeons, experts, video control room, and trainees casts some new light on the instructional character of a multiactivity in which an operation-cum-demonstration is performed.

The instructable way in which relevant moments of the operation are highlighted by seniors (surgeons and experts), as well as the skilled way in which questions are ultimately asked during the procedure, reveal the competences to be learned by the trainees. Asking questions supposes that the trainees watching the video-transmitted operation make sense of the visual features accessible on the screen, and the details of the moment-by-moment organization of the operation, including the manual performance of the surgeon and the interactional coordination of the surgical team. This requires and at the same time constitutes a professional vision (Goodwin, 1994) able to read the anatomical images, to relate the gestures displayed on the screen to routine gestures made in the operating room. Moreover, asking questions also relies on the ongoing understanding of the talk produced during the operation: on the ability to project the announcement of an action to come and the completion of an explanation, but also the ability to understand the exchanges between the surgeon and his team, or the surgeon with the expert, in order to infer his availability and potential moments within this complex management of the multiactivity that will make the question audible. Thus, asking questions during the operation is an action that not only exercises a professional vision, but also an interactional competence, allowing the trainees to navigate multiple participation frameworks and activities. The multiactivity of articulating the operation and its demonstration ultimately enables trainees to be instructed, but also generates specific troubles, making their access to the floor difficult.

The practices and problems studied in this chapter refer more generally to issues of the accountability of actions in complex professional environments, where the successful identification of organizational details rests on linguistic resources, the skilled endogenous analysis of ongoing actions, the skilled use of technology, and the skilled interpretation of images. In this sense, the instruction and the seizure of these moments constitute a pivotal moment in the socialization of novices in the midst of the situated ongoing activity.

References

Clayman, S. (2010). Questions in broadcast journalism. In A. Freed & S. Ehrlich (Eds.), *Why do you ask?: The Function of Questions in Institutional Discourse*. Oxford University Press.

Clayman, S., & Heritage, J. (2002). *The news interview: Journalists and public figures on the air*. Cambride University Press.

De Ruiter, J. P. (Ed.). (2012). *Questions: Formal, functional and interactional perspectives*. Cambridge University Press.

Duran, D., & Sert, O. (2021). Student-initiated multi-unit questions in EMI classrooms. *Linguistics and Education, 65*. https://doi.org/10.1016/j.linged.2021.100980

Enfield, N., Stivers, T., & Levinson, S. (2010). Question–response sequences in conversation across ten languages. *Journal of Pragmatics, 42*(10), 2615–2619.

Frankel, R. (1990). Talking in interviews: A dispreference for patient-initiated questions in physician-patient encounters. In G. Psathas (Ed.), *Interaction competence* (pp. 231–261). University Press of America.

Goodwin, C. (1994). Professional vision. *American Anthropologist, 96*(3), 606–633.

Goodwin, C. (2017). *Co-operative action*. Cambridge University Press.

Haddington, P., Keisanen, T., Mondada, L., & Nevile, M. (Eds.). (2014). *Multiactivity in social interaction: Beyond multitasking*. Benjamins.

Heritage, J. (2012). Epistemics in action: Action formation and territories of knowledge. *Research on Language and Social Interaction, 45*(1), 1–29.

Hindmarsh, J. (2010). Peripherality, participation and communities of practice: Examining the patient in dental training. In N. Llewellyn & J. Hindmarsh (Eds.), *Organisation, interaction and practice* (pp. 218–240). Cambridge University Press.

Hindmarsh, J., Hyland, L., & Banerjee, A. (2014). Work to make simulation work: 'Realism', instructional correction and the body in training. *Discourse Studies, 16*(2), 247–269. https://doi.org/10.1177/1461445613514670

Lindwall, O., Johansson, E., Ivarsson, J., Rystedt, H., & Reit, C. (2014). The use of video in dental education: Clinical reality addressed as practical matters of production, interpretation, and instruction. In M. Broth, E. Laurier, & L. Mondada (Eds.), *Studies of video practices: Video at work* (pp. 161–180). Routledge.

Lindwall, O., & Lymer, G. (2014). Inquiries of the body: Novice questions and the instructable observability of endodontic scenes. *Discourse Studies, 16*(2), 271–294. https://doi.org/10.1177/1461445613514672

Macbeth, D. (2003). Hugh Mehan's "Learning Lessons" reconsidered: On the differences between the naturalistic and critical analysis of classroom discourse. *American Educational Research Journal, 40*(1), 239–280.

Mehan, H. (1979). *Learning lessons: Social organization in the classroom*. Harvard University Press.

Mondada, L. (2003). Working with video: How surgeons produce video records of their actions. *Visual Studies, 18*(1), 58–73.

Mondada, L. (2007). Operating together through videoconference: Members' procedures for accomplishing a common space of action. In S. Hester & D. Francis (Eds.), *Orders of ordinary action* (pp. 51–67). Routledge.

Mondada, L. (2011). The organization of concurrent courses of action in surgical demonstrations. In J. Streeck, C. Goodwin, & C. LeBaron (Eds.), *Embodied interaction, language and body in the material world* (pp. 207–226). Cambridge University Press.

Mondada, L. (2014a). The surgeon as a camera director: Maneuvering video in the operating theatre. In M. Broth, E. Laurier, & L. Mondada (Eds.), *Studies of video practices: Video at work* (pp. 97–132). Routledge.

Mondada, L. (2014b). The temporal orders of multiactivity: Operating and demonstrating in the surgical theatre. In P. Haddington, T. Keisanen, L. Mondada, & M. Nevile (Eds.), *Multiactivity in social interaction* (pp. 33–75). Benjamins.

Risberg, J., & Lymer, G. (2020). Requests and know-how questions : Initiating instruction in workplace interaction. *Discourse Studies*, *22*(6), 753–776. https://doi.org/10.1177/1461445620928239

Roberts, F. (2000). The interactional construction of asymmetry: The medical agenda as a resource for delaying response to patient questions. *The Sociological Quarterly*, *41*(1), 151–170. https://doi.org/10.1111/j.1533-8525.2000.tb02370.x

Sacks, H. (1992). *Lectures on conversation*. Blackwell.

Sacks, H., & Schegloff, E. A. (2007). Two preferences in the organization of reference to persons in conversation and their interaction. In N. Enfield & T. Stivers (Eds.), *Person reference in interaction: Linguistic, cultural and social perspectives* (pp. 23–28). Cambridge University Press.

Sanchez-Svensson, M., Luff, P., & Heath, C. (2009). Embedding instruction in practice: Contingency and collaboration during surgical training. *Sociology of Health and Illness*, *31*(6), 889–906.

Schegloff, E. A. (1968). Sequencing in conversational openings. *American Anthropologist*, *70*(6), 1075–1095.

Schegloff, E. A. (2007). *Sequence organization in interaction: A primer in conversation analysis*. Cambridge University Press.

Schegloff, E. A., & Sacks, H. (1973). Opening up closings. *Semiotica*, *8*(4), 289–327.

St. John, O., & Cromdal, J. (2015). Crafting instructions collaboratively: Student questions and dual addressivity in classroom task instructions. *Discourse Processes*, *53*(4), 252–279. https://doi.org/10.1080/0163853x.2015.1038128

Ten Have, P. (1991). Talk and institution: A reconsideration of the 'asymmetry' of doctor-patient interaction. In D. Boden & D. H. Zimmerman (Eds.), *Talk and social structure* (pp. 138–163). Wiley.

Zemel, A., & Koschmann, T. (2014). "Put your fingers right in here": Learnability and instructed experience. *Discourse Studies*, *16*(2), 163–183.

Zemel, A., Koschmann, T., & LeBaron, C. (2011). Pursuing a response: Prodding recognition and expertise within a surgical team. In J. Streeck, C. Goodwin, & C. LeBaron (Eds.), *Embodied interaction, language and body in the material world* (pp. 227–242). Cambridge University Press.

5 Monitoring, coordinating, and correcting professional conduct

Soliciting absent requests during surgery

Mikaela Åberg and Jonas Ivarsson

Introduction

In this chapter, we report on a collection of recordings from an operating room where interprofessional surgical team members coordinate their work to achieve a critical task – the resumption of a sedated patient's breathing that has been placed on hold. In this setting, teams of vascular surgeons, nurse radiologists, and nurse anesthetists are engaged in an image-guided procedure of abdominal aortic repairs. They perform something called digital subtraction angiographies (DSA) on sedated patients, a procedure involving the surgeon injecting a contrast medium into the patient's aorta as a series of X-ray images are taken. To obtain clear images, the nurse anesthetist must put the sedated patient's breathing on hold – something regularly referred to as apnea. Whenever patient breathing is artificially paused, it must be promptly resumed to ensure the patient's health and safety. The first part of the study presents instances of routine and straightforward communication and coordination in resuming the patient's breathing. The second and third parts of the study present instances in which complications arise. In these instances, the resumption of breathing becomes delayed because of communication problems, which may impact the patient's well-being. Our analysis focuses on episodes in which *requests* to resume the patient's breathing are treated as officially absent. Our main topic is how anticipated but nonpresent requests are addressed and handled by the professionals.

The current study aligns with previous ethnomethodological and conversation analytic (EM/CA) research investigating how members coordinate their work to achieve critical tasks in settings such as underground line control rooms, airplane cockpits, and operating rooms (Heath & Luff, 1992; Hindmarsh & Pilnick, 2007; Nevile, 2007; Melander & Sahlström, 2009; Sanchez Svensson et al., 2009; Zemel & Koschmann, 2016). Even when professionals are engaged in routine work, orderly conduct constantly needs to be produced, coordinated, and maintained on a moment-by-moment basis with an orientation toward responsibilities, risks, and contingencies. For instance, Heath et al. (2002) show "how coordination and collaboration within the operating theatre entails a sensitivity both to the task and responsibilities of others and the ability of others, ongoingly, to undertake their activities" (p. 339). Mondada (2014) demonstrates that "[i]nstructions in the form of directives and requests are mostly done in a routine way, but they can also acquire an urgent character, responding to possible contingencies, unforeseen events and emergence of risks" (p. 132).

DOI: 10.4324/9781003312345-7

In a study of cockpit interactions, Nevile (2007) shows how two pilots mutually monitor each other's conduct and how they interactionally establish *what* is expected to happen next and *when* that action is expected. When some action is deemed relevant and should happen at the current moment but has not yet been initiated by the pilot responsible for it, the matter is treated as an obstacle to the "sequentially implicated next action" (Schegloff et al., 1977, p. 380). More specifically, the establishment of monitoring and prompting actions is made visible by the pilots' use of "and-prefaced talk." By prompting actions with an "and," the copilot can indicate that an action is treated as timely and expected but noticeably absent. In contrast to more traditional work on talk in interaction, the members of Neville's study are not repairing the troubles of speaking or hearing. As sequences of repair, his study shows that "the talk does not repair a progress within or from a current sequence [...] – for example, as the second turn of an adjacency pair—but rather signals progress TO a professionally known and necessary next action that is due but not yet begun" (Nevile, 2007, p. 248, (small) caps in original). In workplace environments such as these, where professional tasks' progression relies on routines, anticipated but nonoccurring actions can become noticeable as being officially absent. When an absence is topicalized, it could be made into a "negative observation" that "announces not only that its speaker has perceived an absence but also, more important, that its absence is a relevant omission" (Jacoby & Gonzales, 2002, p. 131).

In line with Nevile (2007), the present study focuses on how some sets of actions make other actions conditionally relevant (Schegloff, 1968; Schegloff & Sacks, 1973) and, as a result, how the nonoccurrence of a relevant next action is rendered officially and noticeably absent (Schegloff, 1968, p. 1038). In surgical settings, team members are expected to perform and coordinate actions on time. There is a reflexive relationship between professional tasks and the communication that takes place. The work also builds on a clear division of labor (see also Ikeya et al., this volume). Embedded in the setting is the expectation that members should do their part and keep within particular trajectories of actions, depending on their medical specialization. However, although individual team members have specified roles and responsibilities, they must simultaneously monitor ongoing procedures and coordinate their actions with others. The absence of a projected action, stalling, or interfering with the expected progression may jeopardize patient safety and, thus, is not only treated as noticeably absent but may also become professionally accountable (see also Nevile, 2007). Schegloff's (1968) work outlines the paired relationship between observed absent responses (such as answers) that have been made conditionally relevant through prior actions (such as questions). Building on this work, the current study shifts attention to the first pair part of an adjacency pair treated as officially absent.

The empirical case

The present study is situated in a grant-funded research project (financed by the Swedish Research Council) between Gothenburg University and surgeons and radiologists in a Swedish hospital (see also Kuroshima & Ivarsson, 2021). The project was approved by the Swedish Ethical Review Agency (grant No. 2015-03621). All participants gave their consent to participate in the data collection. One of the overarching purposes of the project is to advance patient-centered care in the context of hybrid operating procedures of endovascular aortic repairs (EVAR). To work with patient safety, the members of healthcare teams must continuously analyze and develop their working methods by highlighting both the routine and deviant aspects of their work. During the analytical work of the present study, video-recorded sequences of both smooth and problematic coordination from the operating room were discussed within the project where surgeons and radiologists at the hospital were included. The results of the project have continuously been discussed within the group of practitioners and researchers and have also been presented to surgical nurses as part of their communication training.

The data for the present study consist of video-recorded naturally occurring interactions between interdisciplinary teams during surgeries in the operating room (OR). Altogether, the data consist of 58 hours of video recordings captured with the operating room's ceiling-mounted camera of 12 surgical sessions (lasting between 2 h and 10 h) of endovascular aortic repairs EVAR at a Swedish hospital. In these sessions, the surgical teams' working monitor was also captured. During each recorded session, the targeted task of resuming the patient's breathing took place a minimum of five times; at most, resuming the patient breathing occurred 18 times. In total, we could identify, extract, and transcribe 115 sequences of controlled apnea. Within this entire collection, we also identified a subset of 16 instances in which communicative issues specifically related to resuming patients' breathing were observably treated by the members as deviations from the routine pattern of coordination. These instances were further transcribed with the support of ELAN.

The detailed transcription of verbal interaction is based on Jefferson's (2004) notation system. In addition, the transcription used for multimodal details builds on Mondada's (2018) conventions (see pp. 19–20, this volume). However, the material has limitations in terms of what kind of multimodal analysis can be conducted. The surgeons have surgical caps, eye protection (glasses), and face masks covering their mouths and noses, which sometimes makes it difficult to analyze gaze and facial expressions. Since the operating room camera was mounted in the ceiling in a fixed position, the nurse anesthetists are sometimes hidden behind equipment, safety screens, or machines. Sometimes, the participants move out of view as a safety measure to avoid too much radiation exposure. Therefore, our main analysis is based on the verbal interactions in which multimodal aspects have been included, when possible.

In the transcript, the members are named after their profession: the main surgeon "SU1" (and "SU2" for the assistant surgeon), the nurse anesthetist "ANE," the scrub nurse "NUR," and the radiologist nurse "RAD."

Fragment 1

```
100 SU1:  en apne då tack
          an apnea then please
101 ANE:  apne  nu   †Δ
          apnea now  †Δ
    ane:              † (pauses ventilator)-------->
    su1:                Δ (starts radiation/DSA)---->
102       (5)
```
```
103 SU1:        Δ ja^   andas    igen †
                Δ yea^ breathe again †
    su1: --->> Δ (radiation stops)
    ane: --------------------....>>† (starts ventilator)
104 ANE:                         † andas nu
                                 † breathe now
```

"†--->" marks where the nurse anesthetist pauses the ventilator ("†") and that the patient status (apnea) is continuing ("--->") until the symbol "--->>†," which marks when the nurse anesthetist resumes the patient's breathing by restarting the ventilator. The same conventions are used for starting or stopping radiation; however, here, the surgeon's actions are marked with "Δ." Additionally, in Fragment 13, the symbol "+" marks the nurse anesthetist's other bodily actions, and the symbol "*" marks the surgeon's other bodily actions. The symbol "#" marks the scrub nurse's bodily action, and the symbol "§" marks the assistant surgeon's bodily actions. The symbols "......" show a gesture's preparation (e.g., moving one's hand to a switch, preparing to pull). The symbol ",,,,," shows a gesture's retraction (e.g., moving foot from pedal). The following section will first provide an outline of the entire procedure. Afterward, we focus on the latter part of the sequence – coordinating the ending of the DSA/radiation and the resumption of the patients' breathing/starting the ventilator – which is marked within the black square in Fragment 1.

The surgical procedure and joint tasks

In the investigated episodes, the nurse anesthetists and surgeons are engaged in two related but parallel tasks. One way to describe this is that the nurse anesthetist is tasked with continuously monitoring and caring for the intraoperative well-being of the patient (see anesthetist task in Figure 1). The surgeon carries the overall responsibility for the activity, but also focuses on the surgical operation (see surgeon task in Figure 1). However, at critical points in the procedure, the nurse anesthetist and surgeon need to closely coordinate their ongoing projects (see Figure 1 marks 1 and 2) to perform a "trajectory of task-related actions" (Nevile, 2010, p. 447).

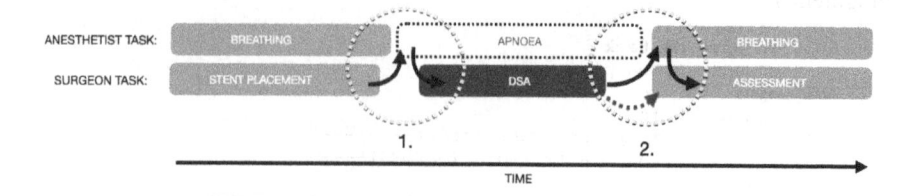

Figure 1 Two related but parallel tasks.

The studied procedure starts with the surgeon introducing a folded stent graft into the abdominal aorta (Figure 1, surgeon task, "stent placement"). During this part of the procedure, the nurse anesthetist is responsible for monitoring the anesthetized patient's vitals. When the stent graft has been put in roughly the correct place and while it is still able to be moved, the surgeon must assess the graft's precise location before it is expanded and becomes fixed. To inform this decision, a DSA is performed. With the DSA, the surgeon injects contrast fluid into the vasculature. As the fluid flows through the blood vessels, images are captured. The relationship between the stent graft and soft tissues can thereby be discerned. This can be performed either when the surgeon is standing in close proximity to the nurse anesthetist or from a distance when the surgeon is standing on the other side of the room. When surgeons are standing in close proximity, they manually control the DSA by having their foot on a control pedal and manually injecting a contrast medium into the blood vessels. As soon as their foot is lifted from the pedal, the DSA stops. When performed from a distance, the surgeon is standing near the radiology nurse control station, and both the DSA and injection of the contrast medium are controlled by the radiology nurse.

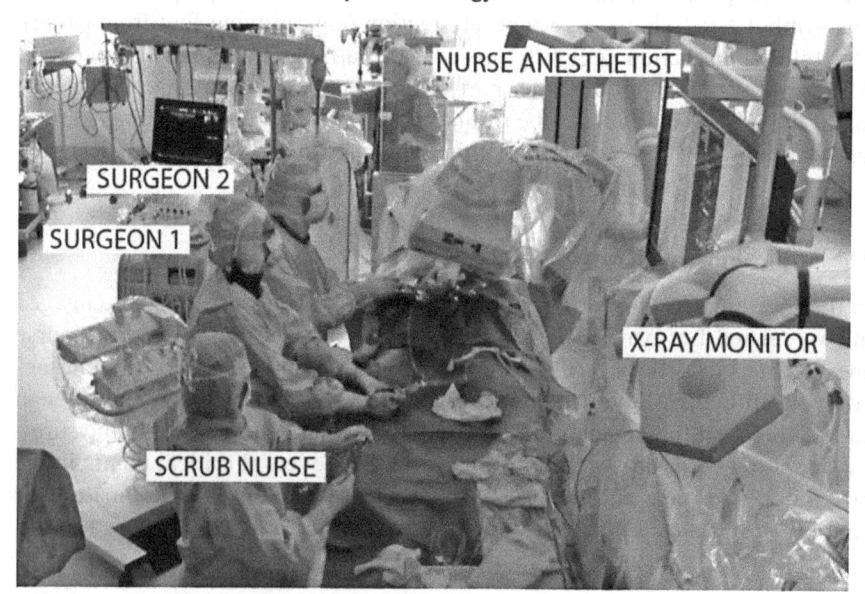

Figure 2 The operating room and participants' positions.

A complication here is that, for DSA imaging to come out clearly, the patient's chest movements must be suppressed. Since the patient is sedated and cannot be asked to hold their breath for the duration of the imaging, the surgeon will ask the nurse anesthetist, who controls the ventilator, to temporarily put the patient's breathing on hold, which is called apnea. The surgeon commonly initiates this point of the procedure by requesting the nurse anesthetist to put the patient's breathing on hold by calling out, for example, "apnea please." The nurse anesthetist commonly confirms this by pausing the patient's breathing and calling out the performed action "apnea." These verbal interchanges could be seen as a *first set of a request–confirmation pair*. The coordination of putting the patient under apnea and starting DSA is the first instance in the procedure (marked with 1 in Figure 1), where the surgeon and the nurse anesthetist need to jointly coordinate their actions; it is also the part where the patient's status changes from breathing to not breathing.

The present study focuses on the procedures and complications that arise at this second juncture. As soon as a patient's breathing is put on hold, this state also makes the resumption of the breathing *conditionally relevant* (Schegloff, 1968); failure to do so would result in asphyxia. It is in this second part (marked with 2 in Figure 1) that the coordination between the surgeon and nurse anesthetist again becomes critical. In the first joint task, the surgeon depends on the nurse anesthetist to put the patient under apnea to start the DSA. However, in the second joint task, the surgeon must also navigate between multiple relevancies. When receiving the X-ray images, the surgeon proceeds to the next stage of the procedure and deals with the outcome of the DSA by performing a retrospective assessment (e.g., of the stent graft's location) and prospective assessment (e.g., of how to continue with the next step of the surgical procedure). This is done by the surgeon on their own or by involving the assisting surgeon. On the other hand, before moving into a closer retro- and prospective assessment, the surgeon preferably should request that the nurse anesthetist resume the patient's breathing and receive confirmation that such action has been taken. These actions could be seen as a *second set of a request–confirmation pair*. There are additional reasons for the sequential structure of this second coordination task. If the nurse anesthetist starts the patient's breathing prematurely before having received a go-ahead from the surgeon, the imaging sequence may be ruined. This should be avoided because retaking the images will expose the patient to additional radiation and contrast fluid. A retake of the images will also prolong the surgical procedure. Although still in charge of the patient's well-being and in control of the ventilator, at this moment, the nurse anesthetist is awaiting the surgeon's explicit request to resume patient breathing.

In the following section, we look at instances in which the team members coordinate the resumption of the patient's breathing. The results are divided into three main parts: the first part focuses on instances *of the orderly management of requests*, the second *when requests are given but not heard*, and the third part *where requests are missing*.

Requests in action

The first part of the results presents excerpts (Fragments 2–7) that illustrate the routine interplay between requests and confirmations and the associated actions connected to these. The instances of communication show how the surgeons' requests and nurse anesthetists' confirmations are carried out in a clear and direct manner (Fragments 2–4). Fragments 5–7 show how the surgeon is addressing the double responsibility of doing an assessment of received X-ray images and coordinating the resumption of the patient's breathing by making a request.

Although this first part of the results works as a backdrop for showing how coordination is routinely done, the second and third parts of the results focus on instances where the collaboration deviates from this routine interplay, along with how this is addressed and handled by the members. In these situations, the team of professionals needs to restore order to secure patient health and safety. These fragments, therefore, highlight the specific order of professional conduct expected in the hybrid operating room. The second part of the results (Fragments 8–9) shows situations when a request is given by the surgeon but is not heard by the nurse anesthetist and how this becomes topicalized as a missing request by the implicated recipient. The final part of the results presents instances where the expected request is not given at a normatively expected time in the procedure and how this trouble is topicalized (Fragments 10–13) by the nurse anesthetist.

Part 1: The orderly management of requests

In Fragments 2–4, requests are given in close juxtaposition to the ending of the DSA and are quickly followed by a confirmation and resumption of the patient's breathing. These instances show the routine interplay and where the second set of request–confirmation pairs was carried out in a clear and direct manner.

Fragment 2

```
200 SU1:  Δ (0.3) andas    igen   tack.
          Δ (0.3) breathe again please.
     su1: Δ (radiation/DSA stops)
201                                    (1.3)↑
     ane: >>----------------------...........↑ (starts ventilator)
202 ANE:                               ↑ andas
                                       ↑ breathes
```

Fragment 3

```
300 SU1:  andas     (0.3) Δ
          breathe (0.3) Δ
     su1: >>---,,,,,,,,, Δ (radiation/DSA stops)
301       (0.7)
302 ANE:                     an↑das
                             brea↑thes
     ane: >>---------------..........↑ (starts ventilator)
```

Soliciting absent requests 137

Fragment 4

```
401 SU1:              tacΔk   (0.4)     anda^st
                      thanΔks (0.4) brea^thet
    sul: >>---,,,,,,,,,,,Δ (radiation/DSA stops)
    ane: >>-----------------------------† (starts ventilator)
402 ANE:                                  † andas
                                          † breathes
```

In Fragment 2, the surgeon (SU1) stops the radiation/DSA before calling out the request to the nurse anesthetist to resume breathing (line 200). The nurse monitors her display and keeps her hand close to the ventilator switch. There is a short pause, during which the nurse anesthetist moves her hand into position before restarting the ventilator (line 201). She then immediately confirms the performed action and the patient's status ("breathes", line 202). In Fragment 3, the surgeon makes the request "breathe" (line 300) and after a short pause, the surgeon completes the action of turning off the radiation/DSA. The nurse anesthetist, who is monitoring the surgeon's conduct, turns his head toward his own monitor and moves his hand to the ventilator switch, and in the middle of the called-out confirmation of "breathes" (line 302), the patient's breathing is resumed. In Fragment 4, the surgeon first calls out a "thanks" (line 401) while simultaneously turning off the radiation/DSA, but the word "thanks" is not treated as a request for action. Instead, the nurse anesthetist continues to monitor the surgeons' conduct while holding his hand on the ventilator switch. When the request "brea^the" (line 401) is produced, the nurse immediately resumes the patient's breathing and verbally confirms the performed action and patient's status (line 402).

These three excerpts illustrate the routine interplay between requests and confirmations and their associated actions. The surgeons' verbal requests are coordinated with their actions in close juxtaposition, even though the performed action of turning off radiation/DSA can be located before (Fragment 2), in the end (Fragment 3), or in the middle (Fragment 4) of the verbal request. When a request is formulated, it is usually quickly responded to and acted upon by the nurse anesthetist. However, as Fragment 4 illustrates, the nurse anesthetist withholds the action until an unambiguous request has been produced.

Dual projects: Assessments and requests

Next, we look more closely at another routine interplay between the surgeons' assessments followed by requests. As previously described, the subsequent step for the surgeon in the surgical procedure is to assess the newly produced X-ray images and request that the nurse anesthetist resume the patient's breathing. In Fragments 2–4, the X-rays are not commented on before the breathing has been resumed.

In Fragments 5–7, an assessment is made by way of a verbal remark, which can involve the assistant surgeon. The assessment and request to resume the patient's breathing could be seen as two separate projects with different orientations: one is related to the surgeon's retrospective and prospective work with the surgical procedure (assessing the X-rays and receiving evidence to move on), while the other concerns the nurse anesthetist and end of the joint task (by requesting the resumption of the breathing). Fragments 5–7 illustrate how surgeons manage these dual orientations.

Fragment 5

```
500 SU1: den ligger alldeles ovanförΔ där tack andas )
         it's positioned right aboveΔ there thanks breathe
    sul: >>---------------------- Δ (radiation/DSA stops)
501      (1.1)
502 ANE: ↑andas
         ↑breathes
    ane: ↑ (starts ventilator)
```

Fragment 6

```
600 SU1: NU:: ä de bra    (.) TACK så mycke      (.) andas igen^
         NO::W it's good  (.) THANK you so much  (.) breathe again^
601      (0.3)
602 ANE: ↑andas    Δ
         ↑breathesΔ
    ane: ↑ (starts ventilator)
    sul: >>-------Δ (radiation/DSA stops)
```

In Fragment 5, the surgeon (SU1) is looking at his monitor and gives the assisting surgeon, who is standing in the background, his evaluation of where the stent graft is located (line 500). This assessment is directly oriented toward the retrospective and prospective continuation of the surgical procedure. Toward the end of this turn, the surgeon terminates the DSA and proceeds by giving the nurse anesthetist the request to breathe again. In response, the nurse anesthetist starts the ventilator and calls out the results of the performed action (line 502).

Prior to the events in Fragment 6, the surgeon (SU1) has struggled to get the projection angle correct for a clear image of the relevant vasculature. As the new images appear, she looks at her monitor and calls out "NO::W it's good", which is almost immediately followed by a "THANK you so much" (line 600). From an analyst's perspective, both of these turn construction units (TCUs) are potentially ambiguous. They could be interpreted as a comment on the stent graft's location, a preliminary for a request, or even a differently formulated request to resume the patient's breathing. However, from the nurse anesthetist's perspective, they are not treated as utterances upon which to act. During these utterances, the nurse anesthetist continues to hold her hand, ready to pull the switch without doing so. In close succession, the surgeon calls out the awaited request "breathe again" (line 600), to which the nurse anesthetist resumes the patient's breathing and then confirms her actions (line 602). In close juxtaposition, the surgeon ends the DSA.

In Fragments 5 and 6, the surgeons offer brief assessments before addressing the nurse anesthetist with a request to resume breathing. In Fragment 7, the surgeon

(SU1) also involves the assistant surgeon (SU2) in the assessment, thereby prolonging the sequence.

Fragment 7
```
700 su1:(radiation/DSA stops)
701     (3.0)
702 SU1: man skulle kunna dra ner den
703     lite egentligen [(ohörbart)
        one could pull that one down a
        bit   actually  [(inaudible)
704 SU2:                [(inaud[iable)
705 SU1:                      [ANdas om  jag  inte sa  de=
                              [BReathe if I didn´t say so=
706 ANE:                                              = ja ↑
                                                      =yeah↑
    ane:                                                  ↑(starts
                                                           ventilator)
707 SU2: det skulle man ku[nna
         one could  do  th[ath
708 SU1:                  [hrm.
```

In Fragment 7, the surgeon (SU1) ends the DSA without any accompanying request to resume the patient's breathing (line 700). This is followed by a longer pause when the surgeon is looking at the monitor (line 701). The surgeon then involves the assistant surgeon (SU2), who is standing next to him, by providing an assessment of the stent graft's position while simultaneously pointing toward the monitor (lines 702–703). In the overlap with the assistant surgeon's response, the surgeon then provides a self-initiated repair "BReathe if I didn't say so=" (line 705). As argued by Schegloff et al. (1977), self-repairs are usually located "within the same turn as [the] trouble source," "in that turn's transition place," or in the "third turn to the trouble-source turn, i.e., in the turn subsequent to that which follows the trouble-source turn" (p. 366). However, what is repaired here is not to be found within the turn or even with a previous turn; instead, the trouble source is the *absence* of a request, which expectedly should occur in close juxtaposition to the ending of the DSA. This self-initiated self-repair also becomes evidence of a departure from the routine order (Fragments 1–6).

In light of this, Fragments 5 and 6 could potentially be considered cases of self-repairs as well. However, unlike Fragment 7, there is no explicit mention of any oversight on behalf of the acting surgeon. Nevertheless, the assessment sequences that are initiated (in lines 500 and 600, respectively) and addressed to the assisting surgeons are momentarily arrested by the interjection of requests that address a different party (the nurse anesthetist).

Part 2: When requests are given but not heard

While the previous part has focused on the routine interplay between requests and confirmations, this section focuses on challenges, looking at those instances where requests are given but not acted upon by the nurse anesthetist. The hybrid operating room is a noisy environment with machines beeping, buzzing, and whistling and where several professional teams verbally coordinate their work across the room. When a request is given (by the surgeon), it can go unnoticed and be treated as missing by the implicated recipient (nurse anesthetist).[1]

In Fragments 8 and 9, these perceived absences are addressed. The fragments also show how the nurse anesthetist monitors the unfolding procedure. In both fragments, the surgeon (SU1) is standing near the nurse anesthetist and controls the DSA using the foot pedal. A scrub nurse (NUR) is also standing close to the surgeon, following the procedure and ready to assist with whatever tools are needed.

Fragment 8

```
800 SU1:  >>   anΔdas<<
          >>breaΔthe<<
     su1: >>----Δ(radiation/DSA stops)
801       #(3.3)
     nur: #(appears on SU1's right side)
802 SU1:  hur gör vi med (ohörbart)
          what about (inaudible)
803 NUR:  vad ska vi ha^
          what should we have^
804 SU1:  eh [ja vill  ] ha-  ja   vill [ha två ]
          eh [I'll-    ] want- I want to [have two]
805 ANE:     [ ska vi- ]  (0.3)         [andas  ] eller^
             [shall we-]  (0.3)         [breathe ] or^
806 SU1:  ja ANdas förlåt    (0.7)↑
          yea BReathe sorry  (0.7)↑
     ane: >>---------------......↑(starts ventilator)
```

Fragment 9

```
900 SU1:  åh^ ANdas:     (1.2) Δ (1.3) så
          and^ BReathe:  (1.2) Δ (1.3) so
     su1: >>-------------- ,,,Δ (radiation/DSA stops)
901       #(2.6)
     nur: # (moves back into position on SU1 right side)
902 NUR:  #räcker påsarna,
          #are there enough bags,
     nur: #(hands over a syringe to SU1)
903       (2.4)
904 SU1:  jepp
          yup
905       (2.9)
906 ANE:  ja vet- ja-  (0.5) ska  vi  an- när få vi andas^
          I dont- yeah-(0.5)shall we bre- when can we breathe^
907 SU1:  ANdas ja^
          BReathe yeah^
908 ANE:  (0.5) ↑ja de är bra om du säger till (.) (ock(h)så)
          (0.5) ↑yeah it's good if you say so (.) (as w(h)ell)
     ane: >>--..↑ (starts ventilator)
909 SU1:  [ja]g tror jag sa  de men   ja sa det för lågt=
          [I]  think I said so but  I said it too low=
910 ANE:  [ja]                                      =jaha jaja
          [yeah]                                    =oh well yeahyeah
```

In Fragment 8, the surgeon (SU1) releases the foot pedal that controls the radiation/DSA. Simultaneously, the surgeon formulates a rushed-through ">>breathe<<" (line 800), and in the middle of the request, he stops the DSA. This request is, however, not confirmed by the nurse anesthetist. In the pause that follows, the scrub nurse (NUR) appears on the surgeon's right side (line 801).[2] Now, turning to her, the surgeon initiates a conversation about what tools to use for the next surgical steps (lines 802–804). The nurse anesthetist, who is holding her hand close to the switch and continuously monitoring the surgeon's conduct, calls out, in overlap with the surgeon's turn, "shall we- (.) breathe or^" (line 805). The first part of this turn overlaps with the first part of the turn produced by the surgeon (line 804), and both parties can be heard cutting off their talk as if in response to the other. However, the surgeon makes a same turn repair by recycling (Schegloff, 2013) the turn's beginning, thereby continuing to address the scrub nurse, not the nurse anesthetist. The second part of the nurse anesthetist's turn (line 805), which contains the words "breathe or", is again produced in overlap with the surgeon's talk. This time, she gets a response. The surgeon aborts his talk with the scrub nurse and – now directed at the nurse anesthetist – he offers the confirmation of "yea BReathe" (line 806). In addition, he also follows up with an excuse of "sorry" to show that he "accepts responsibility for [a] trouble-source" (Schegloff, 2005, p. 470). In the pause that follows, the nurse anesthetist responds by reorienting her hand and pulling the switch, thereby resuming the patient's breathing without any further confirmation.

Even though something that could be understood as a request is provided (line 800), with the "sorry", the surgeon indicates that something he previously said or did can be considered blameworthy. The nurse anesthetist who called out the question ends with the conjunction "eller^" ("or^"). Lindström (1997) has shown that questions that end with the Swedish "eller" are "designed for the social activity of marking the action the turn otherwise engages in as problematic" (p. xvi). In Fragment 8, a called-out question (line 805) from the nurse anesthetist is retroactively being topicalized as something to be accountable for by the surgeon (line 806). However, what is being apologized for is not verbally formulated. One aspect that might be grounds for an apology is that the initial request was obviously not formulated clearly enough.

Fragment 9 begins with the surgeon's (SU1) request to resume the patient's breathing "and^ BReathe:". In the first pause (line 900), the surgeon looks up at his monitor and removes his foot from the control pedal, which stops the emission of radiation. There is then a second pause, during which the surgeon reorients to the patient and the surgical procedure with a "so/så", which in Swedish "takes part in the temporal (or 'aspectual') profiling of the act; marking the shift from its 'ongoing' performance to its status as 'accomplished'" (Andrén, 2012, p. 150). In lines 901–904, the surgical procedure could be seen to be advancing as the scrub nurse moves back into position (line 901) and hands the surgeon a new syringe (line 902). While exchanging the instrument, the scrub nurse also asks if the preparations for setting up the surgical sponge count bags have been sufficient, and she receives a positive confirmation (line 904).

On the other side of the operating table, the nurse anesthetist is still waiting as the patient's breathing is on hold. As the seconds go by, evidence is accumulating that something is amiss. In line 906, some nine seconds after the end of the DSA, the nurse anesthetist begins addressing the problem. This talk is not produced in overlap with any other talk, but the turn is nevertheless filled with several repair initiations. In the recycling and reformatting of the turn, we can witness how the nurse anesthetist struggles to produce something that will be understood correctly. The final formulation "when can we breathe^" could be heard as both topicalizing time ("when") as well as asking for a go-ahead for the relevant action ("can we breathe^"). The surgeon's response is immediate and formulated in the affirmative "BReathe yeah^" (line 907). The nurse anesthetist responds by moving her hand to the switch and resuming the patient's breathing. While confirming her actions with "yeah" she also follows up with an accusatory complaint that specifies that an initial request was found absent: "it is good if you say so (.) (as w(h)ell)" (line 908).

In Fragment 9, lines 906–910 could be classified as a traditional repair sequence where the trouble source is grounded in problems of hearing or understanding. However, in this situation, it is the perceived absence of a request that is raised by the nurse anesthetist as the trouble source "when can we breathe^" (line 906) and in the later complaint "it's good if you say so (.) (as w(h)ell)" (line 908). The complaint also holds the surgeon accountable for wrongdoings; this shows that it is good if a request is formulated in the first place. Instead of an excuse, as in Fragment 8, the direct complaint in Fragment 9 is met by an account from the surgeon (line 909), here specifying that the request was given but it might not have been clear enough, which the nurse anesthetist acknowledges in overlap (line 910).

In both examples, the nurse anesthetists' questions display uncertainty about how to act, and they are being raised as the surgeons and scrub nurses advance the surgical procedure. Such continuations imply that the preliminary assessments of the X-ray images (DSA) are over with. However, from the position of the nurse anesthetists, who have failed to recognize the requests, they correctly await further instructions and continue to suppress the patient's breathing. For surgeons, then, these queries are heard as reports about what is yet to be done: they have failed to secure confirmation that breathing has been resumed. Regardless of the reasons why the nurse anesthetists have not acted on their requests, surgeons are still responsible for ensuring that this happens. In these cases, the nurse anesthetists are not on track, and their need to remind the surgeons of this fact is itself a failure for which the surgeon may apologize or provide an account of.

Part 3: When requests are missing

During surgery, several professionals coordinate a range of different tasks. In the interest of patient safety, it is critical that all members monitor the unfolding procedure and speak up if something is perceived as problematic (Leonard et al., 2004). As shown in the previous section, requests can be perceived as absent, given that they have been made conditionally relevant by specific sequences of actions (apnea). The troubles described in the following section can be understood as being connected to lapses in the timeliness of these kinds of requests.

In the following examples, Fragments 10–13, requests for resuming the patient's breathing are not provided consecutively to the termination of the imaging sequence.

Fragment 10

```
1000  su1:(radiation/DSA stops)
1001       (3.1)
1002  SU1: #ja^ de  va ju-      (.) § de stämde ju va de-
           #yes^ that was (prt)(.) § it §was right (prt) it-
      nur: #-----> (walks toward SU1)
      su2:                          §----->> (walks toward SU1)
1003  SU2: stämde [väldigt fint  ] va
           was    [spot     on   ] then
1004  ANE:        [ANdas igen^   ]
                  [BReathe again^]
1005  SU1: ja      tack (.)↑
           yes please (.)↑
      ane: >>------------↑(starts ventilator)
```

Fragment 11

```
1100  SU1: ÅH^ va bra
           OH^ that's good
1101       (0.6)
1102  SU2: MY:cke* bättreΔ (0.3) fasen
           MU:ch* betterΔ (0.3) damn
      su1: >>--,,,,,,,,,,,Δ (radiation/DSA stops)
1103       (0.8)
1104  ANE: å andas^.
           n' breathe^
1105       (0.9)
1106  SU2: tack^
           thanks^
1107       (0.7)
1108  ANE: +kan vi andas^
           +can we breathe^
      ane: +(leans forward, looks towards SU2)
1109  SU2: ja  ↑tack.
           yes p↑lease.
      ane: >>---↑ (starts ventilator)
1110  SU1: >   jaja[men<
           >that's [fine<
1111  ANE:        [då andas patienten
                  [then the patient breathes
```

In Fragment 10, the surgeon (SU1) is standing next to the patient and, thereby, near the nurse anesthetist. When removing his foot from the pedal, the surgeon terminates the DSA (line 1000); however, he does so without communicating his actions to the nurse anesthetist. Instead, there is silence (line 1001), during which the surgeon puts away the injection syringe and begins to adjust the settings on the operation monitor. He directs a positive assessment of the work performed by the assistant surgeon (line 1002). Both the scrub nurse and assistant surgeon are now approaching the scene (line 1002), and their movements in the room could be seen as indicating that the DSA has stopped. Nevertheless, no request to resume breathing has been issued, and the nurse anesthetist remains on standby. When the assistant surgeon fills in with an upgraded assessment of their work (line 1003), the nurse anesthetist overlaps by calling out "BReathe again^" (line 1004). The format mimics the way that the requests are usually verbalized by the surgeons, and the first surgeon immediately responds with a confirmatory "yes please" (line 1005). In return, the nurse anesthetist resumes the patient's breathing without any further confirmation.

Like Fragment 10, Fragment 11 starts with the first surgeon's (SU1) positive assessment of the visual presentation of her work shown on the X-ray monitor. In overlap with the assistant surgeon's confirming and upgraded assessment, the first surgeon terminates the image acquisition (line 1102). As previously shown, upon the termination of image acquisitions, requests to resume breathing are expected, because there is no further reason to keep the patient under apnea. However, in Fragment 11, the request does not directly follow the termination of the DSA. Instead, the two surgeons remain involved in assessing their own work (line 1103). The nurse anesthetist then questions the absence of any request by calling out "n' breathe^" with a rising pitch (line 1104). After a pause, the response from the assistant surgeon is formulated as "tack^"/"thanks^" (line 1106). In English, stating the word "thanks" indicates a retrospective orientation toward an accomplished action and "yes please" a prospective orientation toward a projective action. In Swedish, however, "tack" covers both uses, which causes vagueness in how to move forward. The "thanks/tack" is more likely responding to the nurse anesthetist's utterance as a description of the status or a confirmation of a performed action rather than as a question. Regardless, this response is not taken as sufficient confirmation to resume breathing. The nurse anesthetist addresses this problem by leaning forward and making eye contact with the assistant surgeon. She reformulates her prior turn as "can we breathe^" (line 1108), thereby specifying that the patient is still under apnea and that no action to change the patient's status has yet been undertaken. The new turn is also formatted as a polar question, with the affirmative as a preferred response. The assistant surgeon looks at the nurse anesthetist and answers with a confirming "yes please." (line 1109), after which the first surgeon chips in with a go-ahead, ">that's fine<" (line 1110). Although none of these formulations match the expected request format, the sequence resolves the ambiguity. The nurse anesthetist immediately resumes the patient's breathing (line 1109) and calls out the action with an embedded complaint: "then the patient breathes" (line 1111).

As shown above, the command "breathe" is the expected format of the request, and when formulated differently, it can be understood as ambiguous. We now turn to additional uses of "tack/thanks" when these are offered in relation to DSA termination.

Fragment 12

```
1200 su1: Δ(radiation/DSA stops)
1201 SU1: ΔDE  var  bra  tack^   jaja    då går den [där nere
           ΔTHAT was good thanks^ yeayea  then it is [down there
1202 SU2:                                            [är det inte
                                                     [isn't it
1203       den som   gick  från (x)
           the one that ran from (x)
1204 SU1: jaja=
          yeayea=
1205 NUR: =vill ni ha den^=
          =do you want this^=
1206 SU1: =.hja =
          =.hyeah=
1207 ANE:       =ska vi andas elle^
                =shall we breathe or what^
1208 SU2: ANdas    JA↑
          BReathe YES↑
     ane: >>---------↑ (starts ventilator)
1209 ANE: ja då andas vi^
          yea then we breathe^
```

Fragment 12 starts with the surgeon (SU1) terminating the image acquisition by removing her foot from the pedal. This is immediately followed by her saying "THAT was good thanks^ yeayea then it is down there" (line 1201). The first part of this utterance, "THAT was good,", is ambiguous; it is unclear whether it is being directed at the nurse anesthetist or if it is an assessment of the work shown on the monitor. The "thanks^" that follows could be seen as a possible go-ahead to resume the patient's breathing directed at the nurse anesthetist. The nurse does not, however, act on this, instead keeping her hand ready to pull the switch. The last part of this utterance, "then it is down there,", is directed at the assistant surgeon and concerns the visual status of an artery's position provided by the series of X-rays shown on the monitor. Both surgeons continue to discuss this topic (lines 1202–1204). When the scrub nurse also asks if the surgeons want a stent graft, the surgical procedure is clearly moving to another phase (lines 1205–1206). In relation to this shift, the nurse anesthetist calls out to question, "shall we breathe or what^" (line 1207). This question shows that the surgeon's initial "thanks^" (line 1201) was not perceived as a go-ahead. On the contrary, in the reminder that she still awaits further instructions, the absence of a request becomes evident. In response, the assistant surgeon answers in the expected format "BReathe YES" (line 1208). This reformulation can be seen as an other-initiated repair, given the now identified trouble of disambiguating the first surgeon's "thanks^" (line 1201). The command is immediately responded to by resuming breathing, and it is followed by an embedded complaint, "yea then we breathe^" (line 1209).

In the fragments above, the nurse anesthetist raises the topic of a missing request to resume the patient's breathing. Below, we present a situation in which a third party – the radiology nurse (RAD) – breaks in to correct the situation. In Fragment 13, the symbol "+" marks the nurse anesthetist's other bodily actions, and the symbol "*" marks the surgeon's other bodily actions.

Fragment 13

```
1300  su1:  (radiation/DSA stops)
1301        *+(5.5)
      su1:  *(takes a step back from the patient, looks at monitor)
      ane:  +(looks at SU1)
1302  SU1:  *blev det bättre,
            *did it get better,
      su1:  *(turns to right, toward su2)
1303  SU2:  §spännande. den är där helt enkelt
            §interesting. that's simply where it is
      su2:  §(walks toward su1)
1304        +(0.3)
      ane:  + (looks towards su1 and su2)
1305  SU1:  +de- den är bara där
            +that- that's just where it is
      ane:  +(looks at her monitor)
1306        +(2.2)
      ane:  +(looks toward rad)
1307  RAD:  andas^
            breathe^
1308        (0.5)
1309  ANE:  +ska vi andas?=
            +shall we breathe?=
      ane:  +(leans toward the surgeons)
1310  SU1:  =JAja:=
            =YEAyea:=
1311  ANE:  =JA::    (.)↑ då    [gör vi det
            =YEAH::  (.)↑ then  [we're doing that
      ane:  >>---------↑(starts ventilator)
1312  SU1:                     [förlåt förlåt
                               [sorry sorry
```

In Fragment 13, the nurse anesthetist (ANE) is holding her hand on the switch and attends to her own monitor when the surgeon ends the DSA (line 1300). Upon ending the DSA, the surgeon (SU1) takes a step back, and the nurse anesthetist shifts her gaze toward him (line 1301). By releasing the foot from the pedal and taking a step away from the patient, he is visibly not continuing the DSA. However, this moment is followed by a long silence (line 1301), during which the first surgeon looks at the X-ray images on his monitor. He then turns to his right and asks the assistant surgeon who walks toward him, "did it get better," a reference to the placement of the stent graft (line 1302). The assistant surgeon answers with a comment on the stent graft's location showing on the monitor (line 1303), which the first surgeon acknowledges (line 1305). During these exchanges between the surgeons and in the following pause, the nurse anesthetist does not establish eye contact with the surgeons;

instead, she shifts her gaze between her monitors and looks toward the radiology nurse, who is standing on the other side of the room. The radiology nurse then calls out "breathe^" with a high-pitched intonation (line 1307).

This utterance could be interpreted as either a request for resuming the patient's breathing or as questioning the absence of a request. With no uptake from the surgeons, the nurse anesthetist responds to the utterance not as an order addressed to her, but as a question directed at the surgeons. This is a recurrent pattern in the materials. When the surgeons initiate the request for putting the patient under apnea, it is also expected that they should give the command to stop apnea. She makes this clear by leaning toward both surgeons and by calling out "shall we breathe" (line 1309), indicating that the patient is under apnea and that a request for changing this status is still missing. This is quickly responded to in the next turn by the first surgeon with a confirmation "YEAyea:=" (line 1310). Immediately after the nurse anesthetist confirms "=YEAH::" (line 1311), she resumes the patient's breathing. Again, this is followed by an embedded complaint, "then we're [doing that" (line 1311). The first surgeon's overlapping response "[sorry sorry" (line 1312) indicates that a mistake has been made and that he is accountable for this inaccuracy.

Discussion

A premise of EM/CA is that social order is continuously produced and maintained in everyday life. With different activities come distinctive orders and orientations. In a surgical setting, the tolerance for some misunderstandings is markedly lower than in, for instance, a mundane conversation, and the accounts for maintaining and reinforcing this professional attitude specifically draw on the notion of patient safety. Under such a regime, if the communication is deemed deficient, members can be observed not only addressing the problems of understanding, but also targeting the very norms regulating their procedures. Thus, formulations about these communicative rules can be seen as a form of professional socialization made in situ.

The current study has addressed a specific moment in the interplay between professionals engaged in a surgical procedure. What is showcased is a complex worksite in which the participants are involved in multiple concurrent tasks that need coordination at regular intervals. Most of this work is carried out very fluently. Some examples in the first part of the study describe the ease with which these interactions can transpire. The first three fragments show instances where joint projects between surgeons and nurse anesthetists are performed within a tight interchange without any complications. The communication and order of requests and confirmations, as well as the associated actions accompanied by these, are done as a matter of routine, all within an expected time frame. To keep patients safe, their breathing should not be paused for longer than necessary. At the same time, surgeons are also responsible for assessing the acquired images to determine the next steps of the surgical procedure. Fragments 4–6 demonstrate how the surgeons visibly juggle these dual orientations and responsibilities, with brief assessments interwoven with the requests directed at the nurse anesthetist. We understand this moment as a taxing and critical task for surgeons because deep involvement with the imaging process may consume their full attention. Fragment 6 is a border case where the delicate matter of delivering the correct instruction – on time – comes through in the surgeon's self-repair ("BReathe if I didn't say so="), topicalizing its tardiness.

In Nevile's (2007) study, the first and second pilots shared both knowledge and experience and, thus, could take over the work if the other should fail. They were also working near each other in a common physical space. In the current study, the operating teams (surgeons, nurse anesthetists, radiologists, and scrub nurses) are linked to different professions and areas of expertise, and they are located at different stations in the operating theater. In other words, separate members have only partial access to each other's work, and the various skills are not fully shared. Within this larger organization, there are also smaller units where the positions are interchangeable. During longer surgeries, intraoperative handoffs between anesthesia and nursing staff can and do occur. The surgeons typically stay put until the end, but like pilots, the two surgeons are both capable of taking the lead when needed. With this potential rotation of individuals for various positions, the organization cannot rely on locally established rules of communication. The patterned orderliness of the situation must outlive the particular persons who staff it.

In the latter parts of the analysis, we target moments of complications in coordination between the different professions. These instances are illustrative because they highlight a specific order of professional conduct. This order comprises a set of expectations that can be spoken of as professional roles and their respective responsibilities. Additionally, there are further expectations regarding the forms of communication and even the formatting of certain expressions. The studied activities operate on a hierarchical structure of responsibilities. Still, the practical actions involved make the monitoring work – and thereby the order in which they are achieved – a shared enterprise (see Heath et al., 2002).

As Schegloff (2007) and others have noted, some first-pair parts can function both as actions in their own right and as vehicles for other actions. In this respect, solicitations for requests delivered by the nurse anesthetists evade univocal classification. In the immediate sense, the sought-for but still absent request to terminate apnea will rectify the unsustainable state in which the patient has been put. Thus, the solicitations are *corrections* of sorts. However, the same actions could also be understood as *reminders*, indicating that something expected has yet to present itself. As soon as the technical reasons for maintaining apnea are no longer present, such as when irradiation has stopped after an imaging sequence, the status of the patient should be adjusted. The absence of timely requests to make this adjustment gives rise to what Schegloff has referred to as "negative observations (observations of and about things that did not happen)" (2007, p. 206). Hence, the sequences concerning absent requests are reminders about missing actions, which are also, by implication, reminding everyone at the scene about the patient's critical state. Instead of simply acting on their own accord to operate the ventilator covertly, the nurse anesthetists work to explicitly reinforce the order of professional conduct. They make witnessable and observable what they expect of the surgeon in charge.

Theoretically, it would be possible to imagine this coordinative work carried out with the help of gazes, nods, or observations of the actions of the other party, a form of complementary actions that Reynolds (1993) has termed heterotechnic cooperation:

> The essence of human technical activity is anticipation of the action of the other person and performance of an action complementary to it, such that the two people together produce physical results that could not be produced by the two actions done in series by one person. I call this process heterotechnic cooperation ("different crafts") to emphasize the complementarity of social roles.
>
> (p. 412)

The studied practice is an exemplary illustration of this form of cooperative labor, with its complementary social roles and distribution of responsibilities for the various technologies involved. The nurse anesthetists also anticipate the upcoming actions of the surgeons. Nevertheless, the safety-critical nature of the activity calls for communication to be done by way of clear verbal commands, so when deviations from this order are observed, the participants have been trained to "speak up."

These remarks about some forms of deviation have led us to the notion of complaints. In studying pilots coordinating their actions, Nevile (2007) shows how some actions were treated as relevant but noticeably absent. However, these absent actions were not oriented as critiques or complaints because "no complaint sequence develops" (p. 254, footnote). In our observations of surgeries, however, the noticings of absences may take on the color of complaints in the same manner as argued by Schegloff (2005), who raises the issue that an utterance such as "you didn't get [an] icecream sandwich" "takes on the color of a complaint, in part by the very insistence on the absent, yet still wanted, target" (p. 468). In situations where problems of coordination occur, the absent yet still timely expected request is explicitly verbalized: "[shall we-] (0.3) [breathe] or^" (Fragment 8), "shall we bre- when can we breathe^" (Fragment 9), "BReathe again^" (Fragment 10), "can we breathe^" (Fragment 11), "shall we breathe or what^" (Fragment 12), and "shall we breathe?=" (Fragment 13). Even if these turns are not explicitly formulated as complaints, they are sometimes followed by excuses (Fragment 8) and, therefore, understood as raising something problematic. Also, the nurse anesthetist can, after resuming the patient's breathing, explicitly formulate a complaint sequence that is met with excuses (Fragments 13) or accounts (Fragment 9). Here, the complaints explicitly topicalize the breached expectations of professional conduct and formal hierarchical responsibilities. The excuses and accounts, in turn, acknowledge and validate the identified problems.

As a matter of sequential organization, the first order of business is clearly to sort out the oxygenation of the patient. However, as soon as this issue has been resolved, the secondary matter of communicating about preferences – how the work should be done – can become relevant. These sequences not only address immediate problems, but they are also simultaneously forward-looking in that they demonstrate or formulate what is expected of future situations. Therefore, the remark explicating that "then the patient breathes" (Fragment 11) can be understood as a method for improving upcoming communications and maintaining patient safety. The accountable nature of the studied sequences also makes them part of an ongoing socialization process. For newcomers and seasoned professionals alike, the order of professional conduct – the surgical practice's expectations and distributed responsibilities – is thereby concurrently exposed and reinforced.

Acknowledgment

This work was supported by the Swedish Research Council (2015-03621). The ethical approval was given by the Swedish Ethical Review Authority (Application id 870-16).

Notes

1 The reason why the nurse anesthetist does not hear the surgeon's request in these situations is not clear to us as analysts.
2 For the duration of the DSA, all staff members (except the nurse anesthetist and the surgeon) should protect themselves from the higher levels of radiation emitted; the common practice is to step back and stand behind protective screens. When the command "breathe" is given, it also indicates that the DSA has stopped and that the staff can move back into position. This also implicates that the action of moving closer to the operating table can be taken as the participant's analysis of the status of the irradiation sequence.

References

Andrén, M. (2012). The social world within reach: Intersubjective manifestations of action completion. *Cognitive Semiotics*, *4*(1), 139–166. https://doi.org/10.1515/cogsem.2012.4.1.139

Heath, C., & Luff, P. (1992). Collaboration and control crisis management and multimedia technology in London underground line control rooms. *Computer Supported Cooperative Work (CSCW)*, *1*(1), 69–94. https://doi.org/10.1007/BF00752451

Heath, C., Svensson, M. S., Hindmarsh, J., Luff, P., & Vom Lehn, D. (2002). Configuring awareness. *Computer Supported Cooperative Work (CSCW)*, *11*(3), 317–347. https://doi.org/10.1023/A:1021247413718

Hindmarsh, J., & Pilnick, A. (2007). Knowing bodies at work: Embodiment and ephemeral teamwork in anaesthesia. *Organization Studies*, *28*(9), 1395–1416. https://doi.org/10.1177/0170840607068258

Ikeya, N., Matsunaga, S., Akutsu, T., Takahashi, S., & Nakazawby, H. (2024). Working out a division of labor in the interprofessional team: Management of prehospital emergency care. In S. Keel (Ed.), *Medical and healthcare interactions. Members' competence and socialization* (pp. 47–72). Routledge.

Jacoby, S., & Gonzales, P. (2002). Saying what wasn't said: Negative observations as a linguistic resource for the interactional achievement of performance feedback. In C. E. Ford, B. A. Fox, & S. A. Thompson (Eds.), *The language of turn and sequence* (pp. 123–164). Oxford University Press.

Jefferson, G. (2004). Glossary of transcript symbols with an introduction. In G. H. Lerner (Ed.), *Conversation analysis: Studies from the first generation* (pp. 13–31). John Benjamins.

Kuroshima, S., & Ivarsson, J. (2021). Toward a praxeological account of performing surgery: Overcoming methodological and technical constraints. *Social Interaction: Video-Based Studies of Human Sociality*, *4*(3). https://doi.org/10.7146/si.v4i3.128146

Leonard, M., Graham, S., & Bonacum, D. (2004). The human factor: The critical importance of effective teamwork and communication in providing safe care. *BMJ Quality and Safety*, *13*, 85–90. https://doi.org/10.1136/qshc.2004.010033

Lindström, A. B. (1997). *Designing social actions: Grammar, prosody, and interaction in Swedish conversation* [PhD Dissertation]. Department of Sociology, University of California, Los Angeles.

Melander, H., & Sahlström, F. (2009). Learning to fly – The progressive development of situation awareness. *Scandinavian Journal of Educational Research*, *53*(2), 151–166. https://doi.org/10.1080/00313830902757576

Mondada, L. (2014). Instructions in the operating room: How the surgeon directs their assistant's hands. *Discourse Studies*, *16*(2), 131–161. http://doi.org/10.1177/1461445613515325

Mondada, L. (2018). Multiple temporalities of language and body in interaction: Challenges for transcribing multimodality. *Research on Language and Social Interaction*, *51*(1), 85–106. https://doi.org/10.1080/08351813.2018.1413878

Nevile, M. (2007). Action in time: Ensuring timeliness for collaborative work in the airline cockpit. *Language in Society*, *36*(2), 233–257. https://doi.org/10.1017/S0047404507070121

Nevile, M. (2010). Integrity in the airline cockpit: Embodying claims about progress for the conduct of an approach briefing. *Research on Language and Social Interaction*, *37*(4), 447–480. https://doi.org/10.1207/s15327973rlsi3704_3

Reynolds, P. C. (1993). The complementation theory of language and tool use. In K. R. Gibson & T. Ingold (Eds.), *Cognition, tool use, and human evolution* (pp. 407–428). Cambridge University Press.

Sanchez Svensson, M. S., Luff, P., & Heath, C. (2009). Embedding instructions in practice: Contingency and collaboration during surgical training. *Sociology of Health and Illness*, *31*(6), 889–906. https://doi.org/10.1111/j.1467-9566.2009.01195.x

Schegloff, E. (1968). Sequencing in conversational openings. *American Anthropologist*, *70*(6), 1075–1095. https://doi.org/10.1525/aa.1968.70.6.02a00030

Schegloff, E. (2005). On complainability. *Social Problems*, *52*(4), 449–476. https://doi.org/10.1525/sp.2005.52.4.449

Schegloff, E. (2007). *Sequence organization in interaction: A primer in conversation analysis* (Vol. 1). Cambridge University Press.

Schegloff, E. (2013). Ten operations in self-initiated, same turn repair. In M. Hayashi, G. Raymond, & J. Sidnell (Eds.), *Conversational repair and human understanding* (pp. 41–70). Cambridge University Press.

Schegloff, E., Jefferson, G., & Sacks, H. (1977). The preference of self-correction in the organization of repair in conversation. *Language*, *53*(2), 361–182. https://doi.org/10.1353/lan.1977.0041

Schegloff, E., & Sacks, H. (1973). Opening up closings. *Semiotica*, *8*(4), 289–327. https://doi.org/10.1515/semi.1973.8.4.289

Zemel, A., & Koschmann, T. (2016). A stitch in time: Instructing temporality in the operating room. *Communication and Medicine*, *12*(1), 85–98. https://doi.org/10.1558/cam.v12i1.25988

6 Teaching and learning how to identify an audible order in traffic

Street-crossing instructional sequences for the visually impaired

Marc Relieu

Introduction

Mobility requires a set of abilities, skills, and competencies that are implemented, at least partially, while moving. As a person moves, she/he generates a changing flow from which she/he sees, discovers, notices, or explores (among other perceptual orientations, see Coulter & Parsons, 1990) many features of the various settings that become available. Some constitutive elements of such settings are themselves produced by other moving entities. For instance, any "vehicular unit" (Goffman, 1971, p. 6) that moves in our surroundings produces visible, audible, and even olfactory tracks to which we can become sensitive.

Although a considerable amount of research since 2000 has been devoted to the study of mobility settings in the ethnomethodological and conversation analytic (hereafter EMCA) traditions, most studies have explored activities based on *visible* features of the environment. In this paper, which is based on a close examination of video-recorded lessons for the visually impaired, we will examine how a trainee learns, with her teacher, how to exercise her listening skills in order to notice a specific type of vehicle in traffic. In particular, we will unpack the configurations within which such learning and teaching activities occur. Instructional sequences play a structuring role in these configurations. Their co-participants are closely oriented to an embodied, situated type of listening that addresses specific unfolding ordered audible features of the traffic. Discussing observations of visually impaired persons in action is also an opportunity to highlight the embodied work embedded in the everyday production and recognition of social order. Such an interest in the embodied, methodical operations that contribute to the "infrastructure" of our common world has always been present in ethnomethodology (see e.g., Garfinkel, 1967, chp 5; Lynch et al., 1983; Sudnow, 1978). It has been considerably extended and sharpened with the development of video-based, CA-inspired studies and the emergence of various cognate theoretical perspectives (Goodwin, 2017; Mondada, 2021; Streeck et al., 2011).

The (a-)theoretical and analytical point of departure in this chapter is the ethnomethodological and conversation analytic (EMCA) research tradition, based on a detailed analysis of collections of recordings of naturally organized activities. We share with this perspective a vivid concern for analyzing all details of the recordings, including the multiple, unexpected bodily features of the voice and other aspects of human conduct, such as those studied by Goodwin (1981), Heath (1986), Luff et al. (2000), Mondada (2007), Streeck (2009), Kendon (1990), and many others. In line with this body of work, our analytical attention will be directed both to the sequentiality of interactional activities (Sacks et al., 1974) and to various mobile features of the material environment (see Streeck et al., 2011). For instance, the direction, pace, and relative position of certain vehicles that circulate on roads close to the participants have been progressively taken into account in the transcription system and our analysis of the video data.

Mobility, instructional sequences, and the learning of abilities

Many years ago, I wrote a paper (Relieu, 1999b) based on a multi-layered embodied analysis of walking with a cane in a corridor, with a special focus on the time-ordered projected features of talk and walking practices, respectively. At that time, I did not anticipate that so much research would be done on mobility, talk organization, and orientations to the material world over the next decade (Haddington et al., 2013). Several studies, based on video recordings of interaction in natural settings, have been done on driving lessons in cars (among others, see Rauniomaa et al., 2018), flight training (Melander & Sahlström, 2009), and horseback riding training (Lundesjö Kvart, 2020). However, most scholars have explored only the various visual dimensions of traffic. A notable exception is a recent paper (Laurier et al., 2020) on the uses of car horns by Indian drivers. The authors show that the drivers produce multiple types of sounds (single, double, or multiple honks) in the traffic in order to perform different actions (offers, requests, appreciations, complaints, etc.). Yet, that paper focused more on the production of the hearable sounds than the listening practices of those who are the intended recipients of the horn sounds.

With a few exceptions,[1] most drivers of motor vehicles contribute to the noise of the traffic[2] through their material conduct without paying attention to it. Yet, the audible traffic sounds and their dynamics, which are the outcome of methodical driving activities in a socially organized material world, are not random. They produce an audible social order whose features are methodically used by visually impaired persons. The audible social order, which is constitutive of our urban lives, provides a vast array of resources for instructing others on how to safely perform many different activities. The instructional sequence we will examine here aims at developing a visually impaired person's ability to independently perform a safe crossing. Our interest in orientation and mobility (hereafter O&M) instruction echoes previous attempts to highlight the practical competencies of various people with disabilities. In his famous studies on aphasia, Goodwin analyzes how Chil who is able "to speak only three words because of a severe stroke, is nonetheless able to position himself as a competent person, indeed a powerful actor, by linking his limited talk to the talk and action of others" (Goodwin, 2004, p. 151) and by the means of a rich ecology of meaning-making practices (Goodwin, 2000). The related field of research on "atypical interactions," as Maynard and Turowetz (2022) recently pointed out, "demonstrate that those with impairments may be using forms of reasoning and communication via other-than-usual or taken-for-granted practices," which "implicates reorganizing the local ecology of sign systems, producing an expansion of common-sense knowledge" (p. 445), to which the present paper aims to contribute.

To some extent, O&M courses share similarities with driver training sessions. Of course, they do not rely on such complex equipment, since O&M training is still based almost exclusively on the methodical use of a long white cane, the adoption of various body orientations, and a set of listening techniques that rely on analyzing the resources that emerge from the environment. Therefore, this training requires both the development of a set of embodied abilities and sensorial exercises and new, specialized knowledge of the organization of the ordered, audible sounds that are found in the traffic (Psathas, 1992).

Whether they occur in cars or other vehicular units (McIlvenny, 2014), these instructional sequences are produced on the move. In this paper, we will focus specifically on a setting in which both the instructor and her students are static, while the students develop an intense focus on the flow of vehicles. There are some parallels with driver training settings, in which the co-participants sometimes orient to the contingencies of the flow of vehicles. However, the relevant focus of attention here has quite distinctive features.

Another common interest with previous driver training studies lies in the organization of the instructional sequences. As De Stefani and Gazin (2014) astutely observed, studies of instructional sequences in EMCA share various theoretical and analytical influences, from Garfinkel's seminal interest in the praxeological gap between instructions and the activity of following instructions (Garfinkel, 2002; Garfinkel & Sacks, 1970) to CA studies of instructional sequences in various educational settings (Mehan, 1979). Roughly speaking, an instructional sequence consists of three interdependent actions. First is the instruction itself, which is an action attached, or at least sensitive, to some membership category, such as "teacher" or "parent" (Rossi & Stivers, 2020). The instruction-giver is supposed to know how this instruction is supposed to be followed (Mehan, 1979). Second is an instructed action, which is performed by the trainee (category-implicative). Correct performance of the instructed action is dependent on the trainee's embodied practical reasoning. Realizing "what the instructions describe depends on the work that we do to find their adequacy. The ability to find that adequacy is, to some extent, what 'skill' is" (Livingston, 2008, p. 100). In their paper on teaching crochet chain stitches, Lindwall and Ekström (2012) add an interesting comment to this same quote. For the novice, who has not yet acquired the required skills, it can be hard to find this adequacy without any help or guidance. In order to proceed, the student needs to consult the materials and the embodied demonstration by the teacher. At the same time, the teacher's verbal directions are central in guiding the student in terms of what to look for. The demonstration builds on the embodied actions in relation to the materials, and the verbal contributions highlight features, distinctions, and contrasts that the student might have trouble seeing in actions and materials.

However, such guidance might be impossible to give when the instructed action is not a manual skill. Finally, assessments, evaluations (Mehan, 1979), and corrections are frequently found in the third phase of a sequence of instructions and have been characterized as "a device for dealing with those who are still learning" (Schegloff et al., 1977, p. 381) and "[seem] tied to a normative order of correct and correctable replies" (Macbeth, 2004, p. 727). Instructional sequences also occur in a serial organization, such as a chain of actions (Goldberg, 1975). Sometimes, a correction is embedded in the building of the next instruction, which becomes what Deppermann (2015, p. 71ff.) has called a "corrective instruction," i.e., an instruction that takes into account the difficulties the student displayed in performing the previous instructed action. Moreover, students not uncommonly have to "unpack" the corrections in order to discover new opportunities for learning (Levin et al., 2017).

Setting, data, and video-recording

The materials come from a video-based EMCA study I conducted in Paris in the late 1990s with the help of two O&M training teachers from the Association Valentin Haüy[3] and the participation of their students. It took me a few months to establish the mutual trust that was necessary before a video camera and wireless audio equipment could be introduced into the courses. I was then able to follow, over a period of one year, a series of courses with six students of various ages and physical conditions. Most of the time, I was recording the courses either in the teacher's office, where some specific training or conversational exchanges took place, or in the various streets or urban configurations that the co-participants selected for the specific training, lessons, and exercises. To be as unobtrusive as possible, I used a basic wireless microphone and a discreet video camera. Depending on the agenda of each course, the microphone was carried either by the student or the teacher. I wore a single earphone, a precious resource to listen to the lessons. As the courses took place on the sidewalk, in the very noisy streets of Paris, this recording procedure was helpful. However, this equipment was not always sufficient to record the complex and strongly spatialized sound patterns to which the students were supposed to attend. The main objective of this recording bricolage was to provide a solution to a complex, multi-layered set of moral and practical constraints and resources: being able to listen to the co-participants' talk, to keep an eye on them and on my surroundings, while tracking with the camera screen the relevant attentional zones that the students were trained to explore. I quickly realized that the challenge for me, as a beginning video practitioner, was to be able to find convenient spots, adjusted to the dynamic, unfolding series of attentional zones that the student and her teacher were exploring. Most courses consisted of training based on a set of practical listening skills. To help them walk straight ahead on the sidewalk, the teacher instructed the students to listen for the sounds that the vehicular units were producing while driving on the road parallel to the sidewalk and to orient their path toward this directional sound "line." Another systematic use of the traffic sounds was connected to the various crossing techniques (see Wiener et al., 2010). These features led me to constantly anticipate the next topography of sound that the student would be trained to attend to. Such anticipations had significant practical consequences for the video-recording process. I had to run ahead to find a spot from which I would be able to frame the relevant zone of action and perception. When arriving at a possible spot, I frequently discovered that vehicular units ended up entering the frame and interfering with the recording, and that I would have to move to another spot. In brief, the specific organization of what a relevant setting meant for the students and their teacher became a set of resources and constraints for the video-recording process. To know what and when to shoot, and how to move from one spot to another, I had to understand the specificities of the practical reasoning and skills that were taught and learned at each street corner. This video recording became a reflexive, pre-analytic training (Relieu, 1999a), which gave me some analytic access into the complexity of this training and some of its organizing practices.

The various excerpts that I will present here were recorded from the same convenient spot I found on the other side of the road that the student was being trained to cross. The frame, a wide shot showing the teacher–student dyad and most of the oncoming traffic on the parallel road, was stabilized manually from the pre-beginning phase of the course and was actively "frozen" until the end of the simulation exercise. The microphone was worn by the instructor, who remained very close to the student. I did not choose to focus or zoom in on their upper bodies because I was already familiar with this type of exercise consisting of listening to the traffic on the parallel road. This is the reason why I selected a wide frame, which encompassed the oncoming vehicles on the parallel road. In order to keep this frame as stable as possible, I had to ensure that my hand-held camera remained oriented to the same direction while keeping an eye on my surroundings to make some minimal adjustments to accommodate oncoming pedestrians. The main difficulty here was to move my lower body slightly to let them pass by while keeping my upper body "frozen" to stabilize the camera and the wide shot. However, such a static, wide-angle video shot prevented me from having visual access to the co-participant's hands, for instance, which might have been relevant in some sequences. The instructor was only visible from behind and the student was mostly hidden behind her teacher. This specific frame, therefore, allowed me to orient my analytical attention to the embeddedness of the instructor–student interaction in the audible environment, to examine the movement of the various vehicles in the traffic in detail, and finally to include them in the transcription. The recording activity helped me to achieve a "weak" form of the "unique adequacy requirement" (Garfinkel, 2002, pp. 175–176), mostly from the teacher's perspective.

How to guide selective listening to the traffic

The activity of crossing streets safely can be taught as a set of listening skills that exploit the audible, organized features of urban traffic. Being able to listen to the traffic going in the same direction and parallel to the student's trajectory is a general instructed practice used to perform various tasks. For example, students in O&M use audible tracks of parallel traffic in order to walk in a straight line. As the car recedes into the distance it projects a straight line ahead. When not attending to the parallel traffic, some students don't walk straight along the sidewalk but zigzag.

Therefore, the traffic provides several resources that can help the student walk in a certain direction without becoming lost. The audible order of the traffic furnishes an organized set of directional sounds that the students use for various practical orientational purposes (Psathas, 1992). To hear these sounds and relate them to her current spatial position, the student must first adjust her/his body in relation to the audible traffic. This adjustment is made through the formation of a specific participation framework with the instructor.

An ecological huddle

Contrary to a car setting, in which the driver and passengers are blocked (see Goodwin & Goodwin, 2012) within the material limits of this physical object, the participants here themselves make up an "ecological huddle" (Goffman, 1964, p. 64), a spatial arrangement in which they orient to each other (see Figure 1) and to the traffic. Before the exercise begins, the instructor approaches her student and stands facing her in close proximity. From this position, she is able to watch the traffic coming down the lane of the parallel road that is nearest them. This position also provides a stable orientation to the student's face and an excellent viewpoint for examining the cars.

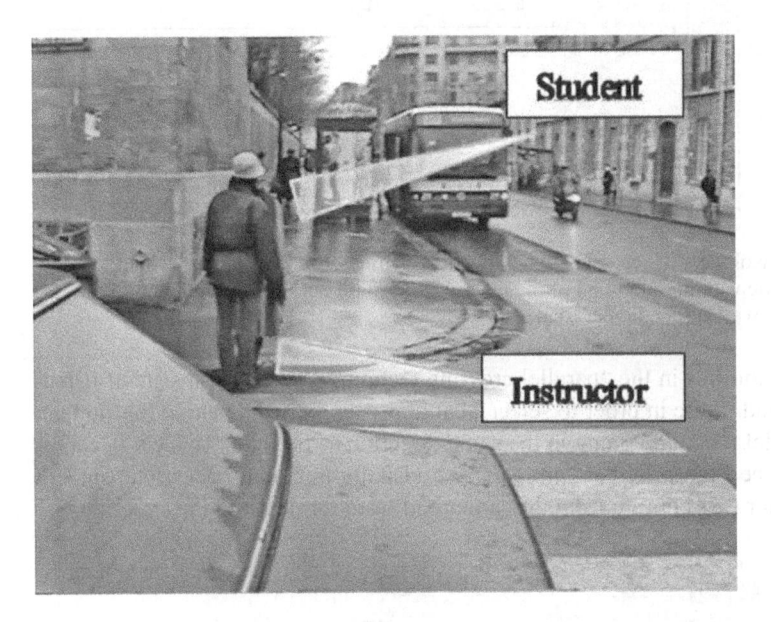

Figure 1 The orientation and mobility instructor and her student stand in close proximity to each other and to the roads.

This huddle provides a participation framework for monitoring the traffic and interacting together. The teacher, who is able to see the oncoming cars, is also in a position to hear the passing cars from very close by her student. She will use this double access to the traffic, both visual and auditory, in building her turns-at-talk.

158 Marc Relieu

The student's position is orthogonal to the traffic on the parallel road. She keeps her line of sight and her shoulder right toward the opposite side of the crossing as if she is about to cross. However, the student can feel the instructor's body, and she is able to listen to what her instructor has to say. From their two perspectives, the two co-participants are able to listen to the oncoming vehicles and talk to each other. Such simultaneous orientations to the traffic, to their mutual words, and to their normative, asymmetric spatial positions (the instructor is blocking her student, who is ready to cross) constitute the basic social infrastructure of this exercise.

The problem and its solution

The problem here is how to cross a simple two-way "T" crossing without taking the risk of being struck (see stars in Figure 2) by a vehicle coming from the parallel, two-lane road.

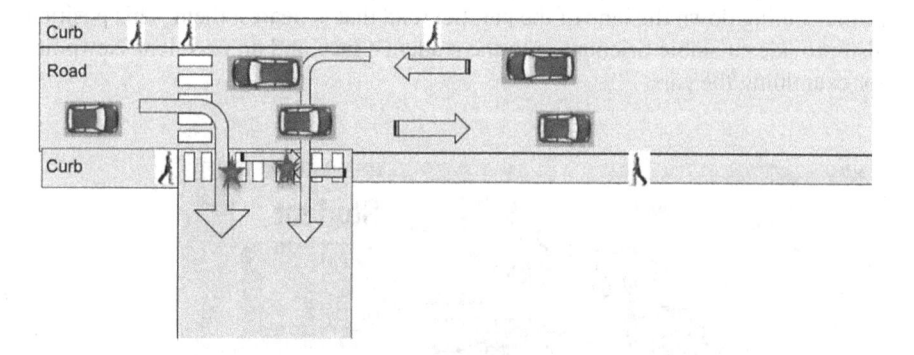

Figure 2 A two-way "T" crossing. The vehicles coming from the two-lane road, parallel to the walking direction of the pedestrian, can hit her/him when they turn into the one-way perpendicular road.

The solution lies in the "parallel crossing technique," which consists of listening to the road traffic in order to select a car approaching from behind the student, on the parallel road, and going in the same direction as her/him. This car becomes a "shield" (see Figure 3) that "protects" the visually impaired pedestrian, since it prevents other cars coming from the same road from turning into the street.

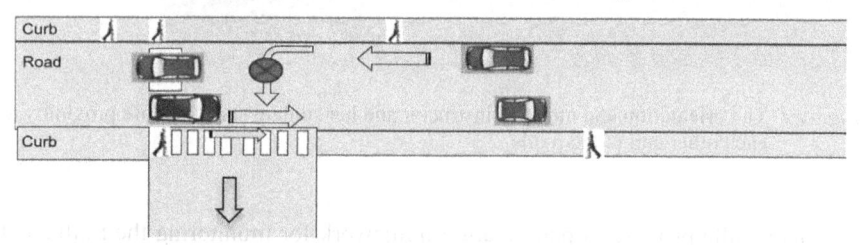

Figure 3 If a pedestrian crosses while a vehicle moves next to her/him on the parallel road, then this vehicle prevents other cars from coming into the perpendicular road and hitting the pedestrian.

How to identify an audible order in traffic 159

In the following excerpt, the instructor gives an overview of this procedure. The overview closes the long preparatory phase of the instructional sequence, during which the instructor has described the problem and introduced the solution, which is this procedure. Suffice it to say that this procedure is circumstantially adequate. In other words, the selection of the "parallel crossing technique" is limited to a previously analyzable, recognizable type of intersection, a particular configuration of roads, lanes, streets, traffic directions, crosswalks, and traffic lights.

Excerpt 1

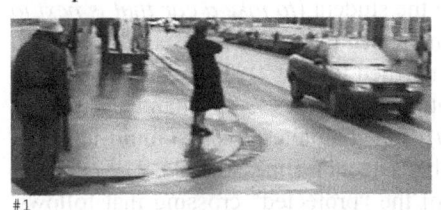

#1

```
1.    I. donc, le but du: du jeu si j'puis di:re, c'est de prendre une voiture,
         so, the goal of the game, if I may say so, is to take a car
2.       qui arrive à votre: hauteur,
         that is next to you
3.    S. oui ::h,
         yes
4.    I. il faut pas que vous la preniez (.) quand elle est au milieu du
         you must not take it when it is in the middle of the
5.       carrefour,
         intersection
6.    S. oui
         yes
7.    I. ni quand elle est. (.) loin derrière vous, c'est quand elle passe à
         nor when it is far behind you it is when it moves
8.       votre hauteur.
         next to you
9.    S. oui.
         yes
10.   I. pour que (.) comme ça que vous vous engagiez, (.) en même temps
         so that like that you start moving at the same time
11.      qu'elle sur la chaussée.
         as it onto the road
12.   S. uhm hum
         uhm hum
13.   I. d'accord ?
         okay?
14.   S. ouais.
         yeah
15.   I. si vous la prenez à votr/ quand elle est à votre: hauteur,
         if you take it next to you when it is next to you
16.   S. uhm.
         uhm
17.   I. ça vous laisse le temps pour vous engagez, et que si une derrière
         that gives you time to start moving, and if another one behind
18.      voulait tourner,
         wanted to turn
19.   S. oui::
         yes
```

```
20.             (.)
21.     S.  elle me voit et [elle
            it sees me and it
22.     I.                   [elle vous voit et que vous soyez déjà à moitié de
                              it sees you and you are already halfway
23.                          votr' traversée.=
                             through your crossing
24.     S.  =ah oui d'accord.
             oh yes okay
25.     I.  d'accord ?
             okay
26.     S.  hé ben !
             uh well
```

The overview of the procedure is given through two multi-unit turns. The instructor first produces a characterization of the procedure (lines 1–2), stressing the relative position of the selected car to the student (*to take a car that is next to you*) and adding two successive exclusions: when the car has passed this position (lines 4–5) and when the car has not yet reached it (line 7). Then, she repeats the first, positive, characterization of the right position (lines 7–8, "quand elle passe à votre hauteur" (*when it moves next to you*)) and completes this first multi-unit turn with an explanation that accounts for such a selection (lines 10–11). The explanation consists of a prospective depiction of the "protected" crossing that follows, based on the formation of a time-sensitive dyad between the visually impaired person and the car next to her/him. Finally, the instructor produces a third repetition of the general characterization of the procedure (line 15) and adds a hypothetical conjecture that enhances the previous explanation and accounts for the procedure's rationality (17–18, 22–23). The repetitions, exclusions, and hypothetical cases all highlight the importance of precise timing: the student has to select a car as it arrives exactly alongside her. During the two multi-unit turns, the student produces several acknowledgment receipts, during turn suspensions (lines 3, 6, 9, 12, 16, 19), as confirmations (line 24), and after verification checks (lines 14, 26). She also completes the instructor's last explicative turn (l.21), a complement that is ratified by the instructor, who echoes it (lines 22–23). In that way, the student displays her continuing attention to the talk and her understanding of the procedure's various characterizations. This selection procedure must now be exercised through methodical listening to the traffic sounds coming from the parallel street.

Producing an assessable listening: "Top"

Since the exercise consists of picking out an audible vehicle from the traffic as it moves up exactly alongside the student, the instructor has to assess something that has been listened to. How can an attempt to pick up an audible mobile "affordance" be made accountable and assessable in interaction (Gaver, 1993; Gibson, 1979)? If the student were to initiate a real crossing, her/his start would display her selection of a specific audible vehicle approaching along the parallel road. However, it might be dangerous to begin crossing immediately in a real setting without any training. To solve this potential issue and to avoid injuries, the instructor adopts a common solution, which consists of a simulation (see Excerpt 2). An ingenious solution to this problem lies in asking the student to utter a specific word that makes the car that she has selected publicly recognizable to the instructor. This word is "top" in French (translated as "go" in the transcripts). "Top" is supposed to be uttered by the student exactly when the approaching "shield" car arrives alongside her. The utterance of this word is a substitute for a real start, a bodily enacted move.

With the utterance of this word, the perceptual selection made by the student in the traffic also becomes a pedagogical object, an item that is projected into the pedagogical interaction and an assessable object that can be corrected by the instructor. In effect, the assessable has a unique character, since it is constituted by the synchronicity of the vocal production with the specific position of the vehicle (next to the student). This connection is locally emergent and evanescent. Unlike instructional activities based on manual gestures (Lindwall & Ekström, 2012), an indexical (Garfinkel, 1967) event cannot be repeated or bodily quoted (Keevallik, 2010). The simulation aims at initiating a training of the student's listening abilities, which she can exercise safely. Using a word to simulate the heard recognition of a vehicle in the correct position presents another practical advantage, since the procedure makes the listening itself recognizable. The instructor is now able to (partly) access and monitor the silent task of listening to the traffic and picking out one particular vehicle. Such features have consequences for the correction opportunities and possibilities that the instructor is able to make use of during the exercise.

In this paper, we will focus on a series of instructional sequences, through which the student practices her skills in the context of this simulation in the field and under the guidance of the instructor, who produces assessments and/or corrections after each attempt, but sometimes intervenes prospectively to prepare the student for the next iteration.

We are interested in (1) how the instructor guides the student's conduct, (2) how the student attempts to follow the instruction, and (3) how both teacher and student assess the student's answers. This setting offers an opportunity to examine how an environment – in this case, a mobile environment – can be locally turned into a pedagogical arena, enabling us to study how detailed features of this mobile environment are transformed into pedagogical, tutorial objects. More precisely, the audible features of a vehicle will here be turned into a pedagogical object. However, this analysis will show that the implementation of the listening exercise into the various components of the instruction sequences will not be easy. On the contrary, this implementation will occasion vivid, locally organized work in order to position the listening display – "top" – in the instruction sequence.

A practical scaffolding

In the following excerpt, the instructor will make use of the possibility of guiding the student's listening attention in advance. Adjusting her talk to the local circumstances as they unfold, she prepares the student to hear a specific vehicle.

162   Marc Relieu

Excerpt 2

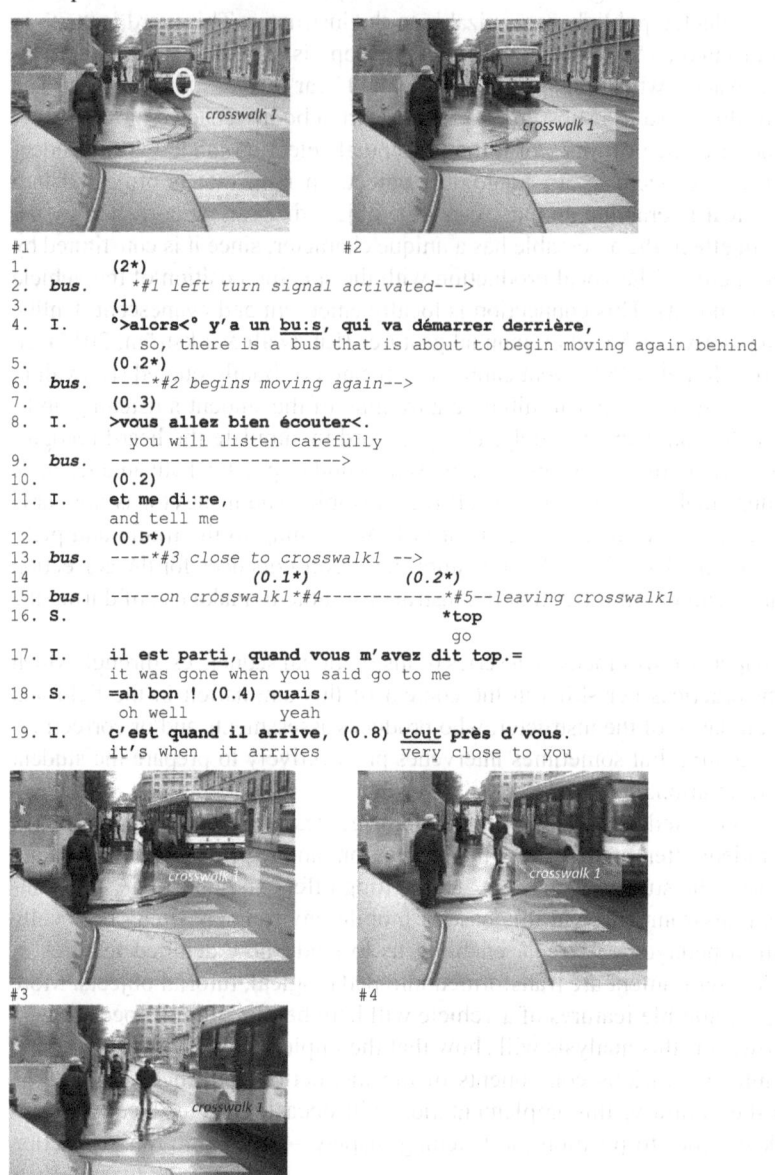

#1 #2

```
1.            (2*)
2.   bus.    *#1 left turn signal activated--->
3.            (1)
4.   I.      °>alors<° y'a un bu:s, qui va démarrer derrière,
             so, there is a bus that is about to begin moving again behind
5.            (0.2*)
6.   bus.   ----*#2 begins moving again-->
7.            (0.3)
8.   I.      >vous allez bien écouter<.
             you will listen carefully
9.   bus.   ---------------------->
10.           (0.2)
11.  I.      et me di:re,
             and tell me
12.           (0.5*)
13.  bus.   ----*#3 close to crosswalk1 -->
14                      (0.1*)          (0.2*)
15.  bus.   -----on crosswalk1*#4------------*#5--leaving crosswalk1
16.  S.                                 *top
                                         go
17.  I.      il est parti, quand vous m'avez dit top.=
             it was gone when you said go to me
18.  S.      =ah bon ! (0.4) ouais.
             oh well         yeah
19.  I.      c'est quand il arrive, (0.8) tout près d'vous.
             it's when    it arrives      very close to you
```

#3 #4

#5

In line 4, the instructor produces an anticipatory announcement of an upcoming event: an imminent move of a specific, potentially recognizable vehicle, a "bus." Note that this event is supposed to be identified by the student from the noise it makes. However, this instruction is grounded on the visual perception of the scene, which places the teacher in a knowledgeable position. The instructor takes the floor back with "alors" (so) and initiates a new turn at talk after she notices that the bus is ready to begin moving again (see Excerpt 2, image #1, the driver's activation of the left turn signal). After this anticipatory announcement, which is designed to direct the student's auditory attention behind her so she can listen for the occurrence of an imminent event, the instructor suspends her turn, while maintaining continuative prosody (line 4).

During the following pause, the bus begins moving again (lines 5–6, image #2). The instructor quickly adds a new turn constructional unit (therefore TCU), an instruction to listen (line 8) and to tell (line 11), which is also audibly unfinished, both on prosodic and syntactic grounds.

The instructor stops talking as the bus moves toward crosswalk 1 (line 13; image #3), then over it (see line 15; image #4). When the bus leaves the crosswalk area (line 15; image #5), the student utters "top" (line 16), which is the instructed word designed to refer to the arrival of the "shield" on the parallel road. The student displays her understanding of the previous turn as an instruction to perform the two successive and interdependent tasks that compose this instructed action: (1) active listening to the passing of the bus, and (2) the vocal production of the expected pre-formatted turn that confirms a positive listening of the relevant event. This attempt receives the following explicative third-turn evaluation from the instructor (line 17): "il est parti quand vous m'avez dit top" ("it was gone when you said go to me"). This turn highlights the lack of temporal simultaneity between the uttered display of recognition and the expected corresponding relative location of the vehicle. The sequential position of this item, produced just after the "top" uttered by the student, confirms that it is an evaluation of what the student has done. In line 18, the student produces a mitigated acknowledgment receipt of this negative evaluation. This reception gives the instructor an opportunity to expand her evaluation with a corrective instruction (line 19), through which she stresses the relevant car's relative expected location. This correction is also interesting in that it invites the student to produce more answers.

Throughout this first excerpt, we have noticed how the instructor progressively orients the student's attention with a prospective description of an upcoming, audible, and recognizable event. This practical scaffolding provides a slot for the production of the silent, instructed listening of this event and the recognition of the named referent, which is conventionally associated with a specific type of sound. To secure this recognition, the instructor organizes her talk in close relation to the traffic: she begins to talk once the bus has activated its turn signal, suspends her turn while the bus moves away from the bus stop to join the road traffic again, and adds a new "listen and tell" instruction, which she also suspends as the bus approaches the crosswalk area. This design of the talk, which is tightly coupled with the movement of a specific type of vehicle, constitutes a resource for instructed listening. By means of this careful construction, the student is progressively directed to the audible traffic and a specific imminent event produced by a specific vehicle. The production of the instruction, the instructed action (*this* listening), and its expected outcome (saying "top") all become pedagogical, publicly available, and witnessable features of the "environmentally-coupled" (Goodwin, 2007) sequence. The sequence consists of a tight co-assembling of the talk's structure and the dynamics of the physical surroundings made relevant by this talk with

164 *Marc Relieu*

the perceptual orientations, both visual (for the instructor) and auditory, of the co-participants.

Moreover, the entire sequence is based on a subtle array of temporal orientations, both prospective and retrospective, that emerge from the preparation phase of the instruction, the instruction itself, the instructed action, and finally its correction, which is designed to improve the quality of the instructed listening during the upcoming rounds.

A final feature of this "first" guided listening should be noted. This attempt is both a singular, locally organized attempt to track a specific hearable vehicle (*this* bus) and a "first" instantiation of what the methodical listening is supposed to be composed of. The student is able to consider what she has done as documenting the method by which she is expected to correctly perform the instructed action: listen for an audible vehicle coming from behind, track it, and finally localize it when it is next to her while simultaneously saying "top." This temporal organization of her listening and telling task provides her with a method for subsequent instruction attempts.

Orienting to the traffic as a continuous flow: A series of listening attempts

The following turns at talk confirm that the student has understood the initial instruction as marking the beginning of a new phase devoted to the remaining instruction. Understanding that the current scene consists of a series of successive attempts to follow the instruction to identify a specific passing vehicle is also made possible by the fact that the traffic is itself continuous. Consequently, the student continues to aurally monitor the traffic in order to pick out a relevant vehicle on the parallel road.

The instruction is not to find a single specific opportunity in the traffic, as has been described in many previous papers on driving, but to make a potentially endless series of repeated listening attempts. Since such attempts can be more successful or less so, the student and her instructor also produce different kinds of accounts, comments, and assessments:

Excerpt 3

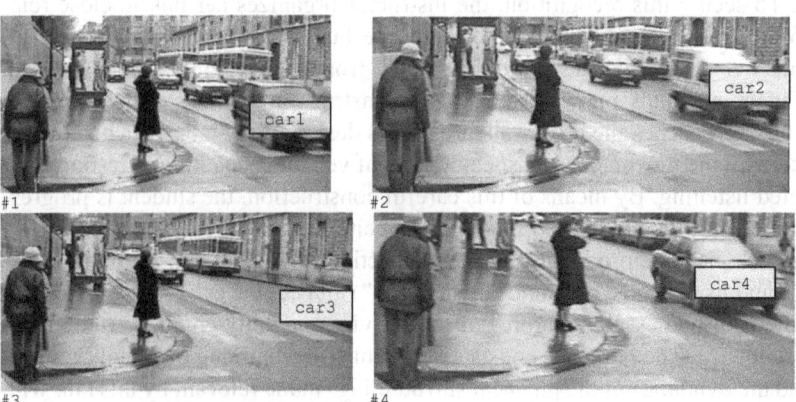

```
30.                (1*)
31.    car1        *#1 moving onto crosswalk1
32.                (0.3*)
33.    car2.         *#2 moving onto crosswalk1
34.                (0.4*)
35.    car3.           *#3 leaving crosswalk1
36.    S.          oh la la:!
                   oh my gosh
37.    I.          c'est dur, hein ?
                   it's hard, huh
38.    S.          *ouais.
                    yeah
39.    car4.       *#4 moving onto crosswalk1
40.                (0.8)
41.    S.          ah oui. >là c'est d'jà trop tard aussi>=
                   eh yes. There it is already too late also.
42.    I.          =oui, là c'est déjà trop tard. .h l'problème, c'est que si
                   yes there it is already too late. the problem is that if
43.                vous la prenez trop tard,=
                   you take it too late
44.    S.          *=top
                    go
45.    moto1.      *#5 approaching crosswalk1
46.                (0.7)
47.    S.          peut-être.
                   maybe.
48.    I.          ouais. c'était c'était mieux.
                   yes. that was that was better
```

#5

The co-participants are not talking, but the absence of talk does not mean that they are not oriented to the same focus. Three cars approach from behind them with an interval of approximately one second (lines 30–35; images #1–3). As the third car is leaving the crosswalk1 area, the student says "oh la la" (line 36), an idiomatic French expression that can be used as a disappointment display. Here, the expression is hearable as a retro-object (Schegloff, 2007) pointing to one or more unsuccessful listening attempt(s). "Oh la la" makes retrospectively publicly available the fact that the student has been involved in trying to pick out the relevant vehicle through her listening. In line 37, the instructor aligns with her and displays a congruent orientation to the relevant audible events. She confirms that she was attending to the same ordered features of the phenomenal world while assessing the difficulty of the listening exercise rather than a previous local performance by the student.

In addition, this second evaluative item offers the opportunity to display a reciprocal affective display with the student (Goodwin & Goodwin, 2006). While the student acknowledges this reciprocal affective display (line 38), a fourth car approaches on the parallel road (image # 4).

After a 0.8-second silence (line 40), the student takes the floor and introduces a second retrospective negative self-evaluation of the absence of the expected "top." Both she (line 41) and the instructor (line 42) notice that the expected but absent

166   *Marc Relieu*

"top" that should have been produced in a specific slot is missing because the student was "trop tard" (*too late*). Both display an agreement on the reason for the failed attempts, the timing of the previous instructed listening, as the student does not manage to adjust to the oncoming vehicle sufficiently in advance.

It is noteworthy here that the repeated evaluative retro-items are produced first by the student (lines 36 and 41), who displays an evaluative orientation toward her own attempts to select a relevant vehicle. Both the student and her instructor share normative expectations about the timely production of iterations of the expected instructed action.

In line 42, the instructor begins to expand her turn with a second TCU that is not completed neither syntactically nor prosodically (l. 43). This second TCU is designed not to comment on the previous single failed attempt, but to introduce an account of a general issue found in the previous desynchronized attempts. This corrective stance confirms that the instructor is coming back to a corrective orientation toward her student's actions. However, the student takes the slot (line 44; image #5) of this second TCU to produce the next "=top". She shows a dual orientation, both to the talk and to the attended-to expected event that she must identify to produce a new assessable in the didactic setting. This new assessable could have been ignored by the instructor, who was producing a spate of talk. Indeed, she does not produce an immediate evaluation of the "top" and the student herself produces a mitigated self-evaluative item (line 47). Finally, the instructor adds a positive evaluation that does not focus on the timing in relation to the expected audible event but instead consists of a general assessment of the learning process (line 48). Saying "ouais. c'était mieux" (*yes, that was better*), the instructor frames the previous performance as a step in a process, a step that is ranked in relation to the others, and this is exactly what she positively assesses.

Guidance and contingencies

To help the student, the instructor returns to the first tactic she used in Excerpt 1: making a practical distinction between listening for a specific, noisy, approaching vehicle (a bus) and the subsequent detection of the unique moment of co-presence between this same vehicle and the student, which should prompt the production of a "top":

Excerpt 4

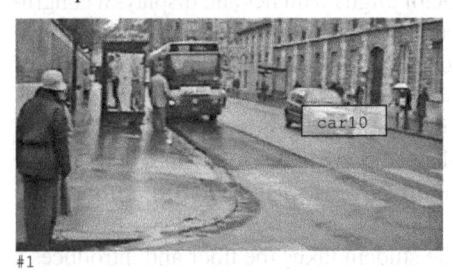

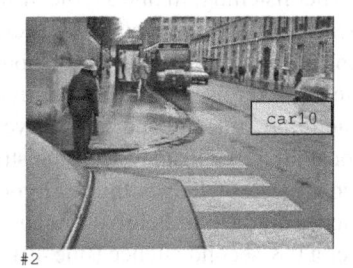

```
49. I.        je sais qu'c'est pas évident. >alors y 'a un autre< bus qui a,
              I know that it's not easy so there is another bus that has
50.           qui va s'arrê:te:r*, et
              that is about to stop and
51. bus2.                    *#1 --->right turn signal on, slows down
52. car10.                   *#1 going into the second lane of parallel road-> 53.
53.           (0.2*)
54. car10.    ----*#2 moving onto the crosswalk
55. S.           *top
                  go
56.           (0.2)
57. I.        >non attendez, quand il va r'déposer ses heu quand y va r'démarrer,
              no, wait, when it will drop off uh when it will start moving again
58.           (5.4)
59.           vous allez essayer de me dire,
              you will try to tell me
60.           (4)
```

In line 49, the instructor mentions a new bus in the surroundings. She refers to this vehicle in two complementary ways. First, she mentions the category of vehicle to which it belongs, a category that has already been used. In the context of the current instructional sequence, the selection of the category projects (in the background) the relevance of a related attribute, which is the recognizable type of sound typically bound to this occasioned (see Sacks, 1972) category of vehicles. Second, she parses this vehicle's activity and says that it is about to stop (line 50). This description highlights a feature of this activity that is also expectably hearable. In other words, the instructor prospectively draws the student's attention to a particular type of sound, the noise produced by a bus slowing to a stop behind her. This prospective description is expressly produced as recipient- and activity-designed.

While the use of "and" indicates that there is a next component to come in the instructor's turn, the student produces a new "top" (line 55) oriented to another possibly relevant event (see car 10 in lines 52 and 54; images #1 and #2). However, in contrast with what happened in the previous excerpt, the student's attempt is not ratified. The instructor does not produce an evaluation. She refuses to accept the previous "top" as a potentially assessable item and stresses that it was misplaced (line 57). Instead, she resumes her previous, unfinished turn and directs the student's attention to the ongoing process. In doing so, she retrospectively indicates that the recognized item (see car 10) was not the expected bus. She parses the audible presence of the bus into two next sub-phases. First, she begins to mention the next sub-phase (the passengers who are getting off the bus), but then interrupts this construction and introduces a new design of her turn, in which she highlights the future move of the bus (line 57). In this way, she structures her student's listening and prepares her to identify a specific phase. In other words, the talk is no longer produced in parallel to the structuring of the attended-to event; through her talk, the instructor proposes making cuts in the audible process. The reflexive link established here between the talk and the audible phenomenon as a temporal process is

168 *Marc Relieu*

supposed to help the student attend to this event and its internal structure in order to produce the recognizable listening. The instructor suspends her turn for several seconds (line 58) before re-introducing the instruction with a prosody indicating a continuation (line 59), after which the student does utter a new "top" (line 61):

Excerpt 5

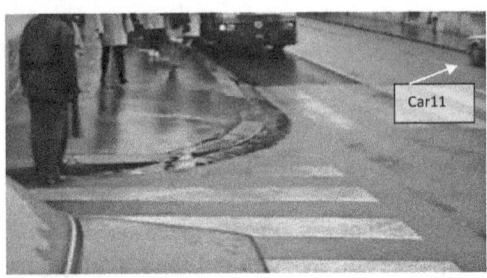

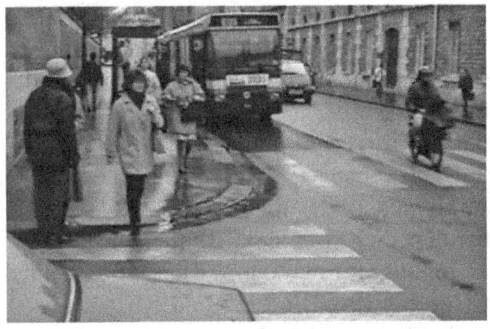

#3

#4

```
61. S.        *top ?[euh:::  non.]
               go      hu::      no
62. car11.   *#3 in the opposite lane moving out of crosswalk
63. I.        [m]mm non. pas dans l'même sens que nous.
              mm. no not in the same direction as us
64. moto.    moving onto crosswalk #4
65. S.       oh la.
             oh boy
```

However, the student quickly realizes that the audible object she has identified is not the right one (line 61), a misidentification that is ratified by the instructor, who adds a corrective characterization of the selected car ("pas dans le même sens que nous.," *not in the same direction as us*, line 63). This remark displays a continuing attention to the traffic by the instructor, who is always orienting to it from the ecological huddle she has set up with the student.

After a new negative self-evaluation from the student (line 65), oriented to the passing of a motorcycle (line 64; image #4), the teacher re-focuses the student's attention on the previous bus (line 67):

Excerpt 6

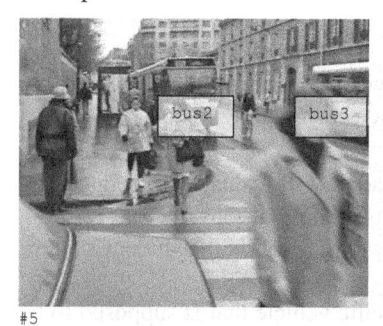

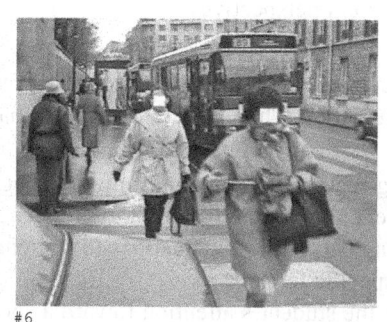

#5   #6

```
66.            (1.4)
67. I.         attendez. écoutez * l'bus,
               wait      listen to the bus
68. bus2.                         *#5 starting to move again--->
69. bus3.                         *#5 moves faster onto the crosswalk in the other lane->
70. S.         top.
               go
71. I.         écoutez l'bus. >l'bus le bus le bus.< (0.4) et dîtes moi::,
               listen to the bus the bus the bus the bus and tell me
72. bus2.      ------------------------------------------------------------>
73.            (0.3*)
74. bus2.          *#6 moving onto crosswalk1-->
75. S.             *top
                    go
76. I.         voi:là.
               yeah
77. I.         d'accord?
               okay
78. S.         oui.
               yes
79. I.         ça va?
               is it okay
80. S.         ouais ouais m'enfin!
               yeah yeah but still
```

The student displays a new recognition of the expected event (line 70), because another bus (3) (line 69; image #5), coming from the other direction, soon moves onto crosswalk1 as bus 2 begins moving again (line 68; image #5). Here, the instructor does not follow with an assessment; she repeats the reference term several times (line 71) and reinitiates the instruction with a directive "dites moi::," (*tell me*). Such repetitions are useful for drawing the student's attention to the upcoming event; finally, the student produces a new "top" (line 75), which receives a positive evaluation (line 76).

Discussion

In his famous ethnomethodological studies on following instructions, Garfinkel (2002) stresses the inevitable features that are missing from instructions and which therefore must be discovered during the activity of turning them into some course of action (see also Livingston, 2008). Here, the student discovers the specific listening work she has to perform – work that is not entirely accessible to the instructor.

- Two different perspectives

The instructor does a considerable amount of work to maintain reciprocity in the ensuing interaction. Three different practices have been highlighted:

- Showing reciprocity and confirming the negative self-evaluations produced by the student after a failed attempt to produce a listening display
- Producing corrective explanations that attend to reorienting the student's attention to specific features
- Guiding the student's attention toward a specific vehicle that is supposed to be easier to track

Despite those attempts by the instructor to display a common orientation to the exercise and therefore shared access to the hearable features of the traffic the student is listening to, the gap between the instruction and the instructed actions, which is constitutive of the process of following instructions itself, does not disappear.

The didactic device, which consists of producing a hearable word in order to make the student's hidden, silent[4] perceptual work recognizable and then assessable, has many implications for the interaction's progressivity. The student is able to identify the next recognizable sound herself and to initiate the next instructed action without waiting for any overt instruction to do it (see e.g., Excerpt 3). Since the instructed action has been sequentially connected to a specific, recurrent environmental audible event (Gaver, 1993), the student is able to re-focus on the traffic at almost any time. This possibility is generated by the intermittent nature of the event she is tracking. These events have to be picked out from the flow of mobile sounds generated by the traffic. The directionality of these sounds matters (see e.g., Excerpts 5–6), as does their spatial proximity relative to the speaker (see e.g., Excerpt 2).

Once she has identified a new possible recognizable audible car, the student can either produce the assessable "top," which is therefore introduced into the ongoing interaction as a new assessable item, or a self-disappointment assessment (see Excerpt 3), making publicly available her failed attempt to utter "top" in time, while the car is still next to her. We have seen that this possibility for the student to self-select in order to produce a new assessable or a self-disappointment assessment is somewhat problematic for the instructor because this production occurs in various sequential, talk-oriented environments. Sometimes, the listening display is produced while the current turn of the instructor is still in progress (see e.g., Excerpt 4). Sometimes, the next listening display is oriented to a different vehicle than the one that has been pre-announced by the teacher (e.g., Excerpt 6).

- Two distinct domains of scrutiny

Another way to understand this difference between the instructor's and the student's perspectives is to focus on the two "domain[s] of scrutiny" (Goodwin, 1994, p. 627) that are relevant for the instruction-giver and the instruction-follower.

The instructor selects a noisy and slow type of vehicle that regularly stops behind them and starts moving again (Excerpts 3 and 5). She instantiates this scaffolding practice with a method for producing a multi-unit turn that is progressively built in a reflexive relationship with the bus. The progression of the turn is thereby co-elaborated with the progression of the bus, in order to attract the student's attention to this specific vehicle. First, the instructor's turn draws the student's attention to a specific vehicle. Second, the instructor's turn projects a temporal space for the expected listening of the coming bus and therefore the production of the display ("top").

However, the student often produces other listening displays, which appear misplaced during the scaffolding episodes because they do not embrace the coupling of the instructor's turn with the progression of the bus. It seems that the student is mostly oriented to another domain of scrutiny, the sequential order of the oncoming new vehicles, which are still arriving at the perpendicular intersection near her. This perspective is not only attentional since it is also embedded in her understanding of the general instruction presented by the instructor before the exercise began (Excerpt 2). This instruction has opened a space of free speech for the student to produce any expected "top." This perspective is therefore consistent with the activity format offered by the instructor. However, this free, self-selecting possibility of producing any "top" that strikes the student as appropriate collides with another, more local configuration, which is instantiated in the two scaffolding episodes. During these local configurations, the student is no longer free to self-select (and thereby to select any approaching vehicle), since she has to wait for the right slot to produce a listening display involving a vehicle that has been selected by the instructor. Finally, in Excerpt 6, the student re-focuses on the instructor's turn at the very moment the bus is approaching them. She, therefore, produces the expected listening display at the right time and her turn receives a positive assessment.

Conclusion

During the first phase of the crossing exercise, the instructor tells the visually impaired student to say a pre-formatted word "top" (*go*) as soon as she identifies a relevant vehicle that can provide protection for safe crossing. This instruction creates a context that prioritizes the achievement of the simulated "go" and involves the student in an identification task focused on the traffic on the adjacent road. However, every utterance of "top" also implies an evaluation task for the instructor: the word becomes an item that can be assessed and has sequential implicativeness for the progression of the didactic interaction.

When a student utters the word "top," she demonstrates that she has identified a nearby and reliable vehicle, excluding any unreliable vehicles in the background. By listening to such sets of moving vehicles, the student reconstructs an involvement in an integrated environment. The relevant vehicle that she listens to projects a trajectory that offers her a prospective crossing. "Top" is a deictic term that locates a momentary configuration between the student's body and an oncoming vehicle. By saying "top," the student emphasizes the salience of this momentary spatial connection between herself, the oncoming vehicle, and any irrelevant vehicle in the background. In other words, each instance of "top" reveals a complex texture of interlaced connections and multiple retrospective and prospective orientations. Saying "top" highlights a retrospective, invisible listening work, emphasizes a specific momentary connection between the student and a single vehicle, and projects a possible crossing.

Each occasioned locally accomplished identification and production of this utterance is understandable by the instructor and her student as a reference to a targeted vehicle. This connection is supposed to become inspectable for the instructor, suitable for some correction, etc. Saying "top" makes the spatiotemporal configuration between the vehicle and the student analyzable. The instructor can thus examine this configuration's correctness and assess the student's listening. However, the instructor is also able to decline the didactic implicativeness of this verbal deictic.

Another feature of this gestalt contexture (Gurwitsch, 1964; Garfinkel & Wieder, 1992) connects or dispels this same word with/from both the organization of the exercise (its initial presentation) and the various talk-based local emergent resources and normative expectations that have been produced by the co-participants. When the instructor uses a scaffolding tactic to facilitate the identification of a specific vehicle (such as a bus), a new contexture is generated. The continuous attempts made by the student to find the relevant velocities of the gestalt contexture she is trying to attend to, through careful listening of the traffic, reveal limited congruencies with the scaffolding tactical orientations.

The learning and teaching of listening abilities, which will ultimately help the visually impaired travel safely, emerge from a complex journey into variously articulated contextures (Garfinkel & Wieder, 1992; Gurwitsch, 1964) of perceptual orientations, normative expectations, talking practices, and socially organized flows of moving vehicles.

Acknowledgments

This work was supported in part by a grant from the MAIF Foundation. I would like to express my sincere gratitude to Louis Quéré (CEMS-EHESS) for his valuable support. I am also thankful to the instructors in orientation and mobility, as well as their students, for generously allowing me to use my video and audio equipment during their training sessions and for taking the time to answer my questions. Finally, I would like to thank Sara Keel and an anonymous reviewer for providing insightful comments on an earlier draft of this paper.

Notes

1 For instance, some drivers would play with the sound of their engine in order to alert others that they are going to make a quick start once the light turns green.

2 The increasing presence of various "quiet" vehicles (electric, hybrid, etc.) obviously challenges such methods based on the perception of the audible traffic, which form the bedrock for the safe autonomous mobility of the visually impaired. However, the sonification of such "silent" vehicles has been discussed (see Sandberg, 2012).
3 The Valentin Haüy Association (France) was founded in 1889 to assist blind and visually impaired people in their daily lives and to facilitate their integration into society.
4 De Stefani and Gazin (2014, p. 67) have also observed that the instructed actions are often done in silence during driving lessons.

References

Coulter, J., & Parsons, E. D. (1990). The praxeology of perception: Visual orientations and practical action. *Inquiry, 33*(3), 251–272.

De Stefani, E., & Gazin, A.-D. (2014). Instructional sequences in driving lessons: Mobile participants and the temporal and sequential organization of actions. *Journal of Pragmatics, 65*, 63–79. https://doi.org/10.1016/j.pragma.2013.08.020

Deppermann, A. (2015). When recipient design fails: Egocentric turn-design of instructions in driving school lessons leading to breakdowns of intersubjectivity. *Gesprächsforschung, 16*, 63–101.

Garfinkel, H. (1967). *Studies in ethnomethodology*. Prentice-Hall.

Garfinkel, H. (2002). *Ethnomethodology's Program: Durkheim's Aphorisme*. Rowman & Littlefield Publishers.

Garfinkel, H., & Sacks, H. (1970). On formal structures of practical action. In J. McKinney & E. A. Tiryakian (Eds.), *Theoretical sociology* (pp. 337–366). Appleton Century Crofts.

Garfinkel, H., & Wieder, D. L. (1992). Two incommensurable, asymmetrically alternate technologies of social analysis. In G. Watson & R. M. Seiler (Eds.), *Text in context: Studies in ethnomethodology* (pp. 175–206). Sage.

Goffman, E. (1964). The neglected situation. *American Anthropologist, 66*(6), 133–136.

Goffman, E. (1971). *Relations in public: Microstudies of the public order*. Harper and Row.

Goldberg, J. A. (1975). A system for the transfer of instructions in natural settings. *Semiotica, 14*(3), 269–296.

Goodwin, C. (1981). *Conversational organization: Interaction between speakers and hearers*. Academic Press.

Goodwin, C. (1994). Professional vision. *American Anthropologist, 96*(3), 606–633.

Goodwin, C. (2000). Action and embodiment within situated human interaction. *Journal of Pragmatics, 32*(10), 1489–1522. https://doi.org/10.1016/S0378-2166(99)00096-X

Goodwin, C. (2004). A competent speaker who can't speak: The social life of aphasia. *Journal of Linguistic Anthropology, 14*(2), 151–170.

Goodwin, C. (2007). Environmentally coupled gestures. In S. Duncan, J. Cassel, & E. Levy (Eds.), *Gesture and the dynamic dimensions of language: Essays in Honor of David McNeill* (pp. 195–212). John Benjamins.

Goodwin, C. (2017). *Co-Operative action*. Cambridge University Press.

Goodwin, C., & Goodwin, M. H. (2006). Concurrent operations on talk: Notes on the interactive organization of assessments. In P. Drew & J. Heritage (Eds.), *Conversation analysis, Volume II. Sequence Organization* (pp. 89–126). SAGE Publications Inc.

Goodwin, M. H., & Goodwin, C. (2012). Car talk: Integrating texts, bodies, and changing landscapes. *Semiotica, 191*, 257–286.

Gurwitsch, A. (1964). *The field of consciousness*. Duquesne University Press.

Haddington, P., Mondada, L., & Nevile, M. (Eds.). (2013). *Interaction and mobility. Language and the body in motion*. De Gruyter.

Heath, C. (1986). *Body movement and speech in medical interaction*. Cambridge University Press.

Keevallik, L. (2010). Bodily quoting in dance correction. *Research on Language and Social Interaction*, *43*(4), 401–426. https://doi.org/10.1080/08351813.2010.518065

Kendon, A. (1990). *Conducting interaction: Patterns of behavior in focused encounters*. Cambridge University Press.

Laurier, E., Muñoz, D., Miller, R., & Brown, B. (2020). A bip, a beeeep and a beep beep. How horns are sounded in Chennai traffic. *Research on Language and Social Interaction*, *53*(3), 341–356. https://doi.org/10.1080/08351813.2020.1785775

Levin, L., Cromdal, J., Broth, M., Gazin, A.-D., Haddington, P., McIlvenny, P., Melander, H., & Rauniomaa, M. (2017). Unpacking corrections in mobile instruction: Error-occasioned learning opportunities in driving, cycling and aviation training. *Linguistics and Education*, *38*, 11–23. https://doi.org/10.1016/j.linged.2016.10.002

Lindwall, O., & Ekström, A. (2012). Instruction-in-interaction: The teaching and learning of a manual skill. *Human Studies*, *35*(1), 27–49. https://doi.org/10.1007/s10746-012-9213-5

Livingston, E. (2008). *Ethnographies of reason*. Ashgate.

Luff, P., Hindmarsh, J., & Heath, C. (Eds.). (2000). *Workplace studies recovering work practice and informing system design*. Cambridge University Press.

Lundesjö Kvart, S. (2020). Instructions in horseback riding. The collaborative achievement of an instructional space. *Learning, Culture and Social Interaction*, *25*. https://doi.org/10.1016/j.lcsi.2018.10.002

Lynch, M., Livingston, E., & Garfinkel, H. (1983). Temporal order in laboratory work. In D. Knorr-Cetina & M. Mulkay (Eds.), *Science observed: Perspectives on the social study of science* (pp. 205–238). Sage.

Macbeth, D. (2004). The relevance of repair for classroom correction. *Language in Society*, *33*(5), 703–736.

Maynard, D. W., & Turowetz, J. J. (2022). Ethnomethodology and atypical interaction: The case of autism. In D. W. Maynard & J. Heritage (Eds.), *The ethnomethodology program: Legacies and prospects* (pp. 442–475). Oxford University Press.

McIlvenny, P. (2014). Vélomobile Formations-in-Action: Biking and talking together. *Space and Culture*, *17*(2), 137–156. https://doi.org/10.1177/1206331213508494

Mehan, H. (1979). *Learning lessons*. Harvard University Press.

Melander, H., & Sahlström, F. (2009). Learning to fly: The progressive development of situation awareness. *Scandinavian Journal of Educational Reseach*, *53*(2), 151–166.

Mondada, L. (2007). Multimodal resources for turn-taking: Pointing and the emergence of possible next speakers. *Discourse Studies*, *9*(2), 194–225. https://doi.org/10.1177/1461445607075346

Mondada, L. (2021). *Sensing in social interaction: The taste for cheese in gourmet shops*. Cambridge University Press.

Psathas, G. (1992). The study of extended sequences: The case of the garden lesson. In G. Watson & R. M. Seiler (Eds.), *Text in context: Contributions to ethnomethodology* (pp. 99–122). Sage.

Rauniomaa, M., Haddington, P., Melander, H., Gazin, A.-D., Broth, M., Cromdal, J., Levin, L., & McIlvenny, P. (2018). Parsing tasks for the mobile novice in real time: Orientation to the learner's actions and to spatial and temporal constraints in instructing-on-the-move. *Journal of Pragmatics*, *128*, 30–52. https://doi.org/10.1016/j.pragma.2018.01.005

Relieu, M. (1999a). Du tableau statistique à l'image audiovisuelle. Lieux et pratiques de la représentation en sciences sociales. *Réseaux, 94*(17), 49–86.

Relieu, M. (1999b). Parler en marchant. Pour une écologie dynamique des échanges de paroles. *Langage et Société, 89*(1), 37–67.

Rossi, G., & Stivers, T. (2020). Category-sensitive actions in interaction. *Social Psychology Quarterly, 84*(1), 49–74. https://doi.org/10.1177/0190272520944595

Sacks, H. (1972). On the analyzability of stories by children. In J. J. Gumperz & D. Hymes (Eds.), *Directions in sociolinguistics: The ethnography of communication* (pp. 325–345). Rinehart and Winston.

Sacks, H., Schegloff, E., & Jefferson, G. (1974). A simplest systematics for the organization of turn taking for conversation. *Language, 50*(4), 696–735.

Schegloff, E., Jefferson, G., & Sacks, H. (1977). The preference for self-correction in the organization of repair in conversation. *Language, 53*(2), 361–382. https://doi.org/10.1353/lan.1977.0041

Streeck, J. (2009). *Gesturecraft: The manufacture of meaning*. John Benjamins Publishing.

Streeck, J., Goodwin, C., & LeBaron, C. D. (Eds.). (2011). *Embodied interaction. Language and body in the material world*. Cambridge University Press.

Sudnow, D. (1978). *Ways of the hand: The organization of improvised conduct*. Routledge & Kegan Paul.

Wiener, W. R., Welsh, R. L., & Blasch, B. B. (Eds.). (2010). *Foundations of orientation and mobility: Volume 1, History and Theory*. APH Press.

7 Instructing and socializing patients with aphasia to gaze at the therapist's mouth to produce speech sounds in language therapy

Sara Merlino

Introduction

This chapter analyzes interactions between speech–language therapists and people diagnosed with aphasia within the health setting of speech–language therapy. This setting is devoted to the recovery of language and communicative abilities that have been impaired by aphasic pathology – that is, a linguistic impairment that can develop following a brain lesion. This paper focuses on the way patients are instructed and socialized by speech therapists in the communicative dynamics of therapy as a specific form of social interaction and, more particularly, in a specific therapeutic technique of scaffolding; this consists of gazing at the therapist's lips/mouth to benefit from a visual cue (the mouth's position) that helps solve difficulties in speech production. This technique is observed during the accomplishment of labeling activities, which consist of naming a referent represented on a card. When the patient is unable to produce the target word, the therapist first deploys a series of verbal and vocal resources to assist them, and then invites them to look at his/her lips to benefit from audio-visual representations of the target sounds and then as a cue for correcting articulatory aspects of the sound production. The instructional and corrective activities then require precise bodily coordination and gaze control.

Speech–language therapy constitutes a specific type of health-related setting in which structural features generally detected in other types of institutional and asymmetric settings of interaction, such as instructional or pedagogical ones (cf. McHoul, 1978; Mehan, 1979), have been observed. The patient is involved in the accomplishment of a performance that is constantly monitored by the speech–language therapist. More generally, the latter organizes therapeutic tasks by soliciting/eliciting the patient's linguistic productions, evaluating/correcting them, helping with different forms of scaffolding, and instructing and correcting the patient's responses. This chapter particularly focuses on the embodied conduct of the patient and on the orchestration of their gaze orientation as relevant for participating, in a proper way, in the therapeutic activity of labeling.

There are two interrelated aspects involved in the way the phenomenon I study here is relevant to issues of socialization. First, like any kind of institutionalized setting of interaction, speech–language therapy requires members to be socialized in its normative principles of interaction, e.g., accomplishing tasks in a structured and ordered way according to the aims of the activity and to the agenda of the professional. Second, given that the aphasic pathology implies a loss of linguistic abilities, the patient (particularly in the initial phase of the pathology) is involved in learning new forms of communication as a result of their language impairment. This means that (s)he is being socialized in different ways of interacting. The work of the speech–language therapist (hereafter, therapist), as I will argue in this paper, also consists of socializing the patient in these new forms of communication, e.g., where looking at the interlocutor's mouth/lips becomes a resource to solve difficulties in speech production.

In the last two decades, several studies have focused on speech–language therapy as a specific setting of interaction (see, for instance, Simmons-Mackie & Damico, 1999; Horton & Byng, 2000; Ferguson & Armstrong, 2004; Wilkinson, 2004; Klippi, 2015; Laakso, 2015). Some studies have underlined the role of embodied resources in the therapeutic process (Laakso & Klippi, 1999; Klippi & Ahopalo, 2008; Wilkinson, 2011; Merlino, 2017, 2018, 2020, 2021a). This chapter contributes to this field of research by focusing on the way in which the patient is socialized in the relevance of visual cues, especially during the very first period of recovery, when aphasia has just occurred, in the early stage of the therapeutic process.

In what follows, I first describe some features of speech–language therapy as a specific instructional setting; I then focus on a specific type of instruction, the correction of speech sounds. I explain why bodily–facial cues are mobilized in these corrective sequences, and I discuss EMCA literature that has focused on instructions and corrections of body movements and on bodily demonstrations. I then move to the description of the data and the method used, particularly discussing the way I reconstructed, through my fieldwork, members' perspectives on the pathological and therapeutic situation and, more particularly, the way they oriented to the therapeutic technique I analyze. I finally move to the analyses, where I address several aspects related to the organization of the corrective sequences, that is, their organization, the specificities of the patient's bodily conduct, the way the therapist instructs them to look at her/his mouth, and, finally, the way the patient initiates this technique by early gazing at the therapist when (s)he encounters a speech difficulty. This will allow me to argue in the conclusion that the patient is involved in a process of socialization and learning of the therapeutic techniques and modes of communication over time.

The instructional dimension of speech–language therapy

Aphasia speech–language therapy is a health-related therapeutic activity devoted to the treatment of a pathology that can take place in different types of clinical contexts, such as hospitals, rehabilitation clinics, or private offices. Pragmatic and conversation analysis research has particularly emphasized the institutional and instructional features of this specific setting of interaction (e.g., Horton & Byng, 2000; Ferguson & Armstrong, 2004; Merlino, 2018).

Therapeutic activities consist of the delivery of a treatment compared to a diagnosis or a prescription, as in other health-related settings. The treatment, aiming at the recovery of linguistic and communicative abilities, requires a specific type of patient participation. The patient is involved in the accomplishment of tasks and performances that are constantly monitored by the therapist. More generally, the latter organizes therapeutic exercises by giving instructions to the patient, soliciting/eliciting their linguistic productions, evaluating/correcting them, and assisting the patient through cueing/scaffolding when needed (see Wilkinson, 2013; Merlino, 2017, 2018).

Consequently, the communicative processes through which rehabilitation takes place show some structural features observed in other types of institutional and asymmetric settings of interaction, such as instructional or pedagogical ones (cf. Mehan, 1979). More specifically, there is an overall structural organization with different phases that are structured according to the therapist's agenda (Silvast, 1991; Horton & Byng, 2000; Ferguson & Armstrong, 2004). Similar to other types of institutional and healthcare therapeutic settings (Maynard, 1991; Ten Have, 1991), therapeutic interactions are asymmetric (Silvast, 1991) and therapist driven (see Simmons-Mackie & Damico, 1999, and Merlino, 2017, for a discussion about patient negotiation of this asymmetry).

Research that has focused on the description of the interactional and sequential organization of speech therapy settings has, for instance, described correction sequences or third-turn evaluations of patients' productions (e.g., Lesser and Milroy, 1993; Damico et al., 1999; Horton & Byng, 2000; Ferguson & Armstrong, 2004; Horton, 2006; Merlino, 2017, 2018; Merlino & Keel, 2017). The techniques used by the therapist to correct the patient in the third turn and to solicit a (new) response have been investigated. The necessity of studying cueing and "what forms they take, their properties as interactional actions, and what effect they have on the PWA [patient with aphasia]'s next try" (Wilkinson, 2013, p. 817) has developed. This is particularly because "the third turn displays the professional practices that are used to support language learning" (Ronkainien et al., 2017, p. 268).

Corrections are indeed an integral part of the therapeutic work of supporting aphasic patients' language recovery. Corrections can be done in an embedded or – more often, in labeling activities – in an exposed way (Jefferson, 1987), that is, by isolating and focusing on the problematic element or trouble source. As discussed later, this is done, for instance, prosodically, by highlighting the correct version of the item with a rise in pitch (see Tarplee, 2010; Ronkainen, 2011; Ronkainen et al., 2017). This is also done through embodied resources that reproduce the articulatory features of the target sound with emphasized lip positions. Together with instructions, corrections are a crucial part of the socialization and learning of the patient in therapy as a specific setting of interaction.

Correcting and instructing speech sounds through embodied resources

Instruction and correction of linguistic units (phonemes or entire words) are typically done within the ongoing instructional activity by producing the target word or part of it, emphasizing the speech sounds through prosodic features, such as volume and stretch. This corrective demonstration[1] of the target sounds works as an instruction (as defined by Garfinkel, 2002), as it makes a second action by the patient relevant, consisting of repeating the target sound produced during the therapist's turn. Nevertheless, when the patient manifests difficulties in repeating the target sounds, the therapist further accentuates her/his performance, emphasizing the position of her/his lips and thus addressing articulatory aspects of sound production.[2] The instructional activity is then organized into a series of sequences (instruction/instructed action or corrective demonstration/response) that are (re) produced until the patient pronounces the target sound correctly and the therapist evaluates this production positively or, alternatively, decides to abandon the task (see also Merlino, 2018, for this type of sequential organization). As a consequence, the instructional activity is realized through the mobilization of audible and visible resources, thus deployed as an embodied activity – an embodied demonstration – that needs to be *seen* by the patient.

In recent decades, research in ethnomethodology and conversation analysis has investigated instructions of embodied skills in several settings in which corporeal practices allow for a competent performance of the activities in question (e.g., orchestral rehearsals, Weeks, 1996; archeology, Goodwin, 2003; surgery, Koschmann et al., 2011; crochet classes, Lindwall & Ekstrom, 2012). Some studies have, more specifically, focused on settings in which physical actions, such as body movements, are trained, for example, in dance classes (Keevallik, 2010, 2013), sport coaching (Evans & Reynolds, 2016), and climbing with visually impaired athletes (Simone & Galatolo, 2020). In instructional activities in which the object of instruction is a bodily practice, the recipient's gaze can be treated as crucial to pursue the activity and deliver an embodied instruction (Sanchez Svensson et al., 2009) or for an "instructed perception" (Nishizaka, 2014). Here, "the request for gaze assumes a prominent function" (see Stukenbrock, 2014, p. 97). As shown in our analyses, gazing at the therapist's face, particularly the mouth, needs to be achieved interactionally.

Within therapeutic settings, instructions and corrections about body movements, although still not largely studied (see Parry, 2005; Martin & Sahlström, 2010), constitute a consistent part of the professional's work. In physiotherapy, for instance, corrections of a patient's body movements can be made to solve troubles with understanding a movement's performance. Previous research has focused on how the therapist formulates corrective instruction verbally and manages issues of physical non-competence by the patient in a delicate manner (Parry, 2005). Martin and Sahlström (2010) focused more on the organization of embodied correction and pointed to issues of bodily coordination (e.g., the use of a gaze-prompting tap on the patient's shoulder or a request to look in the mirror to make the trouble observable and perceptually available, ibid., p. 675). Here, other correction is considered a resource in socialization, as in different settings, and not only educational ones (among which physiotherapy practice), "parties orient to corrections as a central embodied interactional business-at-hand and not just a perturbation of the flow of talk" (Martin & Sahlström, 2010, p. 673). Moreover, through their longitudinal study, the authors showed that learning and socialization can also be explored with reference to repair and correction of movement performance: their results show a change for the patient from other- to self-initiation of repair and correction, and from other- to self-repair and correction.

With reference to speech–language therapy, few studies have explored the way therapists instruct and correct the patient on speech production through visual bodily cues (see Ronkainen, 2011, regarding therapy for children with cochlear implants; Ochs et al., 2005, regarding therapy for children with autism; Merlino, 2021b, regarding therapy for persons with aphasia). However, as far as the relation between visual cues and word retrieval in aphasia therapy is concerned, experimental research has suggested the efficacy not only of therapists' gestures (see, for instance, Rose, 2013) but also of visual cues, such as lip position (what is "technically" called *"visual phonemic cueing"*).[3] My analysis contributes to these findings, showing that therapists mobilize their face, particularly the *mouth's position*, as a hint to assist the person in recognizing and reproducing the target phoneme, as well as finding the target word, with clear effects on the patient's linguistic productions.

Few conversation analytic studies[4] have investigated the individual development and improvement of the patient (see Wilkinson et al., 1998, and Wilkinson et al., 2007, who document changes in the talk of a person with aphasia over time). Nevertheless, *socialization in the practices of the therapy*, although treated through the study of therapeutic interaction (see, e.g., Wilkinson, 2013, for testing activities), to my knowledge, has not been addressed by studies that analyze the communicative conduct of the same participant over time. Through a detailed analysis of participants' embodied conduct of therapeutic sessions taking place with the same patient during the first weeks of his recovery, my study invites reflection on how the patient is socialized in this practice over time and, in the end, needs less support from the therapist to mobilize them.

Data and method

The data analyzed in this study are taken from a corpus of 40 hours of video recordings of speech–language therapy sessions that I recorded *longitudinally* during the six-month recovery period of patients who developed aphasia following a stroke. The recordings took place in several therapeutic settings (hospital, rehabilitation clinic, private speech therapy office, patient's home) and with different speech and language therapists, as I followed the patients along their initial recovery.[5] As a consequence, I collected data both "vertically," that is, over time, and "horizontally," across different settings (for this distinction, see Zimmerman, 1999).

These different therapeutic settings not only make a diversity of therapeutic objectives (e.g., global early recovery versus more targeted therapy for stabilized disease in rehabilitation centers) relevant under the same heading ("speech–language therapy"), they also show a diversity of material and contextual features. For instance, I observed variety in the way participants were positioned (e.g., sitting versus standing, one in front of the other versus side by side) and in the type of artifacts they used (such as objects, cards, documents, or a computer). The features of these ecologies of action have an impact on participants' body conduct, visual orientation, and the organization of the activity itself (Goodwin, 2000). As my analysis indicates, this is deeply intertwined with the way in which the therapeutic process takes place and the therapeutic techniques are implemented in interaction.

Engaging personally, for a long period of time, through the fieldwork and video recordings gave me access to the therapists', the patients', and their families' perspectives – that is, *members' perspectives* on the therapeutic process. Finally, I acquired a deep familiarity with the research setting and "unique adequacy" (Garfinkel, 2002), at least in its weak sense (Ikeya, 2020). More particularly, the topic of progression is highly relevant for both therapists and patients, independent of the medical reasons that might limit progression. One of the patients asked me to look at the video recordings of the early-stage recovery to get a grasp of his own recovery progression.

I also had many exchanges with the therapists, some of whom also had a look with me at some of the video-recorded data. It was through the analysis of the data that I developed an analytic interest in the phenomenon I analyze in this paper, but it was also through discussion with therapists that I came to learn that they often use this therapeutic technique with the patient. According to what they said, this is not an "official" administered technique, but a practice they mobilize in their daily experience because of its efficacy in patients' achievements and progression. My analyses allow me to address different dimensions of progression – not only as progression of linguistic abilities in a person with aphasia but also as progression in the way of responding to and benefiting from a therapeutic technique, with obvious repercussions on the patient's linguistic abilities.

The data presented in this paper were selected from the hospital setting and concerned *one single patient*. Within the entire corpus, the phenomenon I focused on was also observed in the other patients. Nevertheless, systematic documentation of the use of this practice has been realized on only one patient. The patient is a 56-year-old man who was hospitalized following a cerebral infarction that caused the development of aphasia and right hemiplegia. At the hospital, I recorded four sessions with him covering a period of two weeks (in the acute phase of the pathology), from February 20 to March 2. The first data collection took place the day after the patient was admitted to the neurovascular unit (February 19); the last data collection took place the day before he was discharged (March 3). Every extract analyzed in this paper reports the date of the session.

As the sessions took place in the early stages post-stroke, the patient could have significant medical and cognitive complications (e.g., being tired, finding it hard to concentrate). Though I propose an analysis of interaction and I do not discuss the cognitive and pathological reasons for specific embodied conduct (such as closing of the eyes), I am aware that these medical and cognitive factors could encroach on interactional conduct.[6]

Data were collected in France and participants were French-speaking. Interactions were transcribed using the ICOR conventions (inspired by Jefferson, 2004) for the verbal dimension of talk and the conventions developed by Mondada (2018) for the multimodal dimension. Moreover, given the specific focus on issues of pronunciation and articulatory features of the target sounds, IPA conventions for phonetics were used when transcribing specific items in both the patients' and therapists' turns. Nevertheless, for reasons of readability of the transcripts, IPA brackets were not used. Brackets in the transcripts refer to conversation analytic conventions – that is, overlapping onsets in talk. In the transcript, verbal productions were translated from French to English. The vocal productions transcribed with IPA were not translated but just reproduced in the translation line.

Analyses

Corrections of speech production in labeling activities

Labeling or picture naming is a recurrent task in speech–language therapy. It is proposed to the patient to work on different aspects of language production and consists of naming the referent represented on a card. Research on the organization of this activity (see, for example, Wilkinson, 2013; Merlino & Keel, 2017; Merlino, 2018) has identified a specific sequential organization that orients toward a three-part sequence: initiation, response, and evaluation. This sequence structurally defines the boundaries between the different items at the center of the task (a new item is presented only once the previous sequence is closed). Nevertheless, this sequence is quite different from the one observed, for instance, in classroom interactions, as the therapeutic work takes form precisely in the constant reopening – or extension – of the sequence. Following the patient's responses (which can also consist "only" of several hesitations), which indicate different types of difficulties, the therapist gives a hint (that tacitly evaluates the previous answer), and the patient gives a new response, which is either positively evaluated or negatively evaluated through offering a new hint, and so forth.

In my data, these sequences (hint/response) can occupy several turns before the "initial" three-part structure is closed by an evaluation from the therapist and the proposal of a new item/card to be named. This is due not only to the difficulties of the patient in producing the target word but also to the way the therapist treats their productions as not accurate enough in terms of *articulation and pronunciation* (for this type of sequence in children's language acquisition, see Tarplee, 2010). The therapist's turns are indeed oriented toward correcting and modeling the target sounds produced by the patient.

In the following series of extracts, we can see the way the therapist treats the patient's productions by responding in different ways, sequentially, to his difficulties, thus orienting to different types of problems in language production.

In the first extract, the therapist gives a card to the patient (line 1), who takes it and positions it on the table as part of a group of cards related to vegetables (thus showing recognition of the referent and the ability to select a semantic category, line 2). She then asks the patient to name the referent ("poireau", *leek*) by formulating a question ("qu'est-ce que c'est?", *what is it?*, line 4):

Extract (1) (CHU_C_23february. Production of the word: "poireau", /pwaro/, *leek*) (participants: SLT: speech-language therapist; PAT: patient)

```
1            +(5)+
    slt     +gives card to pat+
2   PAT     *hop*
            (interj.)
    pat     *takes card, places on table*
3           (0.6)
4   SLT=>  qu'est-ce que c'e:st?
            what is it?
5           (0.4)
6   PAT     un °°p-°°  (1.3) un (0.2) nap- (0.6) AH::  (0.2) n[e
            a  °°p-°°  (1.3) a  (0.2) nap- (0.6) AH::  (0.2) n[e
7   SLT=>                                                    [un P:WA::r,
                                                              a P:WA::r,
8   PAT     un p- (0.5) pwarœ
            a  p- (0.5) pwarœ
9           (0.2)
10  PAT     [rœ euh
            [rœ eh
11  SLT=>  [pwaRO:
            [pwaRO:
```

The patient aligns with the therapist's action by starting to respond at line 6 with a type-conforming response (Raymond, 2000) ("un p-"); he then immediately repairs his turn by pausing and restarting his production ("un (0.2) nap-"), manifesting frustration ("AH::") and a new try ("ne"). This new try is overlapped by the therapist, who gives a hint; she suggests part of the target word by producing its beginning as an incomplete utterance to be completed – see the volume, the stretch, and the rising intonation (line 7). The patient responds by repeating the determiner, the first sound of the target word, which is self-repaired, and then the entire word, thus completing the therapist's previous suggestion (line 8). This production, nevertheless, is treated by both participants as inadequate; after a short pause, the patient self-repairs by "selecting" the problematic element of his production (the second syllable, line 10). The therapist repeats the word and corrects it by underlining, with the volume, the second syllable and insisting, with stretch, on the vowel sound (line 11).

In the following extract, the response of the patient to the therapist's question is produced with a delay (see the longue pause, line 2) and with a turn-initial device ("alors euh:," *well eh:*, line 3) that projects a possible difficulty in responding to and producing the target word ("camion," *truck*). Indeed, in the subsequent part of the turn, the patient produces several attempts, pauses, and an outbreath (line 3). The therapist restarts the sequence by offering a syntactic hint through an incomplete utterance with rising intonation (line 4).

Extract (2) (CHU_C_23february. Production of the word: "camion", /kamjɔ̃/, *truck*)

```
1  SLT=> qu'est-ce que c'est?
          what is it?
2         (1.3)
3  PAT    alors euh: (1.6) i:- (1.3) h: (0.2)
          well eh: (1.6) i:- (1.3) h: (0.2)
4  SLT=> c'est un:?
          it's a:?
5         (0.3)
6  PAT    .h: (0.2) un kav- -li euh ahr[:.tsk]
          .h: (0.2) a kav- -li eh ahr[: .tsk]
7  SLT=>                               [KA:mi::]jɔ̃=
                                       [KA:mi::]jɔ̃ =
8  PAT    =.h:: (0.6).tsk un (0.2) kavli (.) euh k-=
          =.h:: (0.6).tsk a (0.2) kavli (.) eh k-=
9  SLT=> =KA-MI-JƆ̃
         =KA-MI-JƆ̃
```

The patient's answer (line 6) is pronounced more quickly, recycling the determiner and producing two groups of sounds that are self-repaired by the patient, followed by a hesitation and a manifestation of effort ("ahr" and a dental click, ".tsk" at the end of line 6).

Following this long turn, in line 7, the therapist produces the target word. Nevertheless, the word is not pronounced in an ordinary way, but in a caricaturized and pedagogic way, with stretch and by segmenting it into three syllables. Indeed, the patient interprets it as a hint (versus a closure of the sequence), as he immediately (see the latching) takes the turn (line 8) and tries to repeat it as part of the original task – by producing the determiner – not without difficulty. Following the self-repair, the therapist, line 9, repeats the target word once more by segmenting it again in three units, with high volume and emphasis on the "J" sound, thus showing a focus on the pronunciation and articulation of the word.

These examples provide illustrations of the therapeutic activity and the types of problems addressed by the therapist when dealing with the patient's productions. In all of the examples, we can see how the hints given by the therapist do not only, turn by turn, adjust to what the patient was able to do in the previous turn (thus, very finely tuning to the sounds produced in what could seem, at first glance, only an "inadequate" response), but they also progressively guide the patient to exercising pronunciation and articulation of the target word as part of the task of labeling. Indeed, naming and word production in this context are treated, in a "normative" way, as producing/pronouncing the target word in the best and intelligible way (that is, not for issues of understandability; see also Bloch & Wilkinson, 2011). The activity is then centered on correcting and modeling the patient's speech productions. As the examples show, correction is realized mainly through prosodic means[7] (volume, stretch).

Patient's bodily conduct

Labeling or picture naming is a task situated in a specific ecology of action, which is characterized, among other things, by the use of artifacts, i.e., the cards to be named. Since the word to be produced corresponds to the image represented on the card, the patient generally performs the task by looking at the card. The therapist, instead, looks at the patient, monitoring their conduct and contributing then to defining a specific participation framework and bodily configuration (see Merlino, 2021b). Asymmetry in bodies' disposition and control is further emphasized in the hospital setting, where tasks are performed in the patient's room, while the patient is lying in their bed or sitting on a chair, with the therapist standing or sitting aside (versus in front). As shown later, this configuration does not favor a mutual gaze orientation.

As observed in the previous section, the patient's performance is characterized by several self-repairs and vocal manifestations of effort and/or inability to produce the target word or speech sound (e.g., vocal particles or response cries; Goffman, 1978). As this section underlines, these verbal and vocal productions are accompanied by specific embodied conduct, particularly closing of the eyes and mid-distant gaze in correspondence with self-repairs (cfr. Goodwin, 1983; Goodwin & Goodwin, 1986[8]).

In Extract 3, previously analyzed in its verbal dimension (Extract 1), I now underline some aspects related to the participant's embodied conduct. This extract is taken from a session taking place four days after the hospitalization of the patient. As we see in the multimodal transcription, at the beginning of the sequence, the patient looks at the card (fig. 1) and continues to orient to it during his response, while trying to produce the target word (lines 4–6). The vocal particle of line 6, which signals difficulty, is accompanied by the squeezing of the eyes (fig. 2).

Extract (3) (multimodal transcription of extract 1 - CHU_C_23february, /pwaro/, *leek*)

```
4   SLT   #qu'est-ce que c'e:st?
          what is it?
    pat   >>lks card-->
    fig   #fig.1
5         (0.4)
6   PAT   un °°p-°° (1.3) un (0.2) nap- (0.6)$#AH::$ (0.2) n[e
          a  °°p-°° (1.3) a  (0.2) nap- (0.6) $AH::$ (0.2) n[e
7   SLT                                                    [un P:WA::r,
                                                           [a  P:WA::r,
    pat   ---------------------->lks card->$closes eyes$opens eyes,lks card->
    fig                                    #fig.2
8   PAT   un p- (0.5) pwarœ
          a  p- (0.5) pwarœ
9         (0.2)
10  PAT   [$#rœ euh
          [rœ  eh
          ->$closes eyes-->1.14
    fig   #fig.3
11  SLT   [pwaR:O=
          [pwaR:O=
12  PAT   =£ouais£
          =yeah
          £nods£
13        (0.3)
14  PAT   $#ou[i:£
          ye[s:
```

186 Sara Merlino

```
          $opens eyes,lks card-->
    fig   #fig.4
```

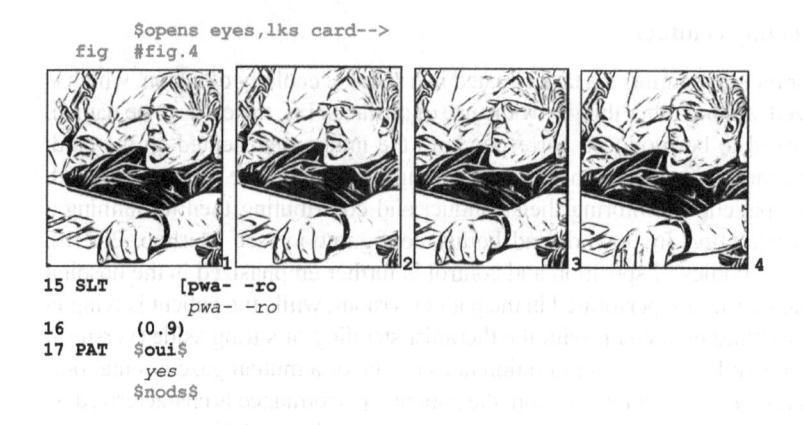

```
15  SLT      [pwa-  -ro
              pwa-  -ro
16           (0.9)
17  PAT      $oui$
              yes
             $nods$
```

The patient continues to look at the card during the turn of line 8, when he recycles the therapist's hint and completes the target word. As previously observed, this word is self-repaired with a repetition of the second syllable (line 10). The self-repair is accompanied by a closing of the eyes (fig. 3). Shortly after, the patient reopens his eyes (line 14, fig. 4), while nodding and acknowledging verbally, for the second time, the therapist's correction of line 11. He continues to look at the card when the therapist offers another correction at line 15. As a result, the suggestions and corrections of the therapist are responded to verbally by the patient and also through nodding but do not occasion a change in his gaze conduct, as he continues to orient toward the card and signals, through his bodily conduct, what he treats as relevant in the ongoing activity – naming a card "autonomously" while being accompanied and scaffolded by the therapist's *audible* suggestions.

Something very similar happens in the next extract, which consists of the multimodal representation of Extract 2, taken again from the same session as Extract 1. Here, the patient is involved in the production of the target word "camion," *truck*. The patient continues to look at the card from the beginning of the sequence (line 1) while trying to respond to the therapist's question (line 3). Moreover, he closes his eyes in correspondence with the self-repair of line 6 (fig. 5) and reopens them following the therapist's correction (line 7). The opening of the eyes coincides with a *mid-distant gaze* (line 8), whose trajectory changes when the patient takes a turn and tries to articulate a new response; here, he gazes at the card again (line 8, fig. 6).

Extract (4) (multimodal transcription of excerpt 2, CHU_C_23february, /kamjɔ̃/, *truck*)

```
1   SLT=>qu'est-ce que c'est?
         what is it?
    pat  >>lks card-->
2        (1.3)
3   PAT  alors euh: (1.6) i:- (1.3) h: (0.2)
         well eh: (1.6) i:- (1.3) h: (0.2)
4   SLT=>c'est un:?
         it's a:?
5        (0.3)
6   PAT  .h: (0.2) un kav- $#-li euh ahr[:$.tsk]
         .h: (0.2) a kav-    -li eh  ahr[: .tsk]
```

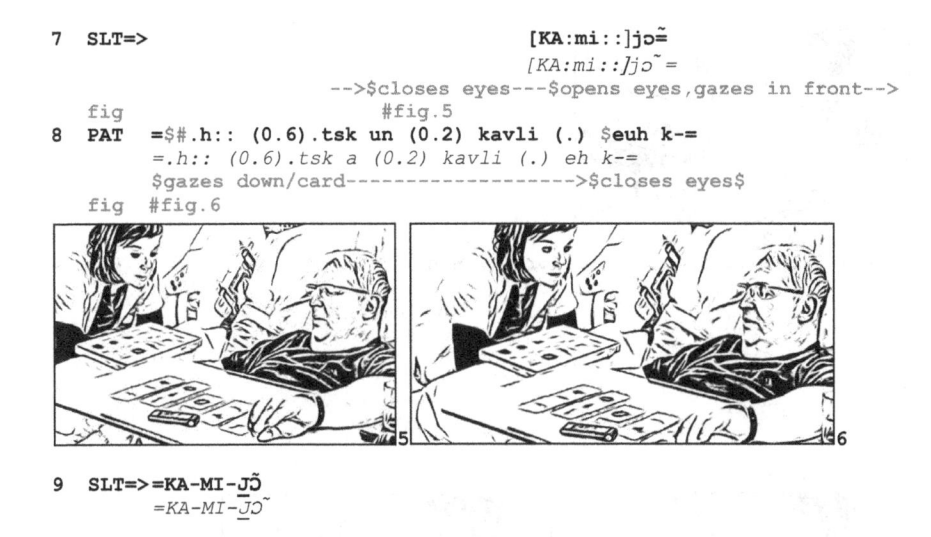

```
7   SLT=>                        [KA:mi::]jɔ̃=
                                 [KA:mi::]jɔ̃=
                         -->$closes eyes---$opens eyes,gazes in front-->
    fig                          #fig.5
8   PAT      =$#.h:: (0.6).tsk un (0.2) kavli (.) $euh k-=
             =.h:: (0.6).tsk a (0.2) kavli (.) eh k-=
             $gazes down/card------------------>$closes eyes$
    fig      #fig.6
```

```
9   SLT=>=KA-MI-JÕ
          =KA-MI-JƆ̃
```

Closing of the eyes as a signal of effort occurs again at the end of line 8, following another try and self-repair. The patient's embodied conduct (particularly gazing at the card, closing of the eyes and gaze withdrawal) accompanies different actions within the process of speech production (articulating, self-repairing, manifesting effort). Globally, the embodied conduct shows that the patient treats the difficulties in producing the target word as something that does not involve orienting to the therapist and soliciting her help.

Indeed, in our data, the patient's solicitation of the therapist's help in labeling activities happens only in specific sequential moments; that is, when the patient does not have any hints about how to respond to the task. In those cases, he mobilizes and solicits the therapist's help through gaze, thus doing something typically observed in both typical and atypical interactions (see Drew & Kendrick, 2018, for embodied recruitments, Goodwin & Goodwin 1986, for ordinary interactions, and Laakso, 2015, for interactions with aphasic speakers).[9]

In the following extract, the patient looks at the card (fig. 7) at the beginning of the sequence (line 1) and until the end of his turn, line 3: after a couple of attempts at producing the target item, he produces a long hesitation and turns his head toward the therapist, looking at her over the pause of line 4 (see fig. 8). This change in body posture results in the therapist's help and hint (line 5, see, for this practice, Merlino, 2018).

Extract (5) (CHU_C_23february, production of the word "cochon", /kɔʃɔ̃/, *pig)*

```
1   SLT      #qu'est-ce que c'e:st?
             what is it?
    pat      >>lks card-->
    fig      #fig.7
```

188 *Sara Merlino*

```
2            (0.2)
3   PAT    .h:: (0.6) .h. °f:: for-° +#euh::
           .h:: (0.6) .h. °f:: for-° +eh::
    pat                            -->+turns head tw,lks slt-->
    fig                                #fig.8
4            (0.6)
5   SLT    +#.tsk un,
            .tsk a,
    pat    +gazes in front/mid-distance gaze-->
    fig    #fig.9
6            (1.6)
7   SLT    Kɔ:
           Kɔ:
8            (0.3)
9   PAT    klɔ- (0.2) .hf:: (0.4)
           klʊ- (0.2) .hf:: (0.4)
10  SLT    ʃ::
           ʃ::
11         Ω(0.4)
    slt    Ωmouth's position on "ʃ"-->l.13
12  PAT    +kɔ-#lɔ- +°euh° non=
           kɔ- lɔ- °euh° no=
    pat    +........+closes eyes,thinking face--->l.17
```

After turning his head toward the therapist and gazing at her, the patient, line 5 (exactly when the therapist gives a syntactic hint), lowers his gaze (fig. 9), thus no longer engaging in mutual gazing anymore. This posture is maintained in the following turns. Indeed, the vocal suggestions/hints offered by the therapist (lines 7, 10) and followed by the patient's attempts at repeating them (lines 9, 12) are produced in a very specific *participatory configuration*; the therapist is constantly gazing at the patient (leaning toward him), and the patient is gazing in front and, when self-repairing (line 12), closes his eyes (line 12) and assumes a thinking face expression (with an embodied manifestation of effort). As a result, despite the cues offered by the therapist "vocally" as audible cues, the patient continues to perform the activity without orienting toward the therapist's body. Gaze orientation toward the therapist is indeed mobilized only at the beginning of the sequence when the patient seems to have no clue about the response and searches for the therapist's assistance. As soon as the therapist responds verbally to his invitation/solicitation by giving a hint, the patient shifts his gaze and either orients to the card or in front of him but not toward the therapist.

Instructing the patient to gaze at the therapist's mouth

As previously stated, following the patient's difficulties in repeating the speech sounds or words suggested by the therapist, the therapist generally modifies the trajectory of the scaffolding and progressively involves the patient in an emphasized production of the target item, which involves not only the audible dimension but also the visual one, through the mobilization of facial cues, such as mouth and lip position. This demonstration requires the patient's visual attention; nevertheless, as observed in the previous section, the patient generally does not orient to the therapist during these tasks. Consequently, the therapist deploys a series of resources to solicit the patient's gaze.

In the following extract, this is done with a *verbal instruction* (the directive "look at me"), which is preceded by a gesture of the therapist's (*grasping of her chin*) that highlights a specific area of the face, *her lips*, as the focus of attention (line 16).

Extract (6) (continuation of extract 5, CHU_C_23february, /kɔʃɔ̃/, *pig*)

```
13 SLT    ⊥=non
          =no
          ⊥...-->
14 PAT    #°euh[: non°
           °eh[: no°
    pat   >>closes eyes,thinking face-->
    fig   #fig.10
```

```
15 SLT            [KƆ:
                  [KƆ:
16          ⊥#(0.1)
    slt   ⊥grasps chin wt hand-->>
17 SLT    >re+gardez-moi<
          >look at me<
    pat   -->+opens eyes-->
```

```
18      +$(0.4)
   pat  +turns head tw,lks slt-->
   pat  $opens mouth-->
   fig  #fig.11
19 SLT  KO::
        KƆ::
   fig  #fig.12
20      $(0.2)
   pat  $rounded lips-->
21 PAT  kɔ::
        kɔ::
```

Before formulating the instruction, the therapist gives (again, as she did in the extract analyzed in the previous section) a vocal hint, as she pronounces, with high volume and stretch, the first syllable of the target word (line 15). The hint is produced while approaching the chin with her hand, thus showing an orientation toward the relevance of her mouth position. Given that the patient, at this precise moment, is not gazing at the therapist and is even closing his eyes (fig. 10), the therapist formulates the instruction "regardez-moi," *look at me* (line 17). The patient immediately opens his eyes and turns his head toward the therapist (fig. 11). Note that, while he changes his posture, he also produces an inbreath in line 18 (which is visible in the video through an opening of his mouth); thus, he projects turn-taking, treating the directive as part of the previous hint ("KO::"), making a response conditionally relevant. This interpretation is nevertheless revised by the therapist's immediate repetition of the first syllable in line 19. The turn of the therapist is characterized by a high volume and stretch of the target sound and is produced with rising intonation. It is performed with an emphasized position of the mouth that allows for underlining the articulatory aspects of the target sound (see fig. 12). Within this *bodily (face-to-face) configuration*, with the patient looking at the therapist's face, the patient achieves the repetition of the target sounds (line 21).

The entire activity (labeling/producing a target word) is then redefined as syllable-by-syllable repetition, guided by the therapist, and continues within this bodily configuration. Following the patient's turn, the therapist goes on not only keeping the same emphasized mouth position (which is mirrored by the patient during the following short pause, see line 22, fig. 13) but also producing a new sound, pronounced with the same lip position (line 23).

Socializing patients in language therapy 191

Extract (7) ("(continuation of extract 6, CHU_C_23february, /kɔʃɔ̃/, *pig*)
```
22      §(0.2)
   pat  §rounded lips-->
   slt  >>grasps chin wt hand-->1.28
   fig  #fig.13
23 SLT  ʃ::
        ʃ::
24      §(0.4)
   pat  §rounded lips-->
25 PAT  ʃɔ̃
        ʃɔ̃
26      £(0.3)⌊£
   slt  £nods£
   slt  withdraws hand⌊
27 SLT  bravo, (0.2) kɔʃɔ̃.
        well done, (0.2) kɔʃɔ̃.
```

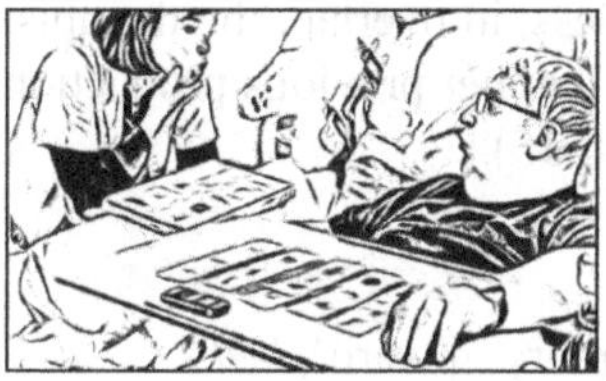

[Figure 13]

The patient responds by repeating the target sound and completing the unit with the nasal vowel (line 25). By completing the unit, the patient shows an orientation toward the original aim of the task, producing the target word and thus showing his capacity to complete the task by himself. The therapist evaluates his production, first by withdrawing her hand and nodding and secondly by formulating a positive evaluation and repeating the target word with a downgrading intonation (line 27).

The relevance of gaze direction is thus introduced by the therapist with an explicit directive (Extract 6, line 17) and a body posture that makes the fact of looking, not only at her face but, more precisely, *at her mouth*, to benefit from the visual cue, together with the audible cue, visible and relevant. The emphasized body position makes the patient's imitation/mirroring of the therapist's mouth relevant and favors the recognition and reproduction of the target sounds. The target word is then produced as part of an exercise of pronunciation, realized progressively, that is, unit by unit and with a specific bodily configuration, in which the patient is oriented toward the therapist.

In this sequence (composed of Extracts 6 and 7), things work quite smoothly, as the request for gaze by the therapist is immediately followed by a change in the gaze orientation of the patient, who continues to look at the therapist until the completion of the sequence, by responding to the embodied instruction in a successful way.

Sometimes, instead, more effort is needed to invite the patient to maintain his visual attention on the therapist's mouth and to align with the type of projected actions. This is related to the fact that this practice needs to be made accountable; that is, gaze solicitation needs to be understood not only as a summoning device by evoking a different participatory framework for solving the task together, but as part of a therapeutic method that consists of gazing at the therapist's lips to solve speech difficulties.

As shown in the following extract, after some attempts by the patient to produce the word "poireau," *leek* (extract previously analyzed), the therapist proposes to restart the sequence (line 19). She offers the beginning of the target word (line 21), which is elongated and pronounced with rising intonation. The patient responds in line 22 not only by repeating this syllable but also by completing it, thus orienting to the production of the entire target word. Nevertheless, in overlap, the therapist produces the second syllable (line 23), thus showing that her previous production was intended as syllable-by-syllable repetition (fig. 14, 15).

Extract (8) (continuation of extract 3, CHU_C_23february, /pwaro/, *leek*)

```
18         (0.4)
19 SLT=> on essaie de redire?
           we try to say again?
20         θ(0.3)
    pat    θopens mouth-->
21 SLT     pθwa:,θ
    pat    θcloses mouthθ
22 PAT     pwa[rœ
           pwa[rœ
23 SLT         [ro.
               [ro.
24         (.)
25 PAT     °rœ°
           °rœ°
26 SLT     ro
           ro
27         θ(0.8)θ
    pat    θarticulates « ro » with the mouthθ
28 SLT=> +regardez-moi,
           look at me,
           +.....................-->
29         $+(0.7)
    pat    $turns head tws SLT-->
    SLT=> +points tws chin-->
30 SLT     r::o
           r::o
31         +(1.0+$0.3)
    slt=> +makes a circle around her lips+
    pat         $nods,turns head in front,lks card-->
32 PAT     +p+wa:- (.) -rœ (.)$ro$
           pwa:- (.) -rœ (.) ro
    slt    +lowers hand+
    pat                      $raises head,gazes up-->
```

In what follows, the patient aligns with the therapist's hint by repeating the target sounds' unit (line 25). Following the new correction of the therapist in line 26, the patient engages in articulatory movements with his mouth (line 27). Note that, up to now, the patient has not gazed at the therapist. The difficulty of articulation (as manifested in the patient's mouth movements) is then addressed by the therapist. She first invites the patient to look at her (line 28) while she starts to point toward her chin (line 29); she then (line 30) engages in a corrective embodied (audio-visual) demonstration of the target sounds.

In the following pause (31), the therapist makes a circle around her lips with her index finger, further emphasizing the target mouth position. Immediately after, the patient nods and turns his head, looking back at the card. He then reengages in the production of the entire word (line 32), again showing difficulty in the articulation of the final vowel (see the self-repair). Note that his gaze direction (from the therapist toward the card and then gazing up as part of the self-repair) indicates the way he treats the therapist's hints. Moving back to his "private" and autonomous resolution of the task of word production, he shows then a preference for producing the target word by himself.

The therapist then reopens the sequence; after a dental click, following which the patient turns his head toward the therapist, the therapist repeats the entire word (line 35) and at the same time points her finger toward her lips again (line 36). The patient interprets the therapist's turn as projecting a completion (as he produces the vowel in overlap with the therapist's turn, 36); he then nods and lowers his gaze, looking back at the card (line 37).

Extract (9) (continuation of extract 8, CHU_C_23february, /pwaro/, *leek*)

```
33 SLT    .tsk
          .tsk
34        $(0.3)
   pat    -->$turns h tws slt-->
35 SLT    +pwa- -r:::[o
          pwa- -r:::[o
36 PAT         [$°°o°°
                [°°o°°
   slt    +pts tws lips-->
   pat                $.........
37        $(0.9)$
   pat    $nods,lowers gaze$
38 SLT    [on essaie >jus[te<
          [we >just< [try
39 PAT    [.h            [ma:
          [.h            [ma:
40        (.)
41 SLT=>regar[dez-moi,
          look at me,
42 PAT         [ah non
                oh no
```

```
43         $(0.8)
   pat    $turns h/lks slt-->
44 SLT    O:
          O:
45         (0.2)
46 SLT=>>essayez< de dire O=
          try to say O=
47 PAT    =o
          =o
48         (0.3)
49 SLT    pwaro
          pwaro
50         (0.3     $1)
   pat    ->lks slt$lks down-->
51 PAT    pwa$rœ
          pwarœ
   pat    -->$lks slt-->
```

Note that despite the withdrawal of gaze, the patient does not abandon the task; his inbreath and the subsequent sound production (line 39) show that he is still engaged in the activity of producing the target word (see the self-repair, line 42). The therapist then again solicits the patient's visual attention with the directive (line 41), to which the patient responds by turning his face toward the therapist again and looking at her (line 43). A new performance of the target sound is realized in line 44; focusing on the single vowel "O=," the therapist asks the patient explicitly to reproduce only the problematic sound (line 46), which is done by the patient by maintaining a mutual gaze (line 47). She then goes back to the production of the entire word (line 49), which is repeated by the patient (line 51). Note that this time, he lowers his gaze during the pause of line 50 and reorients toward the therapist only when producing the final (and problematic) part of his turn.

As a result, the extract confirms that gaze orientation is mobilized by the therapist to assist the patient in speech production by offering a visual cue (lip position) that allows for an audio-visual demonstration of the target sounds. These demonstrations are used when audible demonstrations, as prosodically emphasized repetitions of the target sounds, are not sufficient to help the patient produce them. The extract shows that the use of audio-visual cues in the form of embodied demonstrations requires specific bodily coordination, explicitly solicited by the directives on gaze orientation within a vocal activity and a participatory configuration that, for different reasons, does not favor the patient's gaze orientation toward the therapist. Consequently, the patient *is instructed* to benefit from the therapist's audio-visual hints and to solve speech difficulties collaboratively by maintaining a mutual gaze orientation.

It seems that there is a strict connection between maintaining mutual gaze for accomplishing the task and understanding the therapist's embodied audio-visual performance as a hint for producing the target word or as a request for a unit-by-unit repetition of the single sound units in which the word is decomposed. Indeed, in the previous extract, when solicited to gaze at the therapist, the patient gazed at the therapist during the embodied demonstration but then withdrew his gaze when producing the entire word by himself. When the embodied demonstration is clearly designed as a request for repetition of single vocal units, the patient maintains a mutual gaze.

Indeed, in the following extract, the therapist not only invites the patient to look (line 59), but she also gives instructions about the temporality (line 61) and the turn-taking rules of the activity, which is explicitly designed as repetition (line 63).

Extract (10) (continuation of extract 4, some lines omitted, CHU_C_23february, / kamjɔ̃/, *truck*)

```
52 SLT   M:I
         M:I
53       (0.2)
54 SLT   M[:I
         M:I
55 PAT   [euh
         eh
56       (0.7)
57 PAT   +£#>ah oui<£ (0.3) .h: (0.7) k ø (.) ka- (0.2) mh- va
         >oh yes< (0.3) .h: (0.7) k ø (.) ka- (0.2) mh- va
   pat   +withdraws gaze,lks up--->
   pat   £nods£
   fig   #fig.14
58       +(0.3)
   pat   +lks down--->
59 SLT=>>REGARDEZ<=
         >look<
60 PAT   +=.h::
         .h::
   pat   +lks slt->
61 SLT=>on va le faire doucement.
         we will do it slowly
62       +#(0.4)
   pat   +turns head tws slt->>
   fig   #fig.15
```

```
63 SLT=>vous répétez après moi.=
        you repeat after me.=
64 PAT  =ou[i
        yes
65 SLT     [KA
            KA
66         (0.2)
67 PAT  ka:
        ka:
68      (.)
69 SLT  M:I
        M:I
70 PAT  m:i
        m:i
71      (0.2)
72 SLT  ʒ
        ʒ
73      (.)
74 PAT  ʒ
        ʒ
75      (0.2)
76 SLT  ka:mj:ʒ
        ka:mj:ʒ
77      (0.6)
78 PAT  ka- mi- jʒ
        ka- mi- jʒ
79      *(0.3)*
   slt  *nods*
80 SLT  *+bravo*
        well done
   slt  *nods*
   pat     +turns h in front, gazes down>>
```

Following the therapist's directive, the patient modifies his body posture. He first raises his gaze and looks at the therapist (line 60), then further turns his head toward her (see line 62, fig. 15). He then engages in the activity, repeating the therapist's turns while continuing to look at her (lines 67, 70, 74, 78). The task is then accomplished within a mutual gaze configuration, which is abandoned only after the therapist's non-verbal acknowledgment in line 79.

Finally, audio-visual cues based on the reproduction of the target sound, with a focus on the mouth's position, require a specific bodily configuration, as well as a precise organization of the pair corrective instruction and instructed action. In addition to the crucial role of the audio-visual hints offered by the therapist during the task in assisting in speech production, clear-cut instructions about the procedure of scaffolding (and subsequent modification of the original activity) and segmentation of the speech units are a constitutive part of the instructional work realized by the therapist to guide the patient in the accomplishment of the therapeutic task and to allow him to benefit from the scaffolding audio-visual therapeutic technique.

Gazing at the therapist's mouth to solve speech difficulties: A learned social practice?

In this last section, I analyze a couple of extracts taken from the very last session I recorded at the hospital, which took place the day before the patient was discharged. This is two weeks after the patient was admitted to the neurovascular unit, started his recovery, and went through daily therapeutic sessions. The extracts show that the patient himself, when experiencing a speech difficulty, orients, quite early, and without any instructions, to the therapist, by looking at her face, and solves the speech difficulty by benefiting from the audio-visual cue (mouth position). Although I acknowledge the fact that this change in the patient's conduct could be related to medical/cognitive change (e.g., ability to orientate), the patient seems to have integrated, possibly learned, the social practice of gazing at the therapist's mouth to solve a speech difficulty as part of the process of socialization to which he was exposed during the therapy. Note that the patient in the session analyzed here is sitting on a chair near his bed, so he is less constrained in his movements than in the extracts previously analyzed (where he was lying down in his bed). Moreover, the therapist sits laterally. A different organization of the ecology of the activity could then impact/favor a mutual gaze configuration.

In Extract 11, the participants are again involved in a labeling activity. The word to be produced is "livre," *book*. Following the therapist's request, the patient engages in the search while looking at the card and assuming a thinking posture, with his hand on his forehead (fig.16).

Extract (11) (CHU_C_02March. Production of the word:"livre", /livʁ/, *book*)

```
1  SLT     ⊥#c'est quoi ça?
           what is this?
   slt     ⊥pts on card-->
   pat     >>lks card, hand on his forehead-->
   fig     #fig.16
```

```
2          ⊥(1.3)⊥
   slt     ⊥taps on card⊥
3  PAT     euh:: (.) le:: (0.7)
           eh:: (.) the:: (0.7)
4  SLT     c'est un::?
           it's a?
5          (0.4)
6  PAT     un:: (0.5) °mh° viv:- uhv (0.3)
           a:: (0.5) °mh° viv:- uhv (0.3)
7  SLT     L::
           r..
```

198 Sara Merlino

```
7   SLT         L::
                L::
8               *#(0.2      +£#0.6)
    pat=>       *lks slt-->
    pat=>                   +raises h-->
    slt                     £raises h and opens mouth-->
    fig         #fig.17     #fig.18
9   SLT         l::[:
                l::[:
10  PAT            [l:i- (0.2) *⌊-vʁ.⌋
                    l:i- (0.2)   -vʁ.
    pat                     --->*lowers gaze
    slt                         ⌊nods⌋
```

[figures 17 and 18]

Following the patient's hesitations (line 3), the therapist gives a syntactic cue (line 4) that is recycled by the patient in the following turn (line 6); he produces an item that is immediately self-repaired ("viv – uhv", line 6). Detecting a phonemic problem, the therapist gives a hint, suggesting (and correcting) the first sound of the target word. This hint is produced with high volume and stretching (line 7), as observed in previous extracts. In this case, the patient immediately raises his gaze toward the therapist and continues to look at her throughout the entire pause (line 8), further raising his head (see fig.17). In response, the therapist reproduces the mouth's position of the target sound (see fig.18) and audibly reproduces it in line 9. The patient, in overlap, takes the turn, repeats the sound, and completes the unit by producing the entire target word (line 10). Indeed, the phonemic suggestion allows him not only to repeat the target sound, but also to find the entire target word. Note that the patient continues to look at the therapist's mouth throughout these turns and lowers his gaze only when producing the second syllable of the target word (end of line 10).

In the next and last extract, the patient is involved in a different activity – that is, a conversation solicited by the therapist's questions. She asked what the patient did on the weekend, and he explained that he had some visits from family members. The therapist formulates a question with a known answer (see Macbeth, 2004) by asking who these family members were, and the patient enumerates a list of three members (his wife, his son, and his daughter). As the therapist knows who the patient's family members are (this is ethnographic information I have), she can assist him in the production of the three words designating them (wife, son, daughter). After having named his "wife" and his "son," the patient engages in the production of the word "fille," *daughter*. The production

Socializing patients in language therapy 199

of this word is characterized by typical *searching conduct* (fig. 19): gazing down and doing gestures typically found in connection with word searches (Goodwin & Goodwin, 1986).

Extract (12) (CHU_C_02March. Production of the word "fille", /fij/, *daughter*)

```
1  PAT      [et] (0.4) $*#1- la:
            [and] (0.4) th- the: (fem.)
   pat                  $gazes down
   pat                    *raises and taps hand-->
   fig                      #fig.19
2           (0.5)
3  SLT      et ma,
            and my,
            --->
4           Ω(0.5)
   slt      Ωmouth position on °f°-->
5  PAT      °m-°
            °m-°
6           (0.3*0.3)
   pat      -->*taps on table-->
7  SLT      f:*::-
            f:::-
   pat      --*
8           (0.6)
9  PAT=>    +$oui+
            yes
            +nods+
       =>   $raise head/gaze tws slt-->
   fig      #fig.20
```

10   (0.5)
11 SLT   ma °f:-°
            my °f:-°
12   (0.4)
13 PAT   +fi$j.+
            fij.
            +nods+
            $lowers gaze-->

The turn in line 1 (where the definitive article is produced) is corrected by the therapist (line 3) with the production of the possessive pronoun ("ma"), thus offering a syntactic frame for the word that designates a family member. She then positions her mouth on the target sound "f" without pronouncing it (line

4). After a pause, the patient produces the "m" sound with low volume, while he continues to gesticulate, tapping his fingers on the table (line 6). Once (line 7) the therapist suggests the beginning of the target word audibly (by stretching it), the patient acknowledges the therapist's production; this is done by nodding and raising his head and looking at the therapist (fig. 20). During the following pause (line 10), the patient continues to gaze at the therapist, making her assistance relevant. She then repeats the hint (line 11), emphasizing her mouth's position; this is followed by the patient's production of the target word (line 13). As a consequence, through his embodied conduct – gazing at the therapist *after* this latter has produced a phonemic hint and continuing to look at her throughout the sequence – the patient displays an orientation to a collaborative resolution of the word production and contributes to building the local relevance of the audio-visual hint.

Conclusion

Through scrutiny of the micro-details of interaction, this chapter explored how the instructional dimension of speech–language therapy is accomplished. The chapter took as its point of departure the organization of a specific activity, labeling, which is often used in this therapeutic context to treat and recover, from its very onset, language impairment, such as aphasia. By analyzing the scaffolding resources used by therapists to assist the patient in producing the target words and speech sounds, this chapter focused on the therapeutic practice that consists of gazing at the therapist's mouth to benefit from audio-visual representations – or embodied demonstrations – of the target speech sounds. This social practice requires the patient to address their gaze toward the therapist's mouth; nevertheless, as the analytical sections showed, achieving a mutual gaze configuration in this setting and within this specific type of activity requires some interactional work.

Firstly, the analyses emphasized the organization and the specificities of the task of labeling. Particularly, I showed that the patient's speech productions are generally the object of corrections and modelling (Extracts 1–2). In order to assist the patient in producing the target word in the most intelligible way, the therapist mobilizes different types of resources: (s)he gives the beginning of the target word and isolates and emphasizes, through prosodic means, the target speech sounds. Pronunciation is realized in a pedagogic way so that the patient is progressively guided into exercising articulatory aspects of speech sounds.

Secondly, the analysis focused on participants' bodily conduct and highlighted a general pattern related to the patient's gaze conduct during the accomplishment of these tasks (Extracts 3–5); particularly, a constant orientation toward the card to be named was observed. This orientation is related not only to the aims of the activity, but also to the ecology of action – with the patient lying positioned in his bed and a small table positioned in front of him. While being oriented with his body (particularly face) toward the card, the patient can close his eyes or engage in mid-distant gaze when encountering difficulties and when initiating self-repairs. Modifications of this embodied conduct – particularly, turning toward and gazing at the therapist – are mobilized to solicit help (see Drew & Kendrick, 2018 on embodied recruitments), but quickly "reabsorbed": indeed, once the therapist takes the turn to give a hint, the patient reorients their gaze toward the card and performs repetitions of the therapists' hint in this bodily position. These embodied conducts are coherent with general patterns observed in typical and atypical interactions, in both ordinary and institutional settings of interaction, when dealing with speakers' difficulties in speech production – i.e., where the gaze toward the interlocutor is mobilized for *soliciting help* (see, for instance, Goodwin & Goodwin, 1986, Laakso & Klippi, 1999, Laakso, 2015).

Nevertheless, as the analysis of Extracts 6–10 showed, when the therapist mobilizes specific forms of help such as the facial cues, with embodied demonstrations of the target speech sounds, the patient's gaze toward the therapist's face/mouth assumes a prominent different function: it is treated as a prerequisite to pursue the instructional activity itself (see also Sanchez Svensson et al. 2009, Stukenbrock, 2014). As a consequence, the therapist deploys verbal directives ("look/look at me") and specific professional gestures (grasping of the chin, pointing gestures, see also Merlino, 2021b) in order to focus the patient's attention on their face and lips. Instructions about a specific embodied conduct to be assumed by the instructed person (more than instructions about the task at hand) are then a specificity of this institutional and therapeutic setting of interaction and of the types of tasks that are performed.

Moreover, it seems that there is a strict connection between maintaining mutual gaze for accomplishing the task and understanding the therapist's embodied audio-visual performance as a hint for producing the target word or as a request for a unit-by-unit repetition of the single sound units in which the word is decomposed. When the embodied demonstration is clearly designed as a request for the repetition of single vocal units, the patient maintains a mutual gaze. As a consequence, we observed clear-cut instructions about the "procedure" of scaffolding as part of the instructional work realized by the therapist to guide the patient not only to assume specific bodily conduct, but also in adequately adjusting to the sequential organization of the pair corrective instruction and instructed action. Indeed, during these sequences, the therapist instructs the patient, in relation to both the embodied and temporal organization of the practice, to (1) gaze at the therapist at specific moments (when the therapist's audible hint was not effective), (2) keep their gaze addressed to the therapist's mouth, and (3) repeat (versus complete) the therapist's vocal productions. As a consequence, the patient goes through a process of socialization in the practices (here, in Garfinkel's terms) through which, progressively, they exercise and produce units of speech.

The extracts analyzed in the last analytical section (see Extracts 11–12) allowed me to argue that socialization in visual forms of cues/hints seems to be achieved when, without any instruction, the patient addresses by himself the therapist's face quite early in the sequence. The analyses showed that the phonemic hint produced by the therapist is followed by a modification of the patient's gaze conduct, as the patient orients immediately toward the therapist: the therapist then repeats the previous turn (the phonemic hint) and the patient, while he continues to look at the therapist, repeats the target sound and completes it by producing the entire word. The patient then displays an orientation to the collaborative resolution of speech production and contributes to building the local relevance of the audio-visual hint.

Finally, the analyses of excerpts taken from different sessions with the same patient suggested that this results from the socialization of the patient in the requirements of the therapeutic activity and to the intelligibility of a therapeutic practice for solving speech difficulties. This was sustained by an analysis of the phenomenon over time, as I considered the embodied conduct of the same patient during 4 different therapeutic sessions that took place over 15 days. Though more data are needed to generalize these claims, the results of the analyses underline the necessity of conceiving this health setting as a specific form of social interaction in which members – particularly the patient – are socialized not only to accomplish the tasks in a structured and ordered way but also to adopt new forms of communication that are related both to their new condition (due to the aphasic pathology) and to the instructional dimension of the setting in which they find themselves interacting.

Acknowledgments

I wish to thank the editor and an anonymous reviewer for their careful reading and insightful comments on an earlier version of the text.

Notes

1 Demonstrations are generally defined as "performances of a task-like activity out of its visual context to allow someone who is not the performer to obtain a close picture of the doing of the activity" (Goffman, 1974, p. 66).
2 In L2 classroom interactions, teachers use gestures and mouth positions for teaching the pronunciation of a second language, particularly for the identification of suprasegmental features, such as stress and rhythm (Smotrova, 2017).
3 On the basis of experiences in which the speaker with aphasia is assisted by a computer that provides audible and visible cues, such as mouth shape, Fridriksson et al. (2009) showed, for instance, that audio-visual treatments worked better than audio-only treatments.
4 In aphasiology, longitudinal studies are recurrent, but generally based on *questionnaires* and developed by psychologists and neurologists working with experimental frameworks.
5 In total, 13 patients (with fluent, non-fluent, mixed aphasia) and 9 speech–language therapists were involved in the fieldwork and in the recordings.
6 I thank an anonymous reviewer for raising this point.
7 These means, together with their sequential position, make different types of actions by the patient, either recycling and completing the hint given by the therapist or repeating it, also relevant.
8 Research on word searches in ordinary, typical interactions has highlighted not only their linguistic and collaborative dimension (see, e.g., Schegloff et al., 1977; Lerner, 1991) but also the crucial role played by embodied resources in the searching process and in the organization of the participation framework, by involving or not involving the interlocutors in the search (such as gaze withdrawal, Goodwin, 1983, and "thinking face," Goodwin & Goodwin, 1986, in the initial phase of the search, and gaze shifts, from and toward the interlocutor to solicit interlocutor's participation – see Bolden, 2003; Hayashi, 2003; Iwasaki, 2009; Dressel, 2020).

9 Research on interactions with people with aphasia shows that the collaborative involvement of healthy partners can be solicited by non-verbal means, such as gaze and pointing gestures (Laakso & Klippi, 1999; Helasvuo et al., 2004; Laakso, 2015).

References

Bloch, S., & Wilkinson, R. (2011). Acquired dysarthria in conversation: Methods of resolving understandability problems. *International Journal of Language and Communication Disorders, 46*(5), 510–523. https://doi.org/10.1111/j.1460-6984.2011.00076.x

Bolden, G. B. (2003). Multiple modalities in collaborative turn sequences. *Gesture, 3*(2), 187–212. https://doi.org/10.1075/gest.3.2.04bol

Damico, J. S., Oelschlaeger, M., & Simmons-Mackie, N. (1999). Qualitative methods in aphasia research: Conversation analysis. *Aphasiology, 13*(9–11), 667–679. https://doi.org/10.1080/026870399401777

Dressel, D. (2020). Multimodal word searches in collaborative storytelling: On the local mobilization and negotiation of coparticipation. *Journal of Pragmatics, 170,* 37–54. https://doi.org/10.1016/j.pragma.2020.08.010

Drew, P., & Kendrick, K. H. (2018). Searching for trouble: Recruiting assistance through embodied action. *Social Interaction: Video-Based Studies of Human Sociality, 1*(1). https://doi.org/10.7146/si.v1i1.105496

Evans, B., & Reynolds, E. (2016). The organization of corrective demonstrations using embodied action in sports coaching feedback. *Symbolic Interaction, 39*(4), 525–556. https://doi.org/10.1002/symb.255

Ferguson, A., & Armstrong, E. (2004). Reflections on speech-language therapists' talk: Implications for clinical practice and education. *International Journal of Language and Communication Disorders, 39*(4), 469–477. https://doi.org/10.1080/1368282042000226879

Fridriksson, J., Baker, J. M., Whiteside, J., Eoute, D., Jr., Moser, D., Vesselinov, R., & Rorden, C. (2009). Treating visual speech perception to improve speech production in nonfluent aphasia. *Stroke, 40*(3), 853–858. https://doi.org/10.1161/STROKEAHA.108.532499

Garfinkel, H. (2002). *Ethnomethodology's program: Working out Durkheim's aphorism.* Rowman & Littlefield Publishers.

Goffman, E. (1974). *Frame analysis: An essay on the organization of experience.* Northeastern UP.

Goffman, E. (1978). Response cries. *Language, 54*(4), 787–815. https://doi.org/10.2307/413235

Goodwin, C. (2000). Action and embodiment within situated human interaction. *Journal of Pragmatics, 32*(10), 1489–1522. https://doi.org/10.1016/S0378-2166(99)00096-X

Goodwin, C. (2003). Pointing as situated practice. In Kita, S. (ed), *Pointing: Where language, culture and cognition meet* (pp. 217–241). Lawrence Erlbaum.

Goodwin, M. H. (1983). Searching for a word as an interactive activity. In *Semiotics 1981* (pp. 129–137). Springer.

Goodwin, M. H., & Goodwin, C. (1986). Gesture and coparticipation in the activity of searching for a word. *Semiotica: Journal of the International Association for Semiotic Studies/Revue de l'Association Internationale de Sémiotique, 62*(1–2), 51–76. https://doi.org/10.1515/semi.1986.62.1-2.51

Hayashi, M. (2003). Language and the body as resources for collaborative action: A study of word searches in Japanese conversation. *Research on Language and Social Interaction, 36*(2), 109–141. https://doi.org/10.1207/S15327973RLSI3602_2

Helasvuo, M.-L., Laakso, M., & Sorjonen, M.-L. (2004). Searching for words: Syntactic and sequential construction of word search in conversations of Finnish speakers with aphasia. *Research on Language and Social Interaction, 37*(1), 1–37. https://doi.org/10.1207/s15327973rlsi3701_1

Horton, S. (2006). A framework for description and analysis of therapy for language impairment in aphasia. *Aphasiology, 20*(6), 528–564. https://doi.org/10.1080/02687030600590130

Horton, S., & Byng, S. (2000). Examining interaction in language therapy. *International Journal of Language and Communication Disorders, 35*(3), 355–375. https://doi.org/10.1080/136828200410627

Ikeya, N. (2020). Hybridity of hybrid studies of work: Examination of informing practitioners in practice. *Ethnographic Studies, 17*, 22–40. https://doi.org/10.5281/zenodo.4050533

Iwasaki, S. (2009). Initiating interactive turn spaces in Japanese conversation: Local projection and collaborative action. *Discourse Processes, 46*(2–3), 226–246. https://doi.org/10.1080/01638530902728918

Jefferson, G. (1987). Exposed and embedded corrections. In Button, G. and Lee, J.R.E. (eds.), *Talk and social organization* (pp. 86–100). Multilingual Matters.

Jefferson, G. (2004). Glossary of transcript symbols. In G. H. Lerner (ed.), *Conversation analysis: Studies from the First Generation* (pp. 24–31). John Benjamins.

Keevallik, L. (2010). Bodily quoting in dance correction. *Research on Language and Social Interaction, 43*(4), 401–426. https://doi.org/10.1080/08351813.2010.518065

Keevallik, L. (2013). Here in time and space: Decomposing movement in dance instruction. In *Interaction and mobility: Language and the body in motion* (pp. 345–370). De Gruyter. https://doi.org/10.1515/9783110291278.345

Klippi, A. (2015). Pointing as an embodied practice in aphasic interaction. *Aphasiology, 29*(3), 337–354. https://doi.org/10.1080/02687038.2013.878451

Klippi, A., & Ahopalo, L. (2008). The interplay between verbal and non-verbal behaviour in aphasic word search in conversation. In Klippi, A. and Launonen, K. (eds.), *Research in Logopedics. Speech and language therapy in Finland, Series communication disorders across languages* (pp. 146–171). Multilingual Matters.

Koschmann, T., LeBaron, C., Goodwin, C., & Feltovich, P. (2011). "Can you see the cystic artery yet?" A simple matter of trust. *Journal of Pragmatics, 43*(2), 521–541. https://doi.org/10.1016/j.pragma.2009.09.009

Laakso, M. (2015). Collaborative participation in aphasic word searching: Comparison between significant others and speech and language therapists. *Aphasiology, 29*(3), 269–290. https://doi.org/10.1080/02687038.2013.878450

Laakso, M., & Klippi, A. (1999). A closer look at the 'hint and guess' sequences in aphasic conversation. *Aphasiology, 13*(4–5), 345–363. https://doi.org/10.1080/026870399402136

Lerner, G. H. (1991). On the syntax of sentences-in-progress. *Language in Society, 20*(3), 441–458. https://doi.org/10.1017/S0047404500016572

Lesser, R., & Milroy, M. (1993). *Linguistics and aphasia: Psycholinguistic and pragmatic aspects of intervention.* Longman.

Lindwall, O., & Ekström, A. (2012). Instruction-in-interaction: The teaching and learning of a manual skill. *Human Studies, 35*(1), 27–49. https://doi.org/10.1007/s10746-012-9213-5

Macbeth, D. (2004). The relevance of repair for classroom correction. *Language in Society, 33*(5), 703–736. https://doi.org/10.1017/S0047404504045038

Martin, C., & Sahlström, F. (2010). Learning as longitudinal interactional change: From other-repair to self-repair in physiotherapy treatment. *Discourse Processes, 47*(8), 668–697. https://doi.org/10.1080/01638531003628965

McHoul, A. (1978). The organization of turns at formal talk in the classroom. *Language in Society*, *7*(2), 183–213. https://doi.org/10.1017/S0047404500005522

Mehan, H. (1979). What time is it, Denise?: Asking known information questions in classroom discourse. *Theory into Practice*, *18*(4), 285–294. https://doi.org/10.1080/00405847909542846

Merlino, S. (2017). Initiatives topicales du client aphasique au cours de séances de rééducation: Pratiques interactionnelles et enjeux identitaires. In *Participation et asymétries dans l'interaction institutionnelle* (pp. 53–94). L'Harmattan.

Merlino, S. (2018). Assisting the client in aphasia speech therapy: A sequential and multimodal analysis of cueing practices. *Hacettepe University Journal of Education*, *33*, 334–357. https://doi.org/10.16986/HUJE.2018038810

Merlino, S. (2020). Professional touch in speech and language therapy for the treatment of post-stroke aphasia. In *Touch in social interaction* (pp. 197–223). Routledge.

Merlino, S. (2021a). Making sounds visible in speech-language therapy for aphasia. *Social Interaction. Video-Based Studies of Human Sociality*, *4*(3). https://doi.org/10.7146/si.v4i3.128151

Merlino, S. (2021b). Coordination, visual attention, and professional gestures in the treatment of aphasia. *Langage et Société*, *173*(2), 115–140.

Merlino, S., & Keel, S. (2017), 11–13 May. A fine-grained analysis of therapeutic sequences in aphasia speech therapy sessions. *Intersubjectivity in Action Conference*. University of Helsinki.

Mondada, L. (2018). Multiple temporalities of language and body in interaction: Challenges for transcribing multimodality. *Research on Language and Social Interaction*, *51*(1), 85–106. https://doi.org/10.1080/08351813.2018.1413878

Nishizaka, A. (2014). Instructed perception in prenatal ultrasound examinations. *Discourse Studies*, *16*(2), 217–246. https://doi.org/10.1177/1461445613515354

Ochs, E., Solomon, O., & Sterponi, L. (2005). Limitations and transformations of habitus in child-directed communication. *Discourse Studies*, *7*(4–5), 547–583. https://doi.org/10.1177/1461445605054406

Parry, R. (2005). A video analysis of how physiotherapists communicate with patients about errors of performance: Insights for practice and policy. *Physiotherapy*, *91*(4), 204–214. https://doi.org/10.1016/j.physio.2005.05.004

Raymond, G. (2000). *The structure of responding: Type-conforming and nonconforming responses to yes/no-type interrogatives*. University of California, Los Angeles.

Ronkainen, R. J. (2011). Enhancing listening and imitation skills in children with cochlear implants-the use of multimodal resources in speech therapy. *Journal of Interactional Research in Communication Disorders*, *2*(2), 245–269. https://doi.org/10.1558/jircd.v2i2.245

Ronkainen, R., Laakso, M., Lonka, E., & Tykkyläinen, T. (2017). Promoting lexical learning in the speech and language therapy of children with cochlear implants. *Clinical Linguistics and Phonetics*, *31*(4), 266–282. https://doi.org/10.1080/02699206.2016.1245786

Rose, M. L. (2013). Releasing the constraints on aphasia therapy: The positive impact of gesture and multimodality treatments. *American Journal of Speech-Language Pathology*, *22*(2), 227–239. https://doi.org/10.1044/1058-0360(2012/12-0091)

Sanchez Svensson, M. S., Luff, P., & Heath, C. (2009). Embedding instruction in practice: Contingency and collaboration during surgical training. *Sociology of Health and Illness*, *31*(6), 889–906. https://doi.org/10.1111/j.1467-9566.2009.01195.x

Schegloff, E. A., Jefferson, G., & Sacks, H. (1977). The preference for self-correction in the organization of repair in conversation. *Language: Journal of the Linguistic Society of America*, *53*(2), 361–382. https://doi.org/10.2307/413107

Silvast, M. (1991). Aphasia therapy dialogues. *Aphasiology*, *5*(4–5), 383–390. https://doi.org/10.1080/02687039108248540

Simmons-Mackie, N., & Damico, J. S. (1999). Social role negotiation in aphasia therapy: Competence, incompetence and conflict. In *Constructing (in)competence: Disabling evaluations in clinical and social interaction* (pp. 313–341). Lawrence Erlbaum.

Simone, M., & Galatolo, R. (2020). Climbing as a pair: Instructions and instructed body movements in indoor climbing with visually impaired athletes. *Journal of Pragmatics*, *155*, 286–302. https://doi.org/10.1016/j.pragma.2019.09.008

Smotrova, T. (2017). Making pronunciation visible: Gesture in teaching pronunciation. *TESOL Quarterly*, *51*(1), 59–89. https://doi.org/10.1002/tesq.276

Stukenbrock, A. (2014). Take the words out of my mouth: Verbal instructions as embodied practices. *Journal of Pragmatics*, *65*, 80–102. https://doi.org/10.1016/j.pragma.2013.08.017

Tarplee, C. (2010). Next turn and intersubjectivity in children's language acquisition. *Analyzing interactions in childhood: Insights from Conversation Analysis* (pp. 3–22). Wiley.

Weeks, P. (1996). A rehearsal of a Beethoven passage: An analysis of correction talk. *Research on Language and Social Interaction*, *29*(3), 247–290.

Wilkinson, R. (2004). Reflecting on talk in speech and language therapy: Some contributions using conversation analysis. *International Journal of Language and Communication Disorders*, *39*(4), 497–503. https://doi.org/10.1080/13682820420000226879

Wilkinson, R. (2011). Changing interactional behaviour: Using conversation analysis in intervention programmes for aphasic conversation. In *Applied conversation analysis: Changing institutional practices* (pp. 32–53). Palgrave Macmillan Ltd.

Wilkinson, R. (2013). The interactional organization of aphasia naming testing. *Clinical Linguistics and Phonetics*, *27*(10–11), 805–822. https://doi.org/10.3109/02699206.2013.815279

Wilkinson, R., Bryan, K., Lock, S., Bayley, K., Maxim, J., Bruce, C., Edmundson, A., & Moir, D. (1998). Therapy using conversation analysis: Helping couples adapt to aphasia in conversation. *International Journal of Language and Communication Disorders*, *33*(Suppl.1), 144–149. https://doi.org/10.3109/13682829809179412

Wilkinson, R., Gower, M., Beeke, S., & Maxim, J. (2007). Adapting to conversation as a language-impaired speaker: Changes in aphasic turn construction over time. *Communication*, *4*(1), 79–97. https://doi.org/10.1515/CAM.2007.009

Zimmerman, D. H. (1999). Horizontal and vertical comparative research in language and social interaction. *Research on Language and Social Interaction*, *32*(1–2), 195–203.

8 How to use a mobile app at home

Learning-by-doing introductions in physiotherapy consultations

Sara Keel, Anja Schmid, and Fabienne Keller

Introduction

Our chapter examines video-recordings of naturally occurring interaction in physiotherapy consultations in which the patient is introduced to the mobile eHealth application Physitrack™ (hereafter "the app"). While the physiotherapist and patient discuss app-related issues at various points of the consultation, the patient's introduction to the app constitutes a perspicuous setting for studying how patients are socialized to use the app at home. The physiotherapist's and patient's embodied organization of instructional sequences having to do with the operation of the app, its distinct functions, and the options it offers for supporting and monitoring the therapeutic process plays out in what we have called elsewhere (Keller et al., 2021) a "triangular configuration." In contrast to other studies that examine doctors' use of desktop computers in the presence of patients (see for example the early investigation by Greatbatch et al., 1995), during introductions to the app, the physiotherapist and patient are positioned side by side and their interaction is oriented to the patient's smartphone, on which the app is installed. Both focus on what happens on its screen while they are operating it and thereby achieve "situated learning" (Sanchez Svensson et al., 2009, p. 903), or, as we have glossed it, learning-by-doing introductions to the app.

These learning-by-doing introductions are reflexively adapted to in situ contingencies, such as the app's technological affordances, time constraints inherent to physiotherapy consultations, and patients' displayed understanding of the app. The interactive organization of learning-by-doing activities permits patients to constantly display what they already know about and can do with the app, as well as what still needs to be attended to (Oloff, 2021) if the introduction to the app is to be successful, i.e., if, from a member's perspective, it provides the patient with the "eHealth literacy" (Jimenez et al., 2020) required for them to use the app at home.

Our workplace study on the use of the app in ambulatory physiotherapy was conducted in partnership with Medbase, a large Swiss healthcare provider. Physiotherapists working at Medbase are invited to use the app to compile and distribute individual home exercise programs to their patients, monitor patients' progress over time, and provide them with remote chat/video coaching and educational materials. In Switzerland, the lack of incentives in the national healthcare system and healthcare institutions (e.g., no reimbursement for the use of digital tools outside face-to-face consultations, limited opportunities to acquire the necessary eHealth literacy) puts the main pressure for the adoption of digital tools on individual users and, in particular, physiotherapists. However, a look at the literature unearths only a few studies that look at physiotherapists' and patients' use-in-interaction of digital tools, let alone how, during consultations, patients are instructed and enabled to use tools at home (see Keel et al., 2022, for a more thorough discussion).

Analyzing the ways in which the physiotherapist and the patient organize the introduction sheds new light on patients' socialization. It shows that members "orient[ed]-to and achieve[d]" patients' education in required eHealth literacy not only as one "task" (Greiffenhagen, 2008, p. 36) among others that has to be accomplished efficiently in a 30-minute physiotherapy consultation, but also as a task that has to be constantly adapted within the course of the introduction and reshaped on every following instructional occasion (Sormani, 2010, pp. 183–184).

In what follows, we introduce the notion of eHealth literacy as a concept to describe patients' and therapists' knowledge and skills in using digital tools in healthcare. Further, we outline ethnomethodological and conversation analytic (hereafter EMCA) studies on the use of digital tools in healthcare, the instruction of digital tools in healthcare and beyond, and the sequential organization of instructions more generally. Finally, we briefly present the adopted approach and the collected data on which this study is based, before discussing our analysis on the basis of selected transcribed excerpts.

Digitization in healthcare and eHealth literacy

The ubiquitous digitization in healthcare is transforming healthcare professionals' (HCPs) working practices in profound ways, involving among other things a shift from face-to-face to remote settings, such as telerehabilitation (Konttila et al., 2019), the adaptation of core elements of professional practices (Blixt et al., 2019), and the acquisition of new competences, i.e., eHealth literacy, by both HCPs and patients. eHealth literacy refers to the ability to search for, find, and understand digital health information, to transform and use the knowledge gained to address everyday health problems (Norman & Skinner, 2006), as well as to specific skills and knowledge required for the effective use of eHealth tools (Chan & Kaufman, 2011).

Meanwhile, there is no consistent approach to conceptualizing these required skills (Griebel et al., 2018). In reviews, conceptual works, mixed-methods, or Delphi studies, various domains have been considered, including specific skills required by healthcare members to develop eHealth literacy (Konttila et al., 2019), whereby the focus is on skills required by HCPs and not those required by the patient (Jimenez et al., 2020): (1) digital literacy, which includes the basic knowledge of how to use a computer, mobile phone, or the Internet; (2) knowledge of basic medical informatics and health data analysis; (3) adoption of digital technologies to improve patient care and optimize the provision of healthcare services, e.g., electronic treatment plans; (4) knowledge of assistive technologies or mobile apps for patients' benefit, including digital educational material; (5) health data management, including knowledge of how to access patient data and the ability to read, understand, and forward digital information; (6) knowledge of regulations and laws related to digital tools (Jimenez et al., 2020); (7) awareness, knowledge, and skills to ensure patient safety; (8) social and communication skills associated with tele-technology and awareness of its influence on HCP–patient interaction (Davies et al., 2021); and (9) ethics, including the knowledge of digital inclusion that ensures equitable access to information and communication technologies (Sieck et al., 2021).

It has been argued that there is a lack of professional skill standards to respond to the accelerating developments of digitization in healthcare in practice: many ambiguities, uncertainties, and different expectations exist in general, and in particular at the educational/curriculum level (see Wentink et al., 2019), thus hindering HCPs' development of required digital skills (Butler-Henderson et al., 2020). Furthermore, it has been stressed that digital transformation requires not only the acquisition of specific skills, but also a shift in awareness, new organizational cultures, and everyday professional practices that take empirical knowledge and social realities into account in a compelling way (Samerski & Müller, 2019). Finally, there is a lack of studies on the eHealth literacy patients require to be able to use digital tools in practice (Jimenez et al., 2020) and those required by HCPs to enable patients to do so.

The use of digital tools in healthcare interactions

Unlike the studies cited in the previous subsection, EMCA promotes an approach that considers the use of digital technology in practice. EMCA studies have also highlighted that new technologies are often a challenge for HCPs (Pilnick et al., 2010). At the same time, they stress that the use of technology provides new resources for medical/healthcare practices and training and that challenges can be solved by the participants in disadvantageous but also beneficial ways (Ekberg et al., 2019). It has been shown that the use of technology is not simply determined by its design but that its operation results from an interplay between the affordances of technology, context, and participants' practices (Hartswood et al., 2003; Heath et al., 2003; Mikesell et al., 2018). The methodology of looking at the minute organization of instances of medical/healthcare work and training interactions allows EMCA to reveal how new technologies are effectively handled (Hindmarsh et al., 2007) and how they impact the organization of interaction in both face-to-face (Beck Nielsen, 2019) and remote (Shaw et al., 2020) settings. Most EMCA studies research technologies that are operated by professionals and thus focus on their need for training, e.g., Martin et al. (2007). The few studies on digital tools that are used by patients look for example at how patients exploit affordances of the tool beyond its design (Mikesell et al., 2018) or how home-care workers teach elderly patients how to use a tablet through a combination of explicit educational and motivational work, the importance of the latter often being overlooked (Ertner, 2019).

Instructions concerning digital tools in healthcare specifically may on the one hand be enabled or necessitated by the affordances and constraints of the technology. For example, studies have researched instructions regarding how patients should be placed in relation to the camera in remote medical consultations ("positioning talk") (Shaw et al., 2020). On the other hand, instructions may concern the use of the technology itself, for instance, when a surgeon directs the use of endoscopic and other cameras during an intervention to achieve visibility for the operating team, but also for a remote audience composed of trainees and external experts (Mondada, 2014), or a midwife teaches patients how to read technologically yielded ultrasound images (Nishizaka, 2014). The ways in which patients are instructed to use a digital tool remain underexamined.

The interactive organization of instructional sequences

Meanwhile, instructions related to new technologies are a perspicuous setting not only for analyzing which skills are required to operate a tool (Oloff, 2021), but also for revealing that members do not orient to required skills as set once and for all, but as something that is negotiated throughout a tool's introduction, e.g., in classroom interactions (Greiffenhagen, 2008). Studies have described how adults, in particular the elderly, are instructed to use digital tools and revealed that even commonplace digital actions that are often seen as simple and taken for granted, like pressing keys (Weilenmann, 2010), in fact consist of many small actions that need to be learned and coordinated (Oloff, 2021). Digital actions have been shown to be essentially embodied (Weilenmann, 2010), with learning how to execute them being by preference a haptic process (Råman, 2022). Analyses of video tutorial instructions have revealed that following them involves an alternating organization of watching and pausing the video and thus of controlling the pace at which the instruction is played (Tuncer et al., 2020).

Beyond instructions relating to the use of technology, studies on medical/healthcare educational settings stress that instead of simply being outside observers of professionals' and students' training, patients might contribute to the task at hand (Hindmarsh, 2010). Furthermore, instructions targeting patients' education in therapeutic or readaptation settings, e.g., in speech therapy (Merlino, 2020) or physiotherapy (Martin & Sahlström, 2010), reveal how patients' responses to instructions, i.e., their "instructed actions" (Garfinkel, 2002, p. 197), constitute the bedrock on which professionals build up their next turn and how professionals' and patients' minute organization of instructional sequences constitutes the therapeutic setting as an educational one.

These studies draw on a long tradition of research on face-to-face classroom interaction that provides insight on how instructional sequences are sequentially organized, most notably in three parts: instruction, response, and evaluation (I-R-E) (Lindwall et al., 2015). Its interactive organization relates to the categories of "teachers/instructors" and "students/instructees." "Instructing," "following instructions," and " evaluating instructed actions" are understood as "category-bound activities" through which instructors and instructees display education-in-interaction and make it available for inspection (Keel, 2021). Studies, notably on patients' education in therapy or readaptation (Martin & Sahlström, 2010; Merlino, 2020), stress that the I-R-E organization is not accomplished through interactants' talk alone – in fact, interactants might use touch, gestures, or bodily performance to accomplish instructions and instructed actions and to guide and eventually evaluate these instructed actions.

Researching use of the app in physiotherapy

In our study, we aimed to understand what the introduction to the app and its use implies from the users' perspective, notably with respect to required eHealth literacy. We also sought to achieve the "unique adequacy requirement" – in its "weak sense" (see Ikeya, 2020, pp. 23, 33–34, 36). Starting from a physiotherapist's user interface on the app, we tested what it takes to compile an exercise program for a patient. Furthermore, we explored the app's patient interface by performing an exercise program provided by a Medbase physiotherapist. The first author also used the app as a patient in physiotherapy consultations and at home. To focus on tasks that were considered "topically relevant" by physiotherapists and patients (Garfinkel, 2002, p. 100), we participated in and contributed to two workshops on the use of digital tools in physiotherapy practice organized by and with Medbase physiotherapists. We will touch upon this again in the conclusion.

In line with other EMCA studies on the use of technology, among others, in medical/healthcare settings (Heath et al., 2003), we adopted a workplace study approach (Luff et al., 2000). This approach aims to research how professional practice and collaboration can be achieved through and during the use of technology and other artifacts. As minute actions are essential for both professional work and the efficient use of digital tools, our exploration of the "lived ordering" (Pollner & Emerson, 2001, p. 119) of the app's use in physiotherapy consultations involved three fieldwork phases.

First, we conducted ethnographic fieldwork at two German-speaking Medbase sites from February to June 2020, with an interruption of three months due to COVID-19 restrictions. We shadowed physiotherapists $(N = 13)$ in their daily work to observe their professional practices (therapy consultations, administrative work, and team meetings) and held ad hoc informal interviews with them about their use and perception of the app or other digital tools in physiotherapy practice. In addition, we asked patients $(N = 43)$ about their experience with digital tools in their daily life and/or with the app.

Second, we filmed interactions between physiotherapists and patients in face-to-face (f-2-f) consultations and recorded the screens of the devices that the physiotherapists used during these consultations. As illustrated in Figure 1, we thereby collected video-recordings of consultations in which the app was introduced to the patient for the first time ($N = 8$) or used in follow-up consultations ($N = 19$), involving four physiotherapists (PHYa–d) and eight patients (PATa–h) and amounting to a total of 13 hours and 11 minutes of synchronized video-material. Verbal and multimodal transcriptions of the synchronized video-material were performed, adopting the conventions developed by Jefferson (2004) and Mondada (2018) (for transcription conventions, see this volume, pp. 22–23).

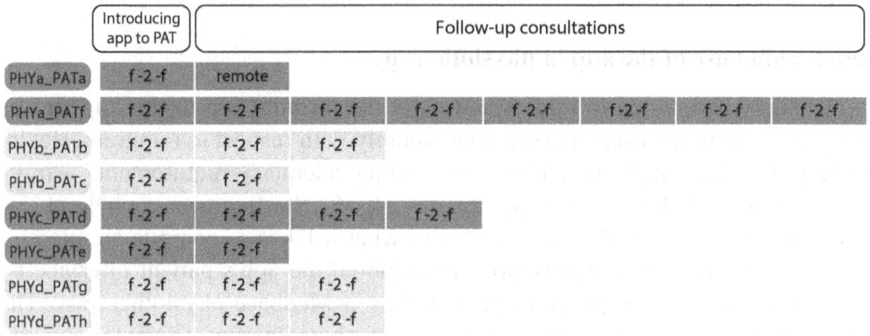

	Introducing app to PAT	Follow-up consultations						
PHYa_PATa	f-2-f	remote						
PHYa_PATf	f-2-f	f-2-f	f-2-f	f-2-f	f-2-f	f-2-f	f-2-f	f-2-f
PHYb_PATb	f-2-f	f-2-f	f-2-f					
PHYb_PATc	f-2-f	f-2-f						
PHYc_PATd	f-2-f	f-2-f	f-2-f	f-2-f				
PHYc_PATe	f-2-f	f-2-f						
PHYd_PATg	f-2-f	f-2-f	f-2-f					
PHYd_PATh	f-2-f	f-2-f	f-2-f					

Figure 1 Video-recorded physiotherapy consultations.

Third, while the follow-up consultations were recorded, our preliminary observations were checked against and/or completed with members' accounts. We conducted semi-structured interviews with participants of phase 2, i.e., physiotherapists ($N = 4$) and patients ($N = 8$), that were audio-recorded and transcribed verbatim, to learn more about how participants perceive using the app.

The patient's introduction to the app in face-to-face physiotherapy consultations

As developed in the background section, introduction activities are a perspicuous, yet under-examined setting. This chapter examines patients' introduction to the app to understand the implication of "situated learning," i.e., learning that is contingent upon the "technological affordances" (Sanchez Svensson et al., 2009, p. 903) of tools as well as time constraints and members' eHealth literacy levels. It is based on video-recordings of face-to-face consultations in which the app was introduced (left column in Figure 1) and in which the introduction to the app involved patients accessing their interface of the app on their smartphones (only PATa–d and f–h). Overall, these consultations lasted approximately 30 minutes each, except the consultation between PHYa and PATa, which lasted 60 minutes, and were composed of distinct activities, such as the opening, anamnesis, and setting of the agenda.[1]

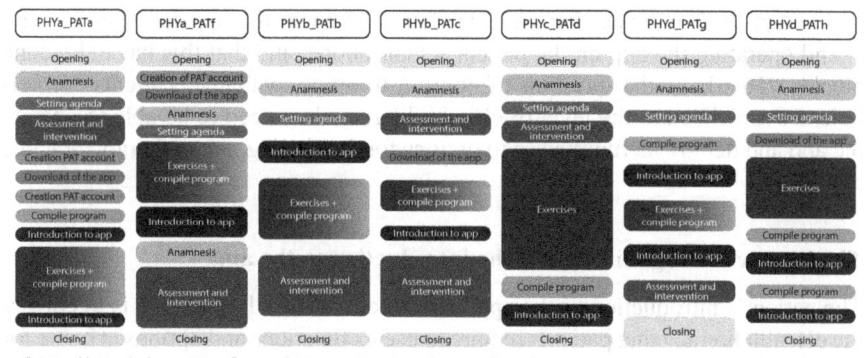

Figure 2 Activity structure of examined consultations.

As illustrated in Figure 2, proportionally, the majority of the time of the filmed consultations was used for the core activities of a typical physiotherapy consultation: assessment, an intervention composed of either physical exercises or passive treatments (e.g., mechanical interventions), and a re-evaluation of these exercises or treatments (Higgs et al., 2001). As a corollary, little time was used for introducing the app to the patient (see the size of the introduction-to-app rectangle compared to the sizes of the rectangles of other activities).

During our ethnographic fieldwork, the physiotherapists stressed that the fact that their work is composed of directly subsequent 30-minute consultations puts them under time constraints. Using the app reinforced this pressure, as it consumed further time (see also Keel et al., 2022). More specifically, patients' introduction to the app were considered important by physiotherapists, but they also pointed out that, due to time constraints, patients needed to acquaint themselves with the tool at home as well (ethnographic fieldnotes; A200617_asc, p. 6).

In line with this observation, before actually beginning to introduce the app in the filmed consultations, the physiotherapists tended to announce that the introduction would be brief:

Excerpt 1 PHYa-PATf

PHYa: you can take your smartphone and have a quick look

Excerpt 2 PHYb-PATb

PHYb: jetz döfet sis mol schnäll ufmache
      now you can quickly open it ((the app))

Excerpt 3 PHYc-PATd

PHYc: let's look at the app\ >very quickly<

214 *Sara Keel et al.*

Excerpts 1–3 indicate that patients' introduction to the app involves looking at and operating the app on the patient's smartphone, and that this has to be done quickly. This begs the question of how, in the time available, patients are sufficiently socialized to the level of eHealth literacy they need to be able to operate the app and deploy its functions and options for facilitating physiotherapy practice at home.

The interactive organization of the introduction to the app

The patient's introduction to the app constitutes a twofold task. This is to convey the eHealth literacy that patients require to use its functions and options at home for supporting the therapeutic process through regular exercise and self-management via the reminder function, the personal exercise program, and the instructive exercise video and text (Figure 3; 1–3); for assessing home exercise, particularly by indicating the frequency and pain involved (Figure 3; 4); for monitoring progress over time (Figure 3; 5); and for accessing therapists' remote coaching, notably via the secure chat functions the app offers (Figure 3; 5; see message symbol highlighted by a circle).[2]

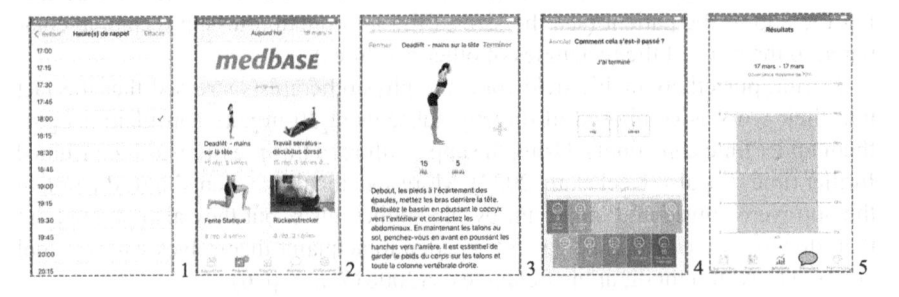

Figure 3 The app's functions and options.

At the same time, the introduction is meant to give the patient the necessary skills for operating the app, e.g., to set the reminder function, to indicate the level of pain involved in exercising, and to click on the message symbol to write the physiotherapist a message (Figure 3; 1, 4, 5). To get an initial idea of how this twofold task is accomplished by the physiotherapist and the patient, we will look at Excerpt 4.

Before Excerpt 4 starts, patient d (PATd) has opened and accessed the app on her smartphone (smph), while physiotherapist c (PHYc) has compiled PATd's exercise program and assigned it to her. Whereas PHYc is sitting in front of his computer (PC1), PATd is standing to his left, both of them busy using their respective devices. Excerpt 4 begins as PHYc has oriented to the patient's smartphone, which is lying on the table, and a triangular configuration between patient, therapist, and smartphone is achieved (fig. 1):

Excerpt 4:

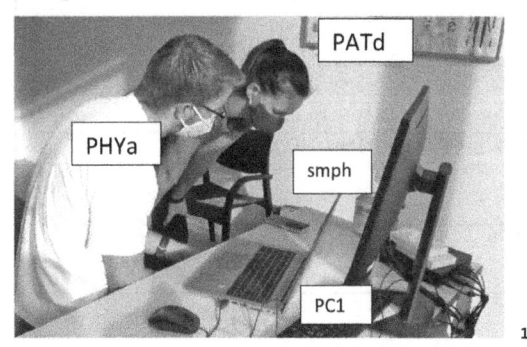

[figure: PHYa, PATd, smph, PC1]

```
1              (4.4)
2   PHYc   okay now # you have to accept the terms?
    fig              # figure 1
3              (1.1)
4          quick, (.) and then (.) press next,
5              (1.8)
6          then you can (.) >decide (an alarm)< if you want
7          to (0.2) have to (0.4) [°uh° remind ↓you]
8   PATd                          [((laughs))]
9   PHYc   like [every morning at six o clock? or fa-]&
10  PATd        [(zack zack pu push:)]
11  PHYc   &four o'clock or whatever?
12             (0.2)
13  PATd   ((laughs))=
14  PHYc   =you can also set it up later [again]&
15  PATd                                 [(°term.°)]
16  PHYc   &or change it later again
17             (0.2)
18  PATd   okay=
19  PHYc   =you can (0.4) put ne:xt
20         and .h: you can: >decide it whether or not you want it<
21         download, (.) I personally wouldn't, because i think
22         it (0.2) (it) uses lot of (0.2) °uhm:° (0.4) capacity .h=
23  PATd   =yeah.=
24  PHYc   =>and then you can< just press (0.5) don:e
25             (0.5)
26         °↑good°
27         now you have your exercise ↑here (0.4)
28         if you click on ↑it
29             (0.9)
30         then: (.) you'll see: (0.2)
31         <just kind of the: overview (0.2)
32         o[ver the ex]ercises ((creaky))>
33  PATd    [<(↑m:hm; ↑a:h yeah) ((affirmative))>]
34             (0.3)
35  PHYc   and then you can (0.6) click on one of the exercise?
36             (2.2)
37         yeah
38             (0.2)
39         and then: (.) you'll [see the video::]
40  PATd                        [is coming the vi]deo=
41  PHYc   =how many tim:es how lo:ng
42             (0.4)
43         >there's a little< description
44             (0.4)
45  PATd   o:[kay.]
```

```
46 PHYc    [uh::]m:(0.3) an:d once you're done with it,
47         you can press comple:te?
48         (0.3)
49 PATd    °o:kay°
50         (0.4)
51 PHYc    so (.) try very quick
52         (0.6)
53         n'then you can set up (0.3) h:ow many times
54         you actually did it?
55         (0.2)
56 PATd    okay?=
57 PHYc    =and if there was any pai:n.
58         (.)
59 PATd    okay.
```

In Excerpt 4, PHYc and PATd on the one hand accomplish a series of instructional sequences that concern the app's operation, e.g., the "terms" and conditions have to be accepted (l. 1–5), a "next" button (l. 4, 19), a "done" button (l. 24–26), a "comple:te" button (l. 46–52), an "exercise" symbol (l. 27–29), or instructive "exercise" video (l. 35) is "just" (l. 24) to be "press[ed]" (l. 4, 24, 47), "click[ed]" (l. 28, 35), "quick," "very quick" (l. 4; 51). On the other hand, the physiotherapist accomplishes a series of instructions that concern the functions and options that the app offers for PATd's home use, e.g., the "alarm (reminder)" function (l. 6–18), the option of "download[ing]" the app's content (l. 20–26), the "overview (0.2) over the exercises," i.e., the patient's exercise program (l. 30–32), the instructive exercise "video::" and "little description" (l. 39–45), the assessment functions: "h:ow many times you actually did [the exercise]" (l. 53–56), and the "pai:n" involved in performing an exercise (l. 57–59).

By and large, the instructional sequences in Excerpt 4 are organized as "adjacency pairs" (see turns marked by boxes, e.g., l. 46–49), composed of two adjacently produced turns (I-R) which form a "minimal conversational unit" between "instructor" and "receiver of instruction" (Goldberg, 1975, p. 276): PHYc produces instructions (I) (see the turns marked in gray) and, apart from one exception (l. 40), PATd responds (R) succinctly, with continuers and confirmation tokens, such as "mmh" (l. 33), "okay" (l. 18, 45, 56, 59), and "yeah" (l. 23, 33) (Goldberg, 1975, p. 277), "laughing" or single words (l. 8, 10, 13, 15), or by embodied means not transcribed in Excerpt 4.

Moreover, PHYc precedes his instructions systematically with a "temporal indicator term" (see Sacks, 1992 Vol 1, pp. 515–522), such as "now" (l. 2, 27), "later" (l. 14, 16), "once you're done" (l. 46), "and then" (l. 4, 24, 35, 39, 53), "then" (l. 6, 30), or the connector "and" (l. 20, 57) (Goldberg, 1975, p. 288). He thus produces instructions as "serially connected turns, joined like links of a chain," in short, as contributing to an "instructional chain" (Goldberg, 1975, p. 269) whose pace of production is set by him. The two-part organization of instructional sequences (I-R) contrasts with the three-part organization (I-R-E) observed in educational settings (Lindwall et al. 2015), in which the instructee's response (R) is either followed by the instructor's positive evaluation (E) that closes the instructional sequence, or an "instructional correction" that provides the instructee with insight regarding how to respond (R) to the instruction in a satisfactory way (Hindmarsh et al., 2014).

Altogether, the concise serially ordered organization treats the "passing of instructional material" (Goldberg, 1975, p. 276) as somehow self-evident. At first sight, one might conclude that the steady pace at which PHYc produces this series of instructions comes at the expense of teaching and learning. Or in other words, that not much pedagogy-in-interaction seems to be taking place here.

However, this judgment misses the point. As stressed by Garfinkel (2002, p. 206), "there is no time out" when it comes to instructing and following instructions. The content and form of the introduction to the app are "oriented-to and achieved phenomena" that are constantly (re-)shaped and (re-)negotiated through participants' actions as accomplished within the contingencies of the moment (Greiffenhagen, 2008, p. 36; see also Sormani, 2010, pp. 183–184). As illustrated in fig. 1, for the task examined here, the physiotherapist and the patient are set up in a triangular configuration that gives them both access to the patient's smartphone and to what is observably happening on its screen, in other words to its technological affordances when operated in situ. Understanding how physiotherapists and patients deploy this triangular configuration to organize the introduction to the app, while operating it and attending to what is visible on the app's interface on the screen, requires further unpacking.

Physiotherapists' and patients' embodied and situated organization of instructions

The embodied organization of physiotherapists' introduction task reveals that physiotherapists and patients accomplish a type of pedagogy that is best glossed as learning-by-doing (Excerpts 5–11) (see also Relieu; Merlino, this volume), notably when the instructions concern what is to be seen and attended to on the smartphone screen (Excerpt 5) or which buttons need to be pressed if one is to operate the app (Excerpts 6–11). At other moments, however, physiotherapists might expand upon their instructions and/or patients might ask questions and elaborate on issues that they deem relevant for using the app to support the therapeutic process (Excerpts 11–14; see also Excerpt 4, l. 6–16).

In the following transcripts, the members' embodied actions are described below the respective lines of talk, and their beginnings and ends are denoted by a symbol in the verbal transcription line. The producer is denoted by the participant's acronym in lower-case letters (phy, pat). The acronyms "appPC" and "appSP" designate screen activities in the app on the PC or smartphone. As an illustration: in line 1 of Excerpt 5, the vertical bar "|" indicates the moment when PHYa starts pointing to the smartphone screen with her right index finger.[3]

Before Excerpt 5 starts, physiotherapist a (PHYa) and patient a (PATa) are at the very beginning of the introduction and are both busy with their respective devices: while PHYa is creating an exercise program for PATa on her tablet, PATa is opening the app on her smartphone for the first time. They are seated some distance from each other. Asked by PHYa if she has managed to open the app, PATa turns her smartphone screen toward her, achieving PHYa's shift of gaze to her smartphone and engendering an embodied instruction from her:

218 Sara Keel et al.

Excerpt 5

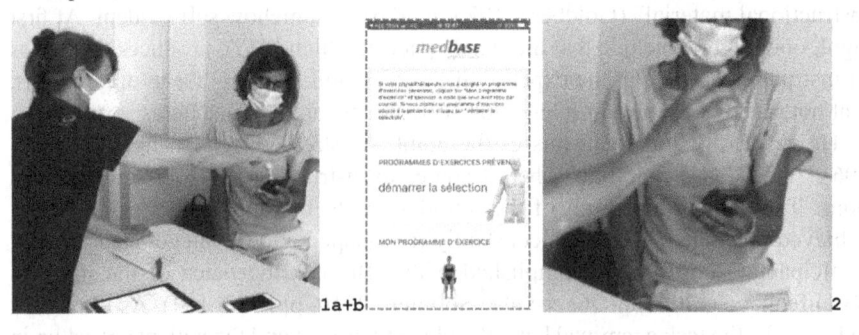

1a+b   2

```
1   PHYa    und (0.4) | (ba-)#
            and       (ba-)
    phya    >>-directs rh toward smph screen and extends index|
    phya           |-rh index points to smph screen->
    fig                 # figure 1a+b
2           da|s progr|amm wo#|n ich für dich zämes|tell
            that program  that  i   compile for you
    phya    >-|lifts rh into air|
    phya          |waves rh|
    phya                  |directs rh toward smph screen, index extended|
    phya                                      |index points to smph screen,
                                                making circular movements->
    fig                   # figure 2
```

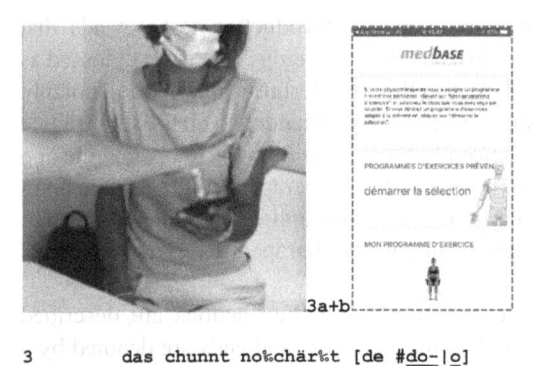

3a+b

```
3           das chunnt no%chär%t [de #do-|o]
            that comes    later  [then here]
4   PATa                         [de #do(|hei]%ne)|
                                 [then herea|bout]
    phya                      >-|-lifts rh in air|-waves rh->>
    pata            %directs lh thumb toward smph screen%
    pata            %points to smph screen with thumb%
    pata                           %retracts lh thumb->>
    fig                       # figure 3a+b
```

As PATa holds her smartphone in front of her, PHYa shows her where "the [exercise] program" (*das programm*), once compiled, is to be found on the smartphone screen (l. 1–3; fig. 1a and b). At the beginning of the first turn constructional unit (TCU) (l. 1), PHYa points to the middle of PATa's smartphone where it says "mon programme d'exercices" (*my exercise program*) (fig. 1a and b). She then retracts her hand (fig. 2), giving PATa full visibility of the screen. Toward the end of the TCU (l. 2), she points again to the middle of the screen, while doing circular pointing (l. 3; fig. 3a and b) throughout the second TCU of her instruction. The embodied instruction works like an invitation for PATa to look at a specific point on the smartphone screen and recognize a relevant item. It enables PATa to produce the end of the instruction "de do-o" (*then here*) in overlap with PHYa, while using her thumb to point to the same space as PHYa (l. 3–4; fig. 3a and b). Through the embodied "choral co-production" (Lerner, 2002), PATa displays understanding of PHYd's instruction, even before PHYd has finished uttering it, instead of merely claiming it (see Goldberg, 1975, p. 277), and thus shows that she is following PHYa's embodied instruction attentively.

Excerpt 5 illustrates how the instruction to look at and recognize relevant items on the patient's smartphone screen is put into action by the patient. In the following Excerpts (6–11), we discuss the ways embodied instructions involve both recognizing and operating relevant visible items on the smartphone screen.

Before Excerpt 6 starts, PHYc and PATd have completed the terms and conditions acceptance step (see Excerpt 4, l. 1–3):

Excerpt 6

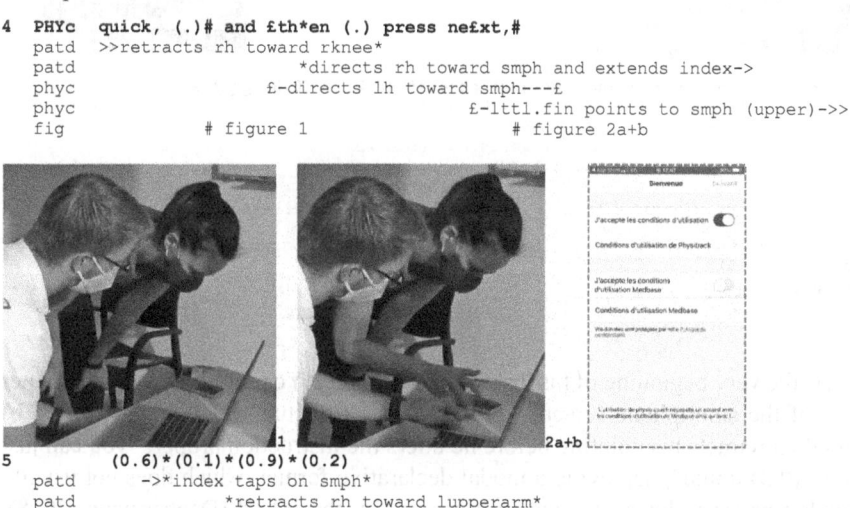

```
4   PHYc     quick, (.)# and £th*en (.) press ne£xt,#
    patd     >>retracts rh toward rknee*
    patd                     *directs rh toward smph and extends index->
    phyc                  £-directs lh toward smph---£
    phyc                                            £-lttl.fin points to smph (upper)->>
    fig              # figure 1                     # figure 2a+b
```

```
5            (0.6)*(0.1)*(0.9)*(0.2)
    patd     ->*index taps on smph*
    patd              *retracts rh toward lupperarm*
    patd                   *rubs lupperarm->>
```

PHYc's instruction, "press next" (l. 4), takes an imperative format. Thus, PHYc encourages PATd to comply with the instruction immediately (Deppermann, 2018). However, PATd has just finished retracting her right hand into "home position" (Sacks & Schegloff, 2002), here her right knee (fig.1), shortly before PHYc utters this instruction. At the same time, PHYc begins directing his left hand, which has so far rested on his knee, toward PATd's smartphone and then uses his little finger to point to the top of it, where it says: "Suivant" (*Next*) (fig. 2a and b). PATc's embodied performance links the instruction reflexively to what is

220   *Sara Keel et al.*

visible on the screen. "As constituents of a unified [learning-by-doing] configuration" (Greiffenhagen & Watson, 2009, p. 67), it engenders an embodied response by PATd clicking on the pointed-to button; she closes the instructional sequence (l. 5). Through her embodied response, PATd again displays "understanding" of PHYc's instruction and the app's design. Retracting her hand into home position immediately after, she moreover displays that she awaits further instructions by PHYc.

In contrast to Excerpt 6, in Excerpt 7, PHYc deploys a modal declarative format, instead of an imperative, while pointing to the referred-to button, i.e., "Effectué" (*Done*), before uttering his instruction and not merely at the end of it:

Excerpt 7

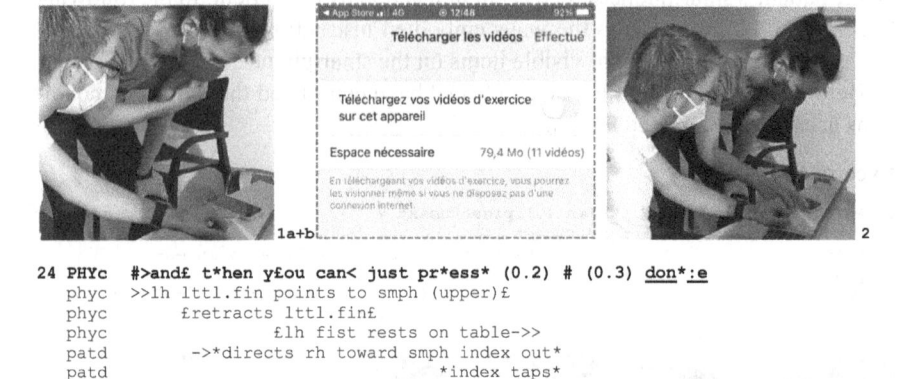

```
24 PHYc    #>and£ t*hen y£ou can< just pr*ess* (0.2) # (0.3) don*:e
   phyc    >>lh lttl.fin points to smph (upper)£
   phyc            £retracts lttl.fin£
   phyc                     £lh fist rests on table->>
   patd            ->*directs rh toward smph index out*
   patd                               *index taps*
   patd                                           *retracts rh toward left wrist->
   patd                                                       *rh on left wrist->>
   fig     # figure 1a+b                          # figure 2
25         (0.5)
26 PHYc    °↑good°
```

At the very beginning of his instruction (l. 24), PHYc points briefly to the upper part of the smartphone screen, where it says: "Effectué" (*Done*) (fig. 1a and b) and then retracts his pointing before he utters the instruction proper: "you can just press (0.3) don:e", deploying a modal declarative format, which does not usually involve pressure for an immediate response by the PATd (Deppermann, 2018). However, the fact that PHYc made the smartphone screen available at the beginning of his instruction invites PATd to direct her right hand to the smartphone, tap on the pointed-to button (fig. 2) in synchrony with PHYc's "press" (l. 24), and immediately retract her hand even before PHYc has finished his instruction. The interactive organization of this instructional sequence is one of the few that contain the typical third part of a pedagogical instructional sequence (Lindwall et al., 2015) while ensuring a steady pace in the introduction: as soon as PATd has fully retracted her hand, PHYc evaluates PATd's embodied response positively in his next turn (l. 26), closes the sequence, and provides for the relevance of the next instruction (omitted for reasons of space).

How to use a mobile app at home 221

In contrast, in Excerpt 8 PHYb's instruction is not only met by PATb's immediate embodied response, but it is also PATb who, after its completion, drives the instructional chain forward:

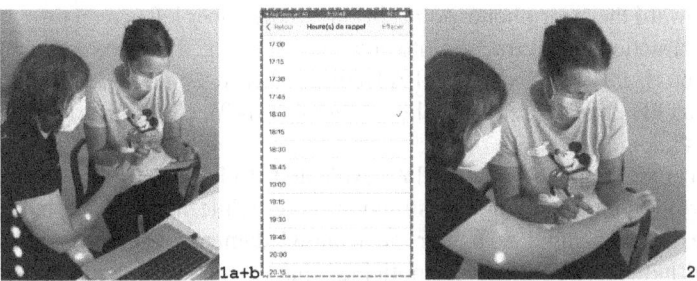

Excerpt 8

```
1   PHYb    #g|enau denn döfed si |#da z|urüc*kch?
             exactly   then you can    here return
    phyb    |-directs rh toward smph---|
    phyb                           |points to screen|
    phyb                                            |retracts rh from smph->
    patb              >>rh index over smph screen*directs rh index toward smph (upper)->
    fig     # figure 1a+b          # figure 2

2           (0.2)#(0.2)
    fig          # figure 3
3   PATb    ah|a* da hat (es
             ah     here (it) has
    phyb    ->|
    patb      ->*taps, then retracts rh->
4           [sich)   sch|*o] e*ingest[ell*t.]
            [(itself) already]    set [in  ]
5   PHYb    [    gena|*u?]       [und*   ] d*an[n |wi#e*der| *wei]ter?|
             [    exactly|        [and  ]  then again        next?|
6   PATb                                        [we|it#e*r:       ]
                                                [next            ]
    phyb          |-directs rh toward smph-----|points to smph|
    phyb                                                      |retracts rh|
    patd          ->*    *directs index to smph*
    patd                                 *moves index to left*
    patd                                                      *directs index to smph>
    fig                                            # figure 4a+b
7           (.)*(0.4)
    patd    ->*taps, then retracts rh index->
8   PHYb    gena*u
            exactly
    patd      ->*
```

Following a confirmation token that closes a previous instructional sequence, PHYb precedes her next instruction with "denn" (*then*) (l. 1). The instruction proper is produced in a modal declarative format and refers to the "zurück" (*retour/return*)-button visible on the screen (fig. 1a and b). Whereas PATb holds her right index over the smartphone, ready to operate it, so to speak (fig. 2), PHYb directs her right hand toward the smartphone, points briefly to the upper left screen toward the end of her instruction, and retracts it into home position (fig. 3) before completing her instruction (l. 1). As in Excerpt 7, PATb directs her index to the referred-to button, as soon as PHYb starts retracting her pointing (l. 1–2), clicks on it (fig. 2), and then retracts her index.

In contrast to Excerpt 7, in which PHYc evaluated PATd's instructed action positively before moving to the next instruction, here, while holding her index ready to operate the app again, PATb utters an acknowledgment token (l. 3) and an indexical spatial indicator "here" before noticing: "hat (es sich) scho eingestellt" (*it has (itself) already set in*) (l. 3–4). PHYb treats PATb's embodied conduct as a summons to move forward (l. 5). In overlap with PATb's noticing, PHYb produces a confirmation, points toward the upper part of the smartphone screen (fig. 4a and b) while uttering: "und dann" (*and then*), and retracts her pointing at the end of the instruction. She thus allows PATb to complete the instruction with "weiter:" (*next*) (l. 6) even slightly prior to PHYb (l. 5) and to operate the referred-to "weiter" ("*Suivant*," *next*)-button (fig. 3a) less than 0.2 seconds after the end of PHYb's instruction.

In the instructional sequences analyzed so far, we have revealed embodied practices through which physiotherapists instruct patients to see and recognize specific visible features of the app's interface on their smartphones (Excerpt 5) and to operate them (Excerpts 6–8). Physiotherapists' instructions most often take a declarative format (Excerpts 5 and 7–8), which usually does not require an immediate response by the instructee (Deppermann, 2018). However, physiotherapists use indexical spatial indicators, such as "here" or the denomination of the app's design features in combination with pointing gestures, and thereby strongly constrain patients' responses. At the same time, patients' gaze at the screen allows them to coordinate their own actions with the unfolding of the physiotherapists' embodied instructions and what happens on the screen. Learning-by-doing thus allows patients to display their understanding of the embodied instructions and the "instructional material" they refer to (Goldberg, 1975, p. 282) as they unfold.

Moreover, whereas physiotherapists' retraction from pointing during or immediately after their instructions invites patients to operate the smartphone on the spot, patients' immediate retraction from operating the smartphone after accomplishing the instructed action provides the physiotherapists with the next opportunity to instruct. Together, physiotherapists and patients thus display their orientation to and constitute the learning-by-doing activities as involving two categories, instructor and instructee, a typical distribution of "rights/obligations" and "category-bound activities" attached to them (Keel, 2021). Whereas the instructor sets the pace of the task at hand, the instructee, by receiving embodied instructions immediately with an embodied response, seizes the learning(-by-doing) opportunity readily and goes along with the set pace or might even take the initiative to set a rapid pace (Excerpt 8).

In spatial configurations in which the patient has better access to the smartphone screen than the professional, the patient may not only anticipate the completion of an instruction, as shown in Excerpt 8, but even produce the instruction. This is the case in Excerpts 9 and 10, in which the patients are just about to access the app on their smartphone. Since the patients are to enter personal data (birthdate; access code) on the smartphone, the physiotherapists might keep a slight distance:

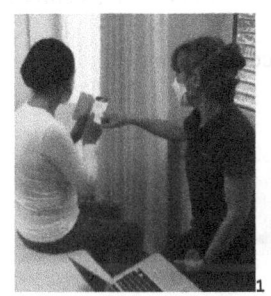

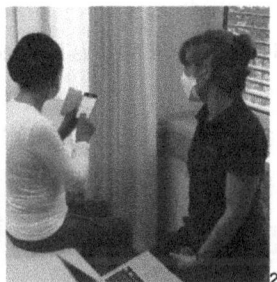

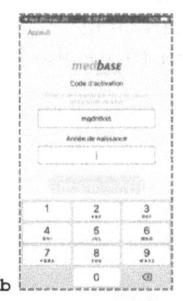

Excerpt 9

```
1           (.)|(0.4)
   phya     |-directs rh toward smph->
2  PHYa     an:d *you |a#d|d you:*r* (.) yea|r
   phya              ->|points to smph screen (middle)|
   phya                               |-retracts rh-----|
   patf     *directs rh index toward smph*
   patf                      *taps on screen (middle)*
   patf                             *retracts index, still directed toward screen->
   fig                  # figure 1
3           (.)
4           on*ly the year #of* (0.2) ↑birth::
   patf     ->*moves index over screen*
   patf                           *taps on smph screen keyboard->
   fig                       # figure 2a+b
5           (1.0)*(0.4)
   patf        ->*directs index to screen (middle)->
6  PATf     ac*c#e[%ss*]
7  PHYa        [%ac*]c%ess* yes::* # h
   patf     ->*index paused over screen (middle)*
   patf                   *-taps-*lowers rh*
   phya              %-nod-%
   fig      # figure 3a+b           # figure 4
8           (2.5)
```

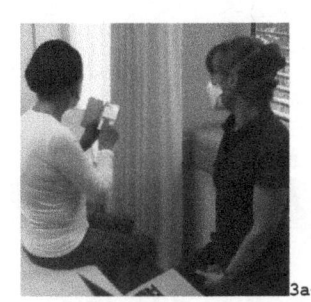

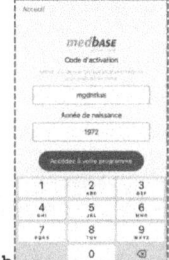

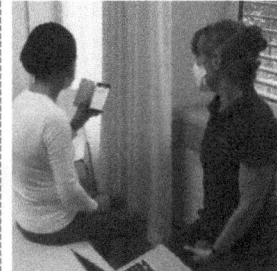

224 *Sara Keel et al.*

In lines 2–4, PHYa monitors PATf's actions and, as in Excerpts 7–8, briefly points to the middle of the smartphone screen (fig. 1a and b) as she begins uttering an instruction. This instruction takes a declarative format: "you add you:r (.) year" and involves a self-repair in line 4 that allows PHYa to modify her instruction to match the indication visible on the screen: "Année de naissance" (*Year of birth*) (fig. 1b), without deploying another pointing to the screen. After a moment of silence (l. 5), the instructional chain continues. After PATf has entered her year of birth, the app's design (fig 3a and b) highlights the button "Accédez à votre programme" (*Access your program*) (l. 6, fig. 3b). In this case, it is PATf and not PHYa who reads the highlighted instruction aloud, using a rising intonation (l. 6), and as soon as she receives PHYa's agreement (l. 7), she taps on it.

In Excerpt 10, we also join PHYd and PATd as they access the app:

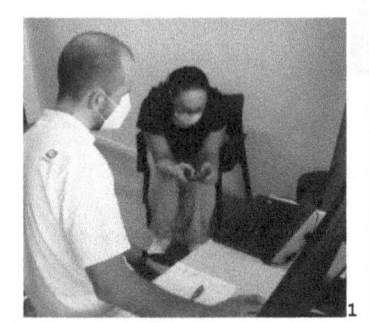

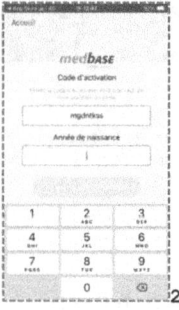

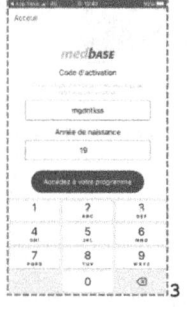

Excerpt 10

```
1   PHYd    #gena*u?
            exactly
    patg    >>---*-tapping on smph screen (lower)->
    fig     # figure 1
2           (0.4)*(1.2)*#(0.4)
    patg    >----*      *taps on screen (middle)
    fig                  # figure 2
3           und s ge*burtsj*ahr#*
            and the year of birth
    patg            *------*----*tapping on screen (lower)->
    fig                          # figure 3
4           (0.4)*(1.3)
    patg    >----*
5   PATg    und dann öffnen °hm?°
            and then access huh
6   PHYd    >genau.<
            exactly
7           (0.3)*(2.3)
    patg            *taps on screen (middle), holds smph in both hands
```

Like in Excerpt 9, having accomplished the instructed activities and entered the access code and her year of birth (l. 1–4, fig. 1 and 2), the patient's next step, highlighted by the app's design (fig. 3), consists of tapping on "Accédez à votre programme" (*Access your program*) (fig. 3). As in the previous excerpt (9), here, it is the patient who vocalizes the next instruction. She deploys a rising intonation (l. 5) while accomplishing the instructed action only after PHYd's confirmation token (l. 6).

In both Excerpts 9 and 10, pressing the "access"-button was recognized by the patient as relevant next step, based on what is provided by the app's design. The distinction between the categories of instructor and instructee and their respective category-bound activities becomes blurred as patients start to predict the instructions themselves. Note, however, that in both excerpts (9 and 10), after tapping on the referred-to button, the patient retracts their hand back into home position to await the next instruction and after confirming the patient's instruction, the physiotherapist utters the next instruction (omitted for reasons of space). As shown throughout Excerpts 5–10, within the instructional sequences examined here, physiotherapists as instructors do not have access to instruction-specific knowledge alone: the patients as instructees concurrently perceive what is going to happen next with the app on their smartphone screens and can thus, like the instructor, continuously react to the app's changing affordances and adapt their display of eHealth literacy accordingly.

In the next excerpt (11), we show how this provides for instruction practices in which physiotherapists might respond to their own instructions on behalf of the patient. Before Excerpt 11 begins, PHYa and PATf have looked at the exercise video and text, when PHYa instructs PATf to move forward in the introduction to the app's functions and the options offered by the tool:

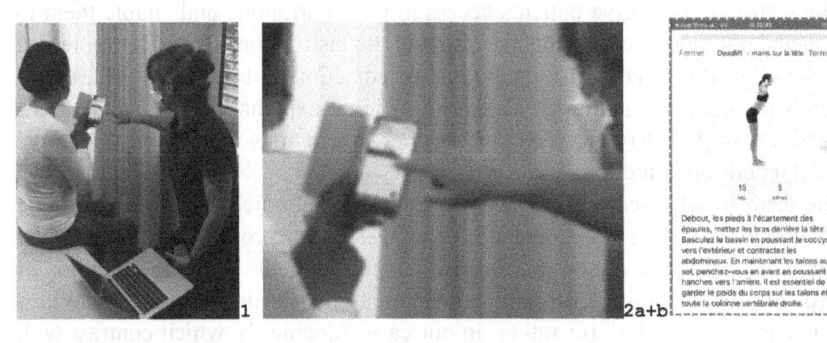

Excerpt 11

```
1   PHYa    u#:hm or you ca|#n type (.)@ comple#te?
    phya    >>rh index points to smph screen|
    phya                     |-taps on complete, keeps index over smph->1.3
    appSP                              @ smph screen changes
    fig     # figure 1     # figure 2a+b       # figure 3a+b
2           (0.3)
```

```
3          mt.h[: |and >you] can actually< (0.5) §i|t s&
4    PATf     [ m|hm]
     phya       ->|-points to smph screen (upper left)|
     phya                                            |-non-pointing gestures->
     phya                      >>looks at smph-§-looks at PATf?->1.6
5    PHYa  &more for (use; you s-; yours-)#
     fig                                  # figure 4
6    i will see §i|t, bu|t it's more| for yourself.
     phya           ->§-looks at smph->>
     phya              ->|rh index points to screen (upper)|
     phya                       |rh gestures|-index points to screen (upper)->>
7    you can go like okay >i did< .h (0.2) this and that
8    ∞much repe↑titio:ns=
     patf  ∞-nods->>
```

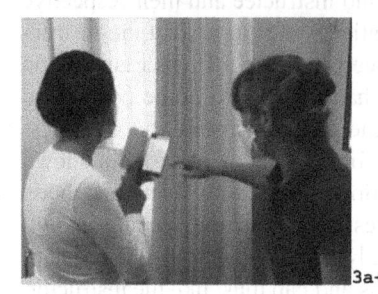

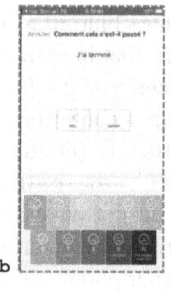

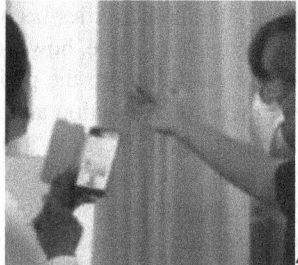

3a+b   4

Before completing her embodied instructions, again taking a modal declarative format (l. 1; fig. 1), PHYa accomplishes the instructed action herself (fig. 2a and b). After a short pause (l. 2), she resumes talking (l. 3–8; fig. 3 and 4). Instead of giving priority to organizational preferences with respect to operating others' devices (Oloff, 2019) and instructees' opportunities for learning-by-doing, PHYa thus focuses foremost on making progress in the introduction to the app and PATf aligns with this approach. Excerpt 11 thus contrasts with the previous excerpts (5–10), in which the physiotherapists retract their pointing while uttering the instructions to give patients access to the smartphone and enable them to display and not merely claim understanding of the instructions. However, note that in Excerpt 11, after accomplishing the instructed action on behalf of PATf, PHYa suspends her next instruction (l. 3) and gives some explanations about the app's interactiveness (l. 5–6) before completing her instructions concerning the app's sets and repetitions function (l. 7–8).

The analysis of Excerpts 5–11 shows how the embodied organization of the instructional sequences examined here provides for a progression through the instructional chain that can be characterized as self-evident. With the exception of Excerpt 11, the physiotherapists and patients treat the learning-by-doing activities as projecting "learnables" (or rather, in our case, "doables"), which contrast with instances in which the instructor of a computer course "solves" the encountered problem on behalf of the "trainee" (Råman, 2022). The interactive organization therefore provides for a rapid pace and the occurrence of learning opportunities that the patient grasps readily.

How to use a mobile app at home 227

Yet, as we will see in the last section, the instructional chain is also organized flexibly, providing for opportunities in which another type of pedagogy-in-interaction might take place. In Excerpt 12 (see also Excerpt 4, l. 53–59), PHYc's expansion (l. 60–63) upon his instruction (l. 57) on the assessment function of the pain level involved in exercising at home engenders PATd's question regarding the app's interactiveness:

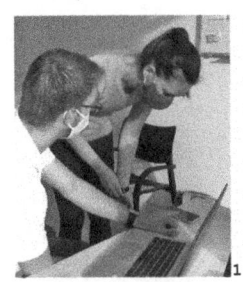

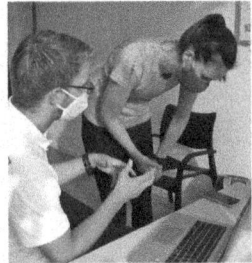

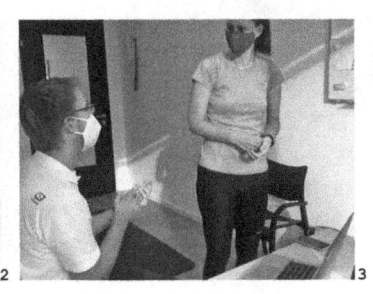

Excerpt 12

```
53 PHYc   n'£then£ you can set up (0.3) h:ow $ many# times
   phyc       £extends lh lttl.fin-£
   phyc           £lttl.fin points to different parts of smph screen->1.59
   phyc                       >>looks at smph$-looks at PATd->
   patf   >>looks at smph->1.62
   fig                                              # figure 1
54         you actually did it?
55         (0.1)$(0.1)
                ->$-looks at smph-> 1.61
56 PATd   okay?=
57 PHYc   =and if there was any pai:n.
58         (.)
59 PATd   ok£[ay.]
   phyc   ->£((lttl.fin not visible))->
60 PHYc   [and] ↑that's .h (.) that's kind of important to me£:
   phyc                                                £retracts lh->
61         just | to see:£ (.) yeah.# (.) how:$ (0.2) we:$ll: (0.5)$
   phyc       ->|lifts rh & gestures in parallel to lh->
   phyc              ->£gestures in parallel to rh->
   phyc                                                   ->$-looks at PATd->
   patd                                  ->$straightens upper body
   patd                                              $-holds position
   fig                          # figure 2
62         the ex$er$¢cise <((creaky)) ↑is for you.>#
   fig                                              # figure 3
   patd        $turns head toward PHYc$
   patd           ->¢looks at PHYc->
63         (0.3)
64 PATd   and [you will] then get: (.) feedback?$ [or:*¢?]
65 PHYc?      [(°xx°)]                           [uhm:] u&
   phyc                              ->$looks at smph->
   patd                                   *directs rh & points to PC1->
   patd                                     ->¢looks at PC1-> 1.81
66         &(0.2)$(0.1) yeah. i *can# look [it $up]
67 PATd                                   [i $sh:]ould show you:.
   phyc   ->$-looks at PC----------------$looks at PATd->
   patd              ->*rh gestures toward PC->
   fig                          # figure 4
68         [or $* is coming    di$*rectly (°to you°)]
```

228   *Sara Keel et al.*

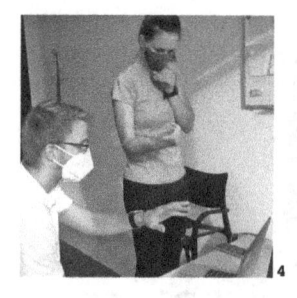

```
69 PHYc   [no.$* (.) i (.) it's $*coming up]=
   phyc   ->$-looks at PC-----$looks at PATd->
   patd     ->*index points toward smph*
   patd                        *retracts rh, keeps it against body->>
70 PATd   =↑o¢:k[ay.]
71 PHYc         [on] my $uh a:h side [↑here]
   patd   ->¢looks at smph->>
72 PATd                        [°ouh] that's really good°=
   phyc         ->$looks at smph->>
```

PHYc's instructional turns (l. 53–54; 57) are connected with an "and" (l. 57) and are accompanied by PHYc's pointings (fig. 1). However, they only engender PATd's claims of understanding (l. 56, 59), while she keeps her hands in home position. In overlap with PATd's second claim of understanding, PHYc begins his next turn with an "and ↑that's .h (.) that's..." (l. 60). By retracting his pointing and using the demonstrative pronoun "that," instead of the typical "[a]n'[d] then" (l. 53), PHYc introduces an expansion that he treats as "kind of important to me:" (l. 60–61). This engenders PATd's shift of gaze away from her smartphone and toward PHYc. Furthermore, instead of uttering a continuer, PATd formulates an understanding check regarding the use of the pain-level function and its relation to the app's interactive functioning more generally (l. 64, 67–68).

In overlap with PHYc's confirming responses (l. 65–66; 69, 71), PATd first produces an understanding token (l. 70) and then evaluates the new knowledge acquired about the app's functioning with a "change-of-state token," "ouh" (Heritage, 1984, p. 299), followed by a positive assessment (l. 72). She thus displays that she "has undergone some kind of change in her locally current state of knowledge, information, orientation or awareness" regarding the app's functioning, while having the necessary "epistemic independence" (Heritage, 2002, p. 198) to assess the newly gained knowledge regarding the app's interactive functions. She thus closes the instructional sequence expanded by PHYc.

In the continuation of Excerpt 11 and before the next excerpt (13) starts, PHYa and PATa have looked at the app's assessment and chat functions. In overlap with PHYa's completion on what they are to do with PATf's comments in the chat (l. 1–3; fig. 1), PATa utters a question about the frequency of exercise training at home (l. 4) while PHYa edits PATf's program on her laptop (PC) (fig. 2):

How to use a mobile app at home   229

Excerpt 13

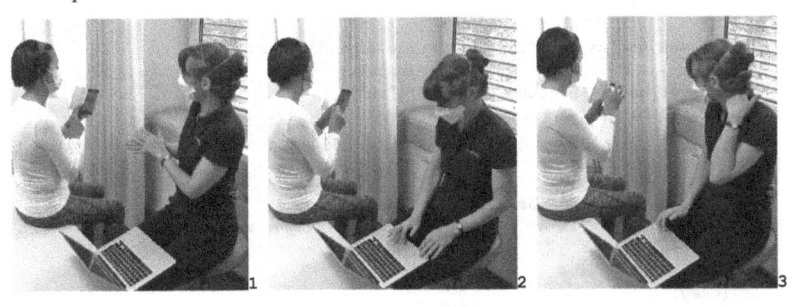

```
1  PHYa   >and then we#¢ look [at it<] §uhm:∞ (too:; to:)| h together#&
2  PATf                           [mhm]
   phya           >>-looks at PATf->§-looks at PC->
   phya                                              |directs hands to keyboard>
   patf    >>looks at PHYa¢
   patf                  ¢-looks at smph->1.6ff.
   patf       >>nods at different intervals-∞
   fig                 # figure 1                          figure 2 #
3  PHYa   &|*onc:e (0.2) .h|@: (.)[we are ba@|ck   he|re    $]
4  PATf                           [>so i hav@|e to do| this<$] ever#y* day thu:=
   phya   >|-moves cursor--|clicks on "close"|-moves cursor|
   phya                                                     ->§-looks at smph->
   patf    *-moves rh fingers over smph screen---------------------*index points->
   appPC                @ window with access code closes
   appSP                                       @ screen lights up
   fig                                                            # figure 3
5  PHYa   =mtsk .h: (0.3) IF PO§SSI↑BL:E [YE§S]:.
6  PATf                                  [(y$eah)]
   phya               ->$looks at PC-$-looks at smph->
          ((34 lines omitted: PHYa uses the app on PATf's smartphone
          to illustrate how to complete an exercise and that this is
          the same for every exercise. Then, PHYa puts away her laptop and turns to
          PATf. She explains that there are similar exercises
          in the program and that PATf should choose the one that she likes
          most and be able to discuss which exercises she liked during the next
          consultation. PHYa and PATf now both look at each other, PATf
          holding her smartphone in her hand.))

40 PHYa   =so (0.3) i al#so need feedba∞ck
```

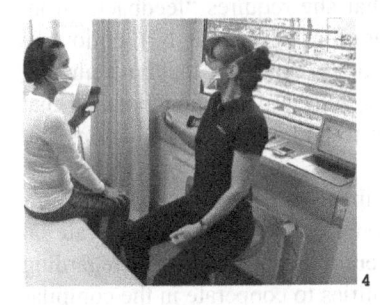

```
           patf                          ∞-nods?->
           fig                 # figure 4
       41         (.)
       42         like (.) ∞oh you kno:w. °th-° exerc∞ise ex-ua:y uhm h∞
           patf  ->nods?-∞                    ∞-nods------------∞
       43         (.) >i never do it< because .h: (0.3) °uh°
       44         >i never< (0.3) get a chance to go∞ down on the floor
           patf                                      ∞-nods->1.48
       45         s[o]
       46 PATf     [m]hm[:]
       47 PHYa         [>it] s just< no possibility: °(but) to do it°
       48         .h (0.2) an∞d i see it as my job to find∞ the right exercise
           patf        ->nods-∞                        ∞-nods->1.52
       49         that [fits for] you:.&
       50 PATf         [okay]
       51 PHYa    &h so- you- (will; we'll)∞ be doing a ↑lot of exer[cise]&
       52 PATf                                                       [yeah]
           patf                 ->nods-∞
       53 PHYa    &.h: >and the two of us we will try to find out<
       54         .h: (0.3) which on:es (.) maybe f:iv∞e or (.) ↑four
           patf                                              ∞-nods->>
       55         exercise(s) in total at the end [will be] (.) &
       56 PATf                                    [mhm]
       57 PHYa    &the right ones for you
       58         (0.2)
       59         okay?
       60         (0.2)
       61 PATf    °yes°$
           phya        ->$-looks at window board->>
       62         (0.4)
```

After PATf's question in line 4, PHYa puts the fast pace of the introduction to the app on hold. She first confirms the question (l. 5) and then explains not only how the exercise video and written description provided by the app is to be handled at home (34 lines omitted), but also that she requires "feedback" from the patient (l. 40) to compile the exercise program for PATf (l. 40–62). Following PATa's question, PHYa thus comes back to the app's functions that have already been addressed by the members before, i.e., the exercise program function and chat function, and thus readily uses PATf's question to address certain functions and options provided by the app in more depth.

As illustrated in Excerpts 12 and 13, participants treat the physiotherapist's expansions and the patient's questions as welcome opportunities to elaborate on the functions and options the app offers, e.g., different feedback practices regarding patients' home exercise (Excerpt 12) or opportunities to cooperate in the compilation of patients' exercise programs (Excerpt 13). Physiotherapists' expansions and patients' questions (see Lindwall & Lymer, 2014, on students' questions during video-broadcasted surgical interventions) are not treated as disturbing the fast pace of the introduction, but rather as providing teaching/learning opportunities. This brings us to the last excerpt (14). Before it begins, PHYd and PATg have already looked at most of the functions the app offers. They have also performed some therapeutic exercises and PHYd has added them to PATg's exercise program via his app interface that runs on his computer.

Excerpt 14

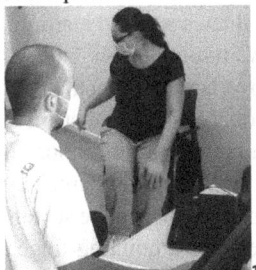

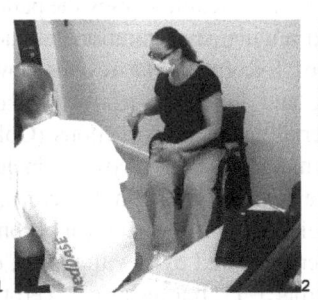

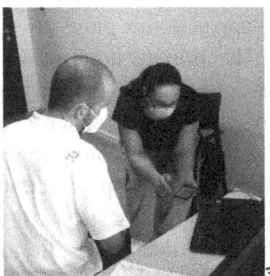

```
1   PATg   ((points to her bag)) jez die# womer jez agluefged hend,
                                  now those  that we looked at now
    fig                           # figure 1
2          ((takes smph out of her bag)) die chan ich jez theoretisch nom#ol?
                                         those i can now theoretically again
    fig                                                                # figure 2
3          (1.4)
4          das spielt jez kei rolle dass jez da
           it's not playing a role now     that now there
5          (1.6)
6          eigentlich absolviert staht.#
           actually is written completed
    fig                              # figure 3
7          (0.5)
8   PATg   denn chame das irgendwie lösche jez.
           then one can  somehow    delete it now
9          (0.6)
10  PHYd   ä:hm nei, ((app is loading on PATg's smph))
           uhm no
11         (1.1)
12         die (0.7) wo:o (3.8) wo:o ((…))
           those     that       that
```

At the beginning of Excerpt 14, PHYd and PATg are seated in front of PHYd's PC (fig. 1). PATg asks an app-related question concerning the exercise program she is to perform at home (l. 1–6), while she takes her smartphone out of her bag and starts opening the app again (fig. 1–3). After line 2, PHYd joins PATg in reinitiating a configuration in which both physiotherapist and patient focus on the patient's smartphone. Readily following PATg's actions, PHYd joins her in the learning-by-doing activity (fig. 1–3) by answering her question (l. 10–12), going through the process of "completing an exercise" on the app, and instructing her in using the app's "general chat" function (l. 13ff., omitted for reasons of space). PATg's questions and opening the app back up thus engender the interactive engagement in a second round of instructions regarding the app's operation and functions for home use.

Conclusion

Our analysis of introductions to the app as naturally occurring interaction in face-to-face physiotherapy consultations describes how physiotherapists and patients accomplish them as a suitable solution for the twofold task at hand: teaching and learning how to operate and use the app's functions and options. We show how patients' "socialization to competence" (Macbeth, 2003, p. 723 cited in Lindwall et al., 2015, p. 142), in our case to the eHealth literacy the patient needs to be able to use the app at home, plays out a triangular configuration that facilitates situated learning.

The minute description of Excerpts 5–11 reveals how, through their embodied achievement, instructing and following instructions overlap with each other. Physiotherapists' concise, serially linked instructions (Goldberg, 1975) most often take a modal declarative format (but see Excerpt 6), include the uttering aloud of features of the app's interface that are visible on the screen, and are accompanied by embodied means, such as brief pointings to what is (or becomes) visible on the screen. The embodied means are then followed by a withdrawal, e.g., of a pointing finger, into the home position (Excerpts 5–11; but see also Excerpt 12). Patients may put the instruction into action on the spot (Excerpts 5–6, 8). Yet they may alternatively do so before completion of the instruction (Excerpt 7), or even read aloud an instruction that is highlighted by the app's design and, after the physiotherapists' confirmation, put it into action (Excerpts 9–10). The distinct categories of instructor and instructee become blurred. Respective category-bound activities are treated as "constituents" that are inextricably "unified" (Greiffenhagen & Watson, 2009, p. 67) and "embedded within a local gestalt contexture (viz: Wieder, 1974, p. 186–94)" (Watson, 2008 [2011], p. 202), which we gloss as a learning-by-doing introduction to the app.

The interactive organization of learning-by-doing activities allows participants to progress rapidly (see the duration of the introduction and treated functions of the app in Figure 4), at least as long as the involved patient displays sufficient eHealth literacy (see the small squares in Figure 4). Yet, as the larger squares in Figure 4 indicate, they can also at any point in the introduction be suspended for instructive expansions by the physiotherapist and/or questions from the patient (Excerpts 11–14) and be taken up again after the participants have accomplished a completely different activity (Excerpt 14).

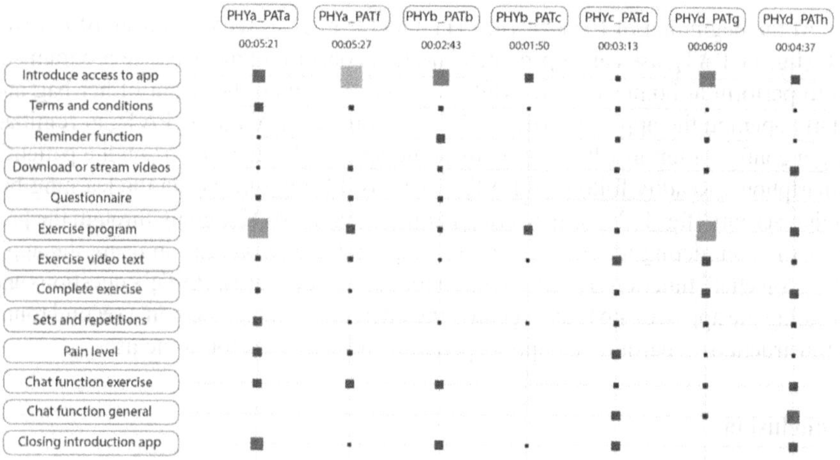

Figure 4 Instructional chains of introductions.

The introduction is thus constantly adapted to patients' displayed (and not merely claimed) eHealth literacy, patients' questions, and physiotherapists' more in-depth explanations of the app's operation, functions, and options. Alternating between learning-by-doing (Excerpts 5–11) and other pedagogical activities (Excerpts 12–14) provides patients with situated learning opportunities. Seizing these opportunities, they acquire the eHealth literacy they need to use the app at home to support self-management, home exercising, and communication with the physiotherapist – in short, the therapeutic process. The introductions to the app described here are thereby treated as sufficient for all practical purposes at hand. In line with Watson (2008 [2011], p. 211), we suggest that although the serially organized instructional sequences examined here display "family resemblances," their local achievement needs thorough examination and unpacking. A more detailed look into the situated and embodied organization of instructional sequences through which introductions are achieved serves as a reminder of this. Statements regarding the pedagogical value of distinct ways of instructing, such as "instructions-as-teaching" versus instructions as "directives" (see Excerpt 6) (Lindwall et al., 2015, pp. 144–145, 153–154), need to be made carefully if they are to match members' understanding.

For instance, the video-recorded physiotherapists and patients in our study were regular users of digital tools in general (for the patients) and of the app (for the professionals) more particularly. This may have consequences for their understanding of the benefits of certain ways of introducing the app to the patient during physiotherapy consultations. For a workshop on the use of digital tools in physiotherapy, organized by Medbase at the end of our research project, we focused on the patient's introduction to the app, using the video-recordings/transcriptions collected during our study. The participating physiotherapists constituted a rather heterogenous group, with some, like PHYa–PHYd, being regular users of the app and others not. The former considered the chosen topic as a relevant one. In contrast to the others, they engaged readily in the data sessions and discussions on the challenges and opportunities involved in introducing patients to the app in face-to-face consultations. For example, they pointed out that for less competent users of eHealth solutions, much more time needs to be allocated to learning-by-doing in introductions, or else they stressed to the contrary that an introduction to the app for less competent users requires too much time. They argued for another solution: skipping the introduction altogether and leaving it to the patient to get acquainted with the app at home.

The physiotherapists' distinct and sometimes even contradictory statements during the workshop prevented us from settling once and for all that the introduction to the app, as described in this chapter, constitutes a "topically relevant" problem of investigation or an instructive "solution" from the practitioners' point of view (Ikeya, 2020, pp. 34–36). We cannot assert that this central requirement of "hybrid workplace studies" is satisfied (Ikeya, 2020, p. 25). However, the physiotherapists' statements remind us that investigating problems and solutions that are relevant to (some) practitioners unavoidably raises a series of questions that need to be addressed empirically. As pointed out above, the serial orderliness of instructional sequences, the level of elaborateness of each instruction, and its pedagogical value are achieved interactively and locally, and are different for every introduction to the app. As our workshop experience with physiotherapists suggests, this also remains true for clarifying whether the problem and solution described here are topically relevant to other practitioners, or in our case, to other users of the app.

Acknowledgments

Our research project is supported by the *Commission scientifique du domaine santé HES-SO*, Switzerland under grant number 95846/S-RAD19-04. The requirement for approval has been waived by the respective Cantonal Ethics Committees and informed written consent from all participating physiotherapists and patients has been obtained.

We thank Medbase for the stimulating collaboration, and Veronika Schoeb for her invaluable support and insight throughout the project. A special thank goes to all participating physiotherapists and patients for making this study possible and Marc Relieu and Philippe Sormani for their insightful and stimulating comments on earlier versions.

Notes

1 Since the consultation between PHYa and PATa took twice the time the other consultations did, its representation was proportionally adapted to match them.
2 While using the app at home, PATa recorded the screen of her smartphone. Apart from these recordings of the patient's app interface, we were not able to record the screens of the patients' smartphones separately. To increase the intelligibility of what happens with the app in our multimodal transcripts, we will provide images taken from the screen-recordings made by PATa and marked with a dashed border.
3 For reasons of space, the descriptions of embodied actions use some abbreviations: l-prefix: left body part, e.g., larm = left arm; r-prefix: right body part, e.g., rwrist = right wrist; lh: left hand; rh: right hand; lttl.fin: little finger; smph: smartphone.

References

Beck Nielsen, S. (2019). Making a glance an action: Doctors' quick looks at their desk-top computer screens. *Journal of Pragmatics*, *142*, 62–74. https://doi.org/10.1016/j.pragma.2018.12.021

Blixt, L., Solbraekke, K. N., & Bjorbaekmo, W. S. (2019). Physiotherapists' experiences of adopting an eTool in clinical practice: A post-phenomenological investigation. *Physiotherapy Theory and Practice*, 1–13. https://doi.org/10.1080/09593985.2019.1681042

Butler-Henderson, K., Dalton, L., Probst, Y., Maunder, K., & Merolli, M. (2020). A meta-synthesis of competency standards suggest allied health are not preparing for a digital health future. *International Journal of Medical Informatics*, *144*, 104296. https://doi.org/10.1016/j.ijmedinf.2020.104296

Chan, C. V., & Kaufman, D. R. (2011). A framework for characterizing eHealth literacy demands and barriers. *Journal of Medical Internet Research*, *13*(4), e94. https://doi.org/10.2196/jmir.1750

Davies, L., Hinman, R. S., Russell, T., Lawford, B., Bennell, K., Billings, M., Cooper-Oguz, C., Finnan, K., Gallagher, S., Gilbertson, D. K., Holdsworth, L., Holland, A.,

Mcalister, J., Miles, D., & Roots, R. (2021). An international core capability framework for physiotherapists to deliver quality care via videoconferencing: A Delphi study. *Journal of Physiotherapy, 67*(4), 291–297. https://doi.org/10.1016/j.jphys.2021.09.001

Deppermann, A. (2018). Instruction practices in German driving lessons: Differential uses of declaratives and imperatives. *International Journal of Applied Linguistics, 28*(2), 265–282. https://doi.org/10.1111/ijal.12198

Ekberg, S., Danby, S., Theobald, M., Fisher, B., & Wyeth, P. (2019). Using physical objects with young children in 'face-to-face' and telehealth speech and language therapy. *Disability and Rehabilitation, 41*(14), 1664–1675. https://doi.org/10.1080/09638288.2018.1482817

Ertner, M. (2019). Enchanting, evoking, and affecting: The invisible work of technology implementation in homecare. *Nordic Journal of Working Life Studies, 9*(Suppl.5), 33–47.

Garfinkel, H. (2002). *Ethnomethodology's program: Durkheim's aphorisme*. Rowman & Littlefield Publishers, Inc.

Goldberg, J. A. (1975). A system for the transfer of instructions in natural settings. *Semiotica, 14*(3), 269–296.

Greatbatch, D., Heath, C., Campion, P., & Luff, P. (1995). How do desk-top computers affect the doctor-patient interaction. *Family Practice, 12*(1), 32–36. https://doi.org/10.1093/fampra/12.1.32

Greiffenhagen, C. (2008). Unpacking tasks: The fusion of new technology with instructional work. *Computer Supported Cooperative Work (CSCW), 17*(1), 35–62. https://doi.org/10.1007/s10606-007-9068-x

Greiffenhagen, C., & Watson, R. (2009). Visual repairables: Analysing the work of repair in human–computer interaction. *Visual Communication, 8*(1), 65–90. https://doi.org/10.1177/1470357208099148

Griebel, L., Enwald, H., Gilstad, H., Pohl, A.-L., Moreland, J., & Sedlmayr, M. (2018). eHealth Literacy Research - Quo vadis? *Informatics for Health and Social Care, 43*(4), 427–442. https://doi.org/https. https://doi.org/10.1080/17538157.2017.1364247

Hartswood, M., Procter, R., Rouncefield, M., Slack, R., Soutter, J., & Voss, A. (2003). 'Repairing' the machine: A case study of the evaluation of computer-aided detection tools in breast screening. In K. Kuutti, E. H. Karsten, G. Fitzpatrick, P. Dourish, & K. Schmidt (Eds.), *Proceedings of the eighth European conference on computer supported cooperative work* (pp. 375–394). Kluwer.

Heath, C., Luff, P., & Sanchez Svensson, M. (2003). Technology and medical practice. *Sociology of Health and Illness, 25*(3), 75–96. https://doi.org/10.1111/1467-9566.00341

Heritage, J. (1984). A change-of-state token and aspects of its sequential placement. In M. Atkinson & J. Heritage (Eds.), *Structures of social action: Studies in conversation analysis* (pp. 299–345). Cambridge University Press.

Heritage, J. (2002). Oh-prefaced responses to assessments: A method of modifying agreement/disagreement. In C. Ford, B. Fox, & S. Thompson (Eds.), *The language of turn sequence* (pp. 198–224). Oxford University Press.

Higgs, J., Refshauge, K., & Ellis, E. (2001). Portrait of the physiotherapy profession. *Journal of Interprofessional Care, 15*(1), 79–89. https://doi.org/10.1080/13561820020022891

Hindmarsh, J. (2010). Peripherality, participation and communities of practice: Examining the patient in dental training. In N. Llewellyn & J. Hindmarsh (Eds.), *Organisation, interaction and practice* (pp. 218–239). Cambridge University Press.

Hindmarsh, J., Hyland, L., & Banerjee, A. (2014). Work to make simulation work: 'Realism', instructional correction and the body in training. *Discourse Studies, 16*(2), 247–269. https://doi.org/10.1177/1461445613514670

Hindmarsh, J., Jenkings, K. N., & Rapley, T. (2007). Special issue: Introduction to healthcare technologies in practice. *Health Informatics Journal*, *13*(1), 5–8.

Ikeya, N. (2020). Hybridity of hybrid studies of work: Examination of informing practitioners in practice. *Ethnographic Studies*, *17*, 22–40. https://doi.org/10.5281/zenodo.405053

Jefferson, G. (2004). Glossary of transcript symbols with an introduction. In G. H. Lerner (Ed.), *Conversation Analysis: Studies from the first generation* (pp. 13–31). Benjamins. https://doi.org/10.1075/pbns.125.02jef

Jimenez, G., Spinazze, P., Matchar, D., Huat, G. K. C., Van Der Kleij, R. M. J. J., Chavannes, N. H., & Car, J. (2020). Digital health competencies for primary healthcare professionals: A scoping review. *International Journal of Medical Informatics*, *143*, 104260. https://doi.org/10.1016/j.ijmedinf.2020.104260

Keel, S. (2021). Membership categorisation and the notion of 'omni-relevance' in everyday family interactions. In R. J. Smith, R. Fitzgerald, & W. Housley (Eds.), *On Sacks. Methodology, materials, and inspiration* (pp. 156–171). Routledge.

Keel, S., Schmid, A., Keller, F., & Schoeb, V. (2022). Investigating the use of digital health tools in physiotherapy: Facilitators and barriers. *Physiotherapy Theory and Practice*, 1–20. https://doi.org/10.1080/09593985.2022.2042439

Keller, F., Keel, S., Schmid, A., & Schoeb, V. (2021). *Introducing a mobile health-application in physiotherapy: Opportunities for patient participation. 2.* Kooperationskongress Smarter Reha [Online].

Konttila, J., Siira, H., Kyngas, H., Lahtinen, M., Elo, S., Kaariainen, M., Kaakinen, P., Oikarinen, A., Yamakawa, M., Fukui, S., Utsumi, M., Higami, Y., Higuchi, A., & Mikkonen, K. (2019). Healthcare professionals' competence in digitalisation: A systematic review. *Journal of Clinical Nursing*, *28*(5–6), 745–761. https://doi.org/10.1111/jocn.14710

Lerner, G. H. (2002). Turn-sharing: The choral co-production of talk-in-interaction. In C. E. Ford, B. A. Fox, & S. A. Thompson (Eds.), *The language of turn and sequence* (pp. 225–257). Oxford University Press.

Lindwall, O., & Lymer, G. (2014). Inquiries of the body: Novice questions and the instructable observability of endodontic scenes. *Discourse Studies*, *16*(2), 271–294. https://doi.org/10.1177/1461445613514672

Lindwall, O., Lymer, G., & Greiffenhagen, C. (2015). The sequential analysis of instruction. In N. Markee (Ed.), *The handbook of classroom discourse and interaction* (pp. 142–157). John Wiley & Sons, Inc.

Luff, P., Hindmarsh, J., & Heath, C. (Eds.). (2000). *Workplace studies: Recovering work practice and informing system design*. Cambridge University Press.

Macbeth, D. (2003). Hugh Mehan's "learning lessons" reconsidered: On the differences between the naturalistic and critical analysis of classroom discourse. *Research in Language and Social Interaction*, *40*, 239–280.

Martin, C., & Sahlström, F. (2010). Learning as longitudinal interactional change: From other-repair to self-repair in physiotherapy treatment. *Discourse Processes*, *47*(8), 668–697. https://doi.org/10.1080/01638531003628965

Martin, D., Mariani, J., & Rouncefield, M. (2007). Managing integration work in an NHS electronic patient record (EPR) project. *Health Informatics Journal*, *13*(1), 47–56.

Merlino, S. (2020). Professional touch in speech and language therapy for the treatment of post-stroke aphasia. In A. Cekaite & L. Mondada (Eds.), *Touch in social interaction. Touch, language, and body* (pp. 197–223). Routledge.

Mikesell, L., Marti, F. A., Guzmán, J. R., McCreary, M., & Zima, B. (2018). Affordances of mhealth technology and the structuring of clinic communication. *Journal of Applied Communication Research, 46*(3), 323–347. https://doi.org/10.1080/00909882.2018.1465195

Mondada, L. (2014). The surgeon as a camera director: Manoeuvring video in the operating theatre. In M. Broth, E. Laurier, & L. Mondada (Eds.), *Studies of video practices video at work*. Routledge.

Mondada, L. (2018). Multiple temporalities of language and body in interaction: Challenges for transcribing multimodality. *Research on Language and Social Interaction, 51*(1), 85–106. https://doi.org/10.1080/08351813.2018.1413878

Nishizaka, A. (2014). Instructed perception in prenatal ultrasound examinations. *Discourse Studies, 16*(2), 217–246. https://doi.org/10.1177/1461445613515354

Norman, C. D., & Skinner, H. A. (2006). Ehealth literacy: Essential skills for consumer health in a networked world. *Journal of Medical Internet Research, 8*(2), e9. https://doi.org/10.2196/jmir.8.2.e9

Oloff, F. (2019). Das Smartphone als soziales Objekt: Eine multimodale Analyse von initialen Zeigesequenzen in Alltagsgesprächen. In K. Marx & A. Schmidt (Eds.), *Interaktion und Medien - Interaktionsanalytische Zugänge zu medienvermittelter Kommunikation* (pp. 191–218). Winter.

Oloff, F. (2021). New technologies – New social conduct? A sequential and multimodal approach to smartphone use in face-to-face interaction. *Bulletin Suisse de Linguistique Appliquée, 1*, 13–34.

Pilnick, A., Hindmarsh, J., & Gill, V. T. (2010). Beyond 'doctor and patient': Developments in the study of healthcare interactions. In A. Pilnick, J. Hindmarsh, & V. T. Gill (Eds.), *Communication in healthcare settings - Policy, participation and new technologies* (pp. 1–16). Blackwell Publishing.

Pollner, M., & Emerson, R. (2001). Ethnomethodology and ethnography. In P. Atkinson, A. Coffey, S. Delamont, J. Lofland, & L. Lofland (Eds.), *Handbook of ethnography* (pp. 118–135). Sage Publications.

Råman, J. (2022). Multimodal negotiation for the right to access digital devices among elderly users and teachers. In J.-P. Alarauhio, T. Räisänen, J. Toikkanen, & R. Tumelius (Eds.), *Shaping the North through multimodal and intermedial interaction* (pp. 67–93). Palgrave. https://doi.org/10.1007/978-3-030-99104-3_4

Sacks, H. (1992). *Lectures on conversations (*Vol. 1 & 2). Basil Blackwell.

Sacks, H., & Schegloff, E. (2002). Home position. *Gesture, 2*(2), 133–146.

Samerski, S., & Müller, H. (2019). Digital health literacy – Thesen zu Konzept und Förderungsmöglichkeiten. In M. A. Pfannstiel, P. Da-Cruz, & H. Mehlich (Eds.), *Digitale Transformation von Dienstleistungen im Gesundheitswesen VI. Impulse für die Forschung* (pp. 35–50). Springer Fachmedien Wiesbaden GmbH, ein Teil von Springer Nature 2019. https://doi.org/https://https://doi.org/10.1007/978-3-658-25461-2

Sanchez Svensson, M. S., Luff, P., & Heath, C. (2009). Embedding instruction in practice: Contingency and collaboration during surgical training. *Sociology of Health and Illness, 31*(6), 889–906. https://doi.org/10.1111/j.1467-9566.2009.01195.x

Shaw, S. E., Seuren, L. M., Wherton, J., Cameron, D., A'Court, C., Vijayaraghavan, S., Morris, J., Bhattacharya, S., & Greenhalgh, T. (2020). Video consultations between patients and clinicians in diabetes, cancer, and heart failure services: Linguistic ethnographic study of video-mediated interaction. *Journal of Medical Internet Research, 22*(5), e18378. https://doi.org/10.2196/18378

Sieck, C. J., Sheon, A., Ancker, J. S., Castek, J., Callahan, B., & Siefer, A. (2021). Digital inclusion as a social determinant of health. *npj Digital Medicine*, *4*(1). https://doi.org/10.1038/s41746-021-00413-8

Sormani, P. (2010). L'ordinaire dans l'« ésotérique » : L'action instruite comme phénomène instructif. In B. Olszewska, M. Barthélémy, & S. Laugier (Eds.), *Les données de l'enquête* (pp. 167–195). Presses universitaires de France.

Tuncer, S., Lindwall, O., & Brown, B. (2020). Making time: Pausing to coordinate video instructions and practical tasks. *Symbolic Interaction*. https://doi.org/10.1002/symb.516

Watson, R. (2008 [2011]). Comparative sociology, laic and analytic: Some critical remarks on comparison in conversation analysis. *Cahiers de Praxématique*, *50*, 203–244.

Weilenmann, A. (2010). Learning to text: An interaction analytic study of how seniors learn to enter text on mobile phones *Proceedings of the SIGCHI conference on human factors in computing*, Atlanta, GA.

Wentink, M. M., Siemonsma, P. C., van Bodegom-Vos, L., de Kloet, A. J., Verhoef, J., Vlieland, T., & Meesters, J. J. L. (2019). Teachers' and students' perceptions on barriers and facilitators for ehealth education in the curriculum of functional exercise and physical therapy: A focus groups study. *BMC Medical Education*, *19*(1), 343. https://doi.org/10.1186/s12909-019-1778-5

9 Socialization and accountability
Instructional responses to peer feedback in healthcare simulation debriefing

Elin Nordenström, Gustav Lymer, and Oskar Lindwall

Introduction

Simulation-based team training is a common feature of healthcare education, offering a safe, ethical, and time-efficient alternative to training with real patients (Issenberg & Scalese, 2008). Debriefing, which takes place after the simulated case, is a central component of such training in which the students' simulation performance is subject to feedback from both instructors and peers. This chapter investigates how the provision of feedback is organized during debriefings and discusses its relevance for professional socialization in healthcare settings. In the following, we first outline how feedback has been conceptualized in the research literature and highlight some findings central to the current chapter. The focus is on the sensitive nature of feedback and the differences between peer and instructor feedback. After introducing the empirical case and setting, we then turn to an analysis of two episodes from post-simulation debriefings. By investigating how feedback from instructors relies on and is responsive to prior talk amongst students, we show how the instructional work accomplished through the instructors' contributions addresses not only simulation performance but also the ways in which performance is accounted for in student talk. The analysis demonstrates how the socialization of members entails an interplay between fostering performative competence through feedback on observable conduct and shaping professional forms of accountability. In the concluding discussion, we return to this observation and its consequences for professional socialization in healthcare settings.

Background

In research on healthcare simulations, debriefing conversations are considered central to simulation training and believed to foster reflection and consolidate the learning of the skills trained (e.g., Dieckmann et al., 2008). Rall et al. (2000), for instance, called debriefing "the heart and soul of simulator training" (p. 517), a description that has been widely cited in the simulation literature. A growing body of studies explores the effectiveness of different ways of eliciting reflection and providing feedback in debriefing to improve learner achievement (see, e.g., Kolbe et al., 2013; Rudolph et al., 2008; Timmis & Speirs, 2015). Meta-analyses have summarized the debriefing literature and identified and discussed features that can impact the effectiveness of debriefing (Tannenbaum & Cerasoli, 2013; Keiser & Arthur, 2021; 2022), including the duration of the debriefing, whether the feedback is individualized or delivered to groups, the amount of structure applied to the debriefing format, the degree of instructor involvement, and the character of the media used to recreate and analyze simulator performances and events (see Keiser & Arthur, 2021).

The terms debriefing and feedback are sometimes used synonymously in the research literature on healthcare simulations (e.g., Chiniara et al., 2013; Issenberg et al., 2005; McGaghie et al., 2010; Motola et al., 2013). Others use "debriefing" for activities where participants and instructors jointly discuss and reflect upon the preceding simulation performance (Eppich et al., 2015), whereas "feedback" refers to the delivery of "[s]pecific information about the comparison between a trainee's observed performance and a standard, given with the intent to improve the trainee's performance" (Eppich et al., 2015, p. 1501). The conceptualization of feedback as the one-way transmission of information from a sender to a recipient (see Chiniara et al., 2013; Sawyer et al., 2016; van de Ridder, 2008; Waznonis, 2014) can be contrasted with the understanding of feedback as a more interactive process that is predominant in contemporary educational research literature (Evans, 2013). In line with this view, feedback is typically used as an umbrella term for evaluative, corrective, recommending, and instructive conversations between two or more parties aimed at improving one party's understanding and/or performance of a task (e.g., Evans, 2013; Hattie & Timperley, 2007; Sadler, 2010).

In this chapter, the term "debriefing" is used to designate the encompassing activity or context in which feedback sequences occur. In parallel with the educational research literature, feedback is used to refer to sequences constituted by various types of actions, including corrections, assessments, and advice. This is also in line with prior conversation analytic studies on feedback, which have treated feedback as compound turns that include "contextualising, evaluative and recommending elements" (Vehviläinen, 2009, p. 187). There is some prior research on simulation-based professional training that outlines the function of debriefing in relation to the scenario (e.g., Hontvedt, 2015; Sellberg, 2018; Roth, 2015), how debriefing can be supported by various tools such as video recordings and other visualizations (Roth & Jornet, 2015; Nordenström et al., 2017; Sellberg et al., 2021), and how the simulation performance in various ways are linked to professional practice (Hindmarsh et al., 2014; Sellberg, Lindwall & Rystedt, 2021). Given the investigated phenomena, however, it is also relevant to mention studies of post-performance feedback talk in other academic contexts that explicitly deal with the sensitive nature of feedback and the difference between feedback from instructors and peers before returning to feedback specifically aimed at professional practice.

As shown in conversation analytic research on various ordinary and professional settings, the production and reception of corrections, negative assessments, and advice tend to be interactionally delicate and coupled with tensions and resistance (e.g., Heritage & Sefi, 1992; Jefferson, 1987; Pomerantz, 1984; Pomerantz & Heritage, 2013). To some extent, this holds true for educational interactions as well, even though critical feedback is typically an expected part of such activities.

With respect to the sensitive nature of feedback, there are systematic differences in the ways in which feedback is delivered by teachers and student peers. Copland (2011) investigated the "negotiation of face" in post-teaching feedback meetings for teacher trainees. She argues that the trainers, although sensitive to issues of "face-threatening acts" or "politeness," largely orient to critical feedback as an interactionally unproblematic activity associated with their institutional role. Peer feedback, in contrast, tends to take the form of descriptive comments and positive evaluations. The rare instances of negative feedback are "unelaborated, hedged, and often linked by the trainee delivering the feedback to a weakness in his/her own performance, as if somehow to share responsibility for the weakness" (p. 3838).

The observations made by Copland (2011) are repeated in other studies (e.g., Park, 2014; Waring, 2007; 2012) and peer feedback seems to be systemically couched with downgrades, hedges, accounts, or other minimizing features to a greater extent than feedback from teachers. These differences are associated with locally relevant categorial relations and entitlements, which potentially shape the ways that actions are produced and responded to. Svinhufvud (2015) noted further differences in terms of turn-taking and turn-allocation: student discussants provide feedback on the reviewed manuscript, primarily in response to invitations or prompts from the supervisor. The supervisor, by contrast, recurrently self-selects to provide feedback, both on the manuscript and on the discussant's prior feedback, in some cases aligning with peer feedback and in other cases objecting to it or prompting further elaboration.

Other studies engage with the instructional significance of teacher feedback by pointing out how student performance during a simulated scenario is linked to disciplinary and professional standards, norms, and principles to demonstrate "the deeply reasoned and skilled practices that characterize professional conduct" (Sellberg et al., 2021, p. 321). In the context of simulation-based dental education, for instance, Hindmarsh et al. (2014) found that tutors' instructional corrections are routinely coupled with accounts that serve to demonstrate the relationship between students' simulation performance and "real" situations and contingencies from work in clinical settings. As emphasized by Hindmarsh et al. (2014), these accounts serve an important instructional function in invoking "situations and contingencies from work in real clinical settings and with human patients […] that they [the students] have not yet experienced" (p. 256), thereby broadening "the horizon of the student's actions […] holding them accountable to issues that are relevant when engaging in professional practice" (p. 256). Similarly, Waring (2017) demonstrated how mentors providing feedback to teacher trainees invoke larger disciplinary and pedagogical principles to frame problems in the trainees' teaching as "not isolated and idiosyncratic, but violating some fundamental understanding of the profession" (Waring, 2017, p. 23). This practice of "going general" serves to establish "the severity of the problem, opening up spaces for exploring principled understandings, and socializing the teacher into important disciplinary and pedagogical conduct and conceptualizations" (Waring, 2017, p. 30).

In sum, the work outlined in this section has demonstrated differences in both interactional organization (e.g., mitigation strategies) and the instructional character of teacher–student and student–student feedback. Our chapter extends previous work by further examining the sequential embeddedness of instructor contributions in relation to peer-feedback interactions. Specifically, the chapter demonstrates how peer feedback, in conjunction with the recipient's uptake, is used as a basis for instructional expansions. First, we show that these expansions can serve to *generalize* prior peer-feedback talk, the latter tending to be locally oriented and particularized. While Waring (2017) examined the practice of "going general" in the context of instructor feedback on practical performance, we explore how generalization may also function as an operation on the immediately preceding talk. Second, our analyses aim to qualify the image of peer feedback as locally oriented and particularized, and teacher feedback as providing generalizations by pointing out the relevance of students' accounting practices in the delivery and reception of feedback.

The case

The investigated simulation training was part of two one-day sessions on interprofessional[1] collaboration for medical students and nursing students in the final stages of their educational programs at a Swedish university. The students were divided into mixed groups of approximately ten medical and nursing students who rotated between different exercises, of which one was based on a full-scale computerized patient simulator. This exercise aimed to train students in communication and interprofessional teamwork in line with the principles of the crisis resource management (CRM) system:[2] a set of 15 principles for individual and team behavior aimed at promoting patient safety in both ordinary and crisis situations. The exercise involved three steps: briefing (short introduction to the simulated case), scenario (performance of the simulated case), and debriefing (follow-up conversation including feedback). Due to the large group size, not all students could take part in the scenario. Therefore, about half of the group observed the scenario through a one-way window from an adjacent control room. Prior to the start of the scenario, the students who were to perform the case received brief background information about the patient. The students also decided on the work distribution, which involved decisions regarding which of the medical students should have the role of the doctor in charge, which student should be the assisting doctor, and what tasks the nurses should perform. The observing students were told to pay careful attention to the course of events to learn as much as possible from their peers' simulation performance and to be able to provide peer feedback in the subsequent debriefing.

The scenario was conducted in a simulation room designed to resemble an authentic hospital wardroom with standard medical equipment and supplies. Two instructors, who were medical doctors, monitored the patient simulator from the control room, and a third instructor, who was a nurse, was present in the simulation room to assist with the equipment. Immediately after the scenario, all instructors and students went into another room to have a debriefing conversation that lasted approximately 15 minutes. In some educational contexts, debriefing is a highly structured event organized according to a predefined template that includes several scripted questions (see Johansson et al., 2017), whereas in other contexts it involves a more loosely structured discussion (see Nyström et al., 2016). The debriefings examined in the present chapter did not follow any predetermined debriefing template and instead took a loosely structured format. In the eight investigated debriefings, the discussion was initiated by one of the instructors, inviting the students to comment on anything they felt like discussing. The opening phrase was similarly formulated across all debriefings, e.g., "You're welcome to speak freely. What do you want to say more? Spontaneously? Everyone? Actors as well as observers." The discussions that followed included both students and instructors commenting on various aspects of the simulation performance, both in positive and critical terms.

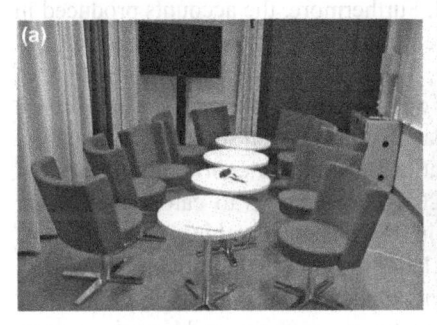

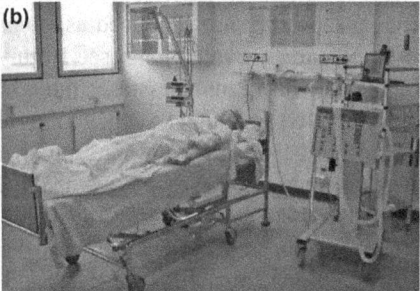

Figure 1 A debriefing room and a simulation room with a patient simulator. Picture from the data.

The analyzed data consisted of video recordings of eight student groups performing the same simulation exercise during two training days (see Figure 1). The briefings, observing students, and debriefings were video-recorded with one video camera with an external microphone, and the scenarios were captured with two cameras with external microphones. The data collection was undertaken as part of a larger research project financed by the Swedish Research Council that explored how simulation-based learning environments could support the training of interprofessional collaboration and teamwork skills for healthcare students and professionals.[3]

Analysis

As part of the analytical work for the study reported in this chapter, all the recordings of the eight simulation exercises were reviewed to gain an understanding of the course of events and the organization of the simulation training. The debriefing conversations were subject to more detailed reviews and transcription,[4] which resulted in the identification of ten episodes initiated by a student providing critical feedback on the simulation performance of one or more student peers, followed by a response by the addressee and concluded by an uptake of the feedback by an instructor. The ten identified episodes demonstrate the same overall sequential organization, although there are substantial variations among them. In this chapter, we focus on two episodes. The first shows a comparatively simple example of the basic episode we are dealing with, to open a discussion of the ways in which instructional interventions are produced as responsive to prior talk. The second episode is more complex and involves more extensive accounting work on the part of the students and a more elaborate response from the instructor.

In line with observations made by Hindmarsh et al. (2014) and Waring (2017), the analyzed cases show how accounts that accompany the delivery and reception of peer feedback are not merely mitigating devices but display "moral and practical reasoning" (Buttny, 1993, p. 49). More specifically, these accounts involve generalized understandings of how a "failure event" (Buttny, 2004, p. 3) noted in critical feedback can relevantly be understood. Furthermore, the accounts produced in these episodes are not produced as isolated utterances; instead, they rely on and seek out hearers' evaluations (see Buttny, 1987). By implication, expressions of alignment or disalignment can be thought of as conditionally relevant in response to a formulated account. To specify the relationship between students' and instructors' accounts, we draw on conceptualizations of both categorial and sequential orders of interaction (see e.g., Watson, 2015). References to categorization are mainly used here to characterize the ways in which student and instructor accounts are constructed, respectively, and how the latter respond to the former. We take an interest in the membership categories and action descriptions (see also Lindwall & Lynch, 2021) that undergird the accounts' status as an excuse and how these same categorial orders are transformed in the instructors' interventions. Specifically, we examine the latter for the ways in which a *professional* frame of reference or "logic of action" is installed and the instructional significance of the contrasts between student and instructor accounts thereby achieved.

Going general in response to peer-feedback talk

The transcribed interaction in Extract 1 involves two medical students and one instructor. It occurs about 1 minute and 20 seconds after the instructor's opening phrase that initiates the start of the debriefing, which occasions positively oriented evaluative comments from several students in the group. Thereafter, a medical student (FPM) who observed the scenario self-selects to proceed. Turning toward the medical student who acted as the doctor in charge (FAM), FPM starts by providing a general positive appreciation of his performance, claiming that it was magnificent. FPM then opines that there is room for improvement and that she has written down a few things that she will now go through quickly, after which she proceeds to address the observations written down on a piece of paper (eight items in total). After addressing the first list item, which concerns FAM's method of giving orders to the other students taking part in the scenario, FPM turns her gaze down toward the paper and takes a deep breath, seemingly preparing to address the next item on the list. At this point, she is interrupted by the instructor (INS), who, after requesting permission to "stop there," invites the other students who took part in the scenario to comment further on the issue addressed by FPM. The way in which the instructor stops the progression of FPM's list construction to initiate further discussion is repeated after the delivery of each of the following items on the list and is thus a distinctive feature of the feedback episode. The episode is too long to show in its entirety, and only the delivery and uptake of the second list item are provided in Extract 1.

Extract 1

```
101   FPM:    åttife:m de e inte pulsen de e mapp
              eighty five that's not the pulse it's map
      fpm:    >>looks at FAM---->
      fam:    >>looks at FPM---->
      ins:    >>looks at FAM---->
102           (0.8)
103   FAM:    +m: ja såg@ de sen  [(att de)    (xxx)]
              m: I saw that later [(that it)   (xxx)]
104   INS:                        €[EH-HEH-HE    +€] men de e jätte-
                                   [EH-HEH-HE      ] but that's very-€
      fpm:             @looks down at notes---->
      fam:    +looks in front------------------+looks at INS---->>
      ins:                        €throws head back, looks at stud to her
                                  left-----------€looks at FAM---->
105   INS:    å bara där om €ja får bara @kommentera .hh (0.3) €ha som vana
              and just there if I may just comment .hh (0.3) have as a habit
      fpm:                                @looks at INS---->
      ins:                      €looks at FPM---------------------€looks at
                                                                  students
                                                                  sitting
                                                                  opposite--->
106   INS:    (.)@när ni ska börja jobba nu på (.) vilka kliniker de än är
              (.)when you'll start working now at (.) whatever clinic it is
      fpm:        @looks down at notes---->>
107   INS:    se till att ni e väl förtrogna me den utrustning som ni
              make sure that you're well acquainted with the equipment you
108   INS:    ska använda bara en sån enkel €grej€
              will be using just such a basic thing
      ins:                                  €looks at FPM€
```

The episode begins with FPM providing a correction of FAM's interpretation of a number displayed on the patient monitor[5] in the preceding simulation scenario (line 101, Extract 1): the number 85 was not a measure of the patient's pulse, as FAM took it to be, but a measure of the *mean arterial pressure* (MAP). Identifying an error in the use of a specific medical device and contrasting this correctable with the proper alternative, the correction is local, specific, and retrospectively oriented, features that characterize many of the students' feedback contributions in the other extracts that have been analyzed as well.

The correction by FPM is followed by a gap of 0.8 seconds (line 102), after which the addressed student, FAM, begins to formulate a response: an affirmative token is followed by a claim of having noticed the error "later" in the scenario (line

103). The response is interrupted as the instructor bursts into loud laughter and turns toward the students sitting next to her, as if to invite them to laugh along with her (line 104). As Glenn (2003) notes, "laughter is *indexical*; it is heard as referring to something, and hearers will seek out its referent" (Glenn, 2003, p. 48). Due, in part, to laughter's lack of adherence to any systematic linguistic code, the referent of individual instances of laughter will, by default, be sought in its immediate proximity. That is, laughter will routinely be heard as a response to the last utterance, or in the case of interruptions, to the "current state of development" (Sacks, 1974, p. 348, cited in Glenn, 2003, p. 48) of the utterance in progress. Of course, speakers can overcome this local referential range by explicitly tying back to earlier events in ensuing talk. Here, however, the instructor's laughter is produced at a transition-relevant point, just after the completion of "I saw that later," thereby overlapping further talk by FAM, and no ensuing attempt is made at locating the laughable elsewhere. Thus, we could relevantly hear the instructor's laughter as responsive to FAM's utterance in line 103. Since there are no prior efforts by FAM to invite a non-serious orientation, the instructor's laughter, in being a "first laugh" targeting someone other than the speaker, thereby displays a *disaffiliating stance* to the prior turn (see Glenn, 2003). What exactly about line 103 warrants such expressed disaffiliation is not immediately apparent. The instructor's ensuing remarks, however, can be heard an indirect elaboration on this issue.

The initial "but", followed by the emphasized indexical "that" (line 104), projects a contrast that can be heard as an elaboration on the laughter. However, the utterance is then aborted and restarted, with "and just there" signaling *continuation* and *expansion* rather than contrast (see Bolden, 2010). Thus, the instructor self-repairs, possibly as a way of downplaying prior laughter by not procccding with further talk in direct connection to it. Subsequently, after a request for permission to interject, a formulation of advice (lines 105–107) is produced. Proposing that the students should make a habit of familiarizing themselves with the equipment available in future workplaces, the instructor's contribution is designed to solve the problem identified by FPM and is thus clearly responsive to the topic raised in the feedback turn.

While the instructor's uptake aligns with the prior feedback, building on and further expanding it, there are several significant differences regarding the design and focus of the student's and instructor's contributions. First, in contrast to the student's correction, the instructor's uptake does not concern the use of a specific medical device but indicates equipment in general. Second, the uptake does not point to what should have been done in the preceding scenario but to what should be done in future work practice. Third, it is not solely directed at the student who made the mistake but addresses all students in the room (note the use of "ni"/plural "you"). Thus, the advice not only serves to demonstrate to FAM how his local educational achievement forms a relevant experience for future professional practice but also provides the entire group of students with a general lesson.

Notably, the advice, albeit not in explicit terms, invokes one of the CRM principles for team behavior to be practiced in the simulation exercise: *know the environment*. It is of vital importance for healthcare practitioners to be familiar with the specific working environment, including personnel, equipment, and supplies (Miller et al., 2014, p. 121). Hence, in addition to demonstrating how the simulation performance is relevant to future work practice, the advice also indexes a model for team behavior, further emphasizing the generalizing thrust of the instructor's remarks. The uptake, in encouraging "an orientation and production of the talk 'as if' it was undertaken in a clinical setting" (Hindmarsh et al., 2014, p. 265), thus has an obvious instructive function in relation to the professional competencies being practiced and learned. In sum, to characterize the instructional intervention as an operation on the prior feedback turn, a local, specific, and retrospectively oriented correction of a peer student's simulation performance is elaborated through generalized and future-oriented advice directed at the entire group of students.

The question of how we might consider the possibility that the instructor's remarks are also oriented to FAM's brief account in line 103 remains. Here, it is helpful to point out the *categorial* order at work in the noted contrasts between the instructor's response and the prior talk. In shifting the address term from the singular (Sw. "du") to the plural (Sw. "ni") in conjunction with the reference to "work" and "clinic", the instructor does not merely expand the set of relevant addressees to include the group of overhearing students – she also invokes a *professional* social organization in which students are addressed as (future) incumbents of professional roles. While this error was made by an individual acting in the simulation, the advice concerns professional practice in general. Moreover, this professional categorial order also reframes the boundaries for assessing the relevance of *accounts*, which is significant for understanding the instructor's disaffiliating laughter. For a professional role incumbent acting under the jurisdiction of the principle to know the environment, "I saw that later" would be a problematic – and at best peripherally relevant – response to the error of mistaking one vital measure for another. The *categorial shift* in the instructor's response can thus be heard as dealing with the everyday, or specifically nonprofessional, character of the feedback recipient's response, in addition to "going general" (Waring, 2017) in relation to the individualized and particularized character of the feedback turn.

These final considerations raise the possible relevance of feedback recipients' responses and accounts more generally for analyzing instructional follow-up interventions. Any determinate analysis of the instructor's intervention as responsive to the detailed construction of FAM's account is, however, compromised by the latter's brevity. In the next extract, we hope to demonstrate such responsiveness more clearly.

The generalizing character of accounts

In Extract 1, both the feedback and the account produced in response are brief and unelaborated. They are also locally and individually oriented in targeting events within the prior scenario. Consequently, the instructor's contribution can be described as an instance of "going general" (Waring, 2017) and doing so *first*, in a sequential context characterized by prior individualized orientations. The accounting work done in peer-feedback talk, however, is not always locally and individually oriented in such a clear-cut way, as the following extract illustrates. The episode shown in Extracts 2a and 2b is taken from another debriefing session led by the same three instructors, but with a different group of students.[6] Prior to the episode, one of the medical students who took part in the preceding scenario (FAM) commented on his own performance in critical terms by saying that he was uncertain about his responsibilities as an assisting doctor and that he was unsure about whether to remain by the head end of the patient's bed to monitor breathing and other vital parameters. In response, FPM – the student who played the role of the doctor in charge in the scenario – delivers feedback beginning on line 201.

Extract 2a

```
201   FPM:   ja tror liksom man vill ju inte störa den som
             I think somehow one doesn't (PRT) want to disturb the one who
202          ä:r (0.6) ledaren (0.3) e läkar (.) ansvarige så att
             is (0.6) the leader (0.3) uh the doctor (.) in charge so to
203          säga men de hade ju: (0.7) de hade nog vart bra alltså (.)
             speak but it had (PRT) (0.7) it had probably been good then (.)
204          [å de e väl de          ]
             [and it's the thing]
205   STX:   [ja:                    ]
             [yeah               ]
206   FPM:   att vi känner ju (.) inte varandra jättebra
             that we don't know (PRT) (.) each other very well
207          [heller sådär    ]
             [either like that]
208   FAM:   [nä:             ]
             [nah             ]
209   FPM:   sen tidigare men (.) har man jobbat ihop då kanske du
             since earlier but (.) has one worked together then maybe you
210          hade sagt så här a men har du tänkt på du kanske
             had said like this yeah but have you thought about maybe you!
211          borde gå igenom (.) de [här ]
             should go over (.)     [this]
212   FAM:                          [a:  ]
                                    [yeah]
213   FPM:   ibland så (.) hakar man ju upp sig lite å fastnar å
             sometimes so (.) one gets caught up a little and gets stuck and
214   FAM:   (xxx)=
215   FPM:   =ja försökte få kontakt me dej nån gång men (.) j↑a=
             =I tried to get in touch with you at some point but (.) yeah=
216   FAM:   =a=
             =yeah=
217   FPM:   =ja va nog inte så tydlig heller     [där liksom    ]
             =I was probably not that clear either [there somehow]
218   FAM:                                         [nä            ]
                                                   [nah           ]
219   FPM:   att (0.3) du hade ju kunnat stötta
             that (0.3) you could (PRT) have provided support
```

```
220   FAM:  a: (.)    [jo å de va nåra           ]
            yeah (.)  [yeah and there were a few]
221   FPM:            [(xxx)                     ]
222   FAM:  gånger som de (.) va i mitt huvud nu borde ja kanske säga de
            times that it (.) was in my head now maybe I should say
223         här men-
            this but-
224   FPM:  a:
            yeah:
225   FAM:  sen lät ja dej (.) [göra din grej (xxx)         ]
            then I let you (.) [do your thing (xxx)         ]
226   FPM:                     [nä precis asså de e ju svårt ] å veta
                               [nah exactly so it's (PRT) hard] to know
227         va man (.) vilken typ av roll man har där
            what one (.) what kind of role one has there
228   FAM:  m:
229   STX:  °m°
```

As in Extract 1, the student delivering the feedback in Extract 2a provides a correction of the peer student's simulation performance. On line 219, FPM contrasts the somewhat passive behavior pointed out by FAM himself in his preceding self-critique with a preferable course of action: "you could (PRT) have provided support". Note, however, that the correction in Extract 2a is not direct and overt, as in Extract 1, but *embedded* (Jefferson, 1987) – it is incorporated into a stretch of talk that includes accounts justifying both the criticism (line 213) and the criticized behavior (lines 201–202; 206), evidentials and modifiers ("Jag tror"/"I think", "probably", "maybe"), mitigators ("a little"), and longer within-turn pauses (line 202, 203) that serve to downplay the criticism and mark it as interactionally delicate (Pomerantz, 1984; Pomerantz & Heritage, 1984). Further, similar to what Copland (2011) noted in the context of feedback conversations involving teacher trainees providing feedback on each other's teaching, FPM links the correctable to his own performance, thus assuming part of the responsibility for the problematic behavior (line 217: "I was probably not that clear either there somehow"). Thus, in line with much prior research on peer feedback, the delivery of peer feedback is marked by a set of mitigating devices. We would like to highlight here, however, a further aspect of the use of *accounts* in this episode. In prior research on feedback interactions, accounts have been placed under the rubric of mitigating devices, along with hedges, evidentials, modifiers, etc. Not denying the fact that accounts do have such an interactional function, they also invariably embody some form of substantive formulation regarding the *significance* of the "failure event" (Buttny, 1993). As Buttny notes, "social accountability practices reflect a person's moral or practical reasoning for action" (Buttny, 1993, p. 49). An account's transformative power to "recast the pejorative significance of an event" relies on the ways in which it refers to a putatively shared social and moral order and the degree to which it will gain acceptance for the relevance of the particular "folk logic of action" (Buttny, 1993) it invokes.

What this means is that there is invariably a generalizing component to accounts in the ties they make with shared moral orders for justification and excuse. Two aspects of FPM's feedback delivery can be highlighted: first, the various *generalizing* devices employed; and second, the *everyday* character of the folk logic of action (see Buttny, 1993) invoked. Recurrently, a generic "one" is used (Sw. "man"). See, for instance, lines 201–202, in which a generalized statement that "one does (PRT) not want to disturb the one who is the leader" prefigures the critical comment in line 203. The Swedish epistemic particle "*ju*" ties the statement to something putatively shared and taken for granted (Heinemann et al., 2011). The following rule-like formulation invoked as an explanatory resource for the noted lack of communication also implies generalization: FPM notes that "we don't know each other very well" (line 206) and that "has one worked together then maybe you would have said..." (lines 209–210). The general observation that "sometimes so (.) one gets caught up a little" (line 213) offers an additional normal and reasonable explanation, this time of a more cognitive nature. Finally, FPM concludes that "it is hard to know [...] what kind of role one has there" (lines 226–227).

Throughout, FPM does extensive work to frame the criticized performance as reasonable and normal in relation to an everyday logic of social interaction and cognition. When the professional situation is made relevant, it is in connection with considerations of tact and deference (e.g., knowing one's "role" and not wanting to disturb "the leader"). This logic is offered as an organizing principle for producing accounts and as an explanatory frame of reference for understanding the "failure event" (see Buttny, 1993). The offer is accepted by FAM, who produces tokens of affirmation throughout (208, 212, 216, 218), and (line 220) an "accept with account" (Waring, 2007), which aligns with the social-relational logic set up by FPM's prior accounting work: FAM claims to have noted the possible relevance of "saying something" on several occasions, but decided in the end not to: "but- [...] then I let you (.) do your thing" (lines 223–225). Not speaking when it would have been relevant is thus framed as an active choice; moreover, with FPM as a benefactor, the formulation alludes to something akin to "negative face" as described by Goffman (1982), in indexing a reluctance to impose on FPM's personal domain of action. As already pointed out, FPM concludes by responding affirmatively and in overlap with reference to a role-related uncertainty.

In sum, the episode so far partly echoes the observations regarding peer feedback made in prior research: criticism of performance has been delivered in a downplayed and mitigated manner. In addition to this achievement, however, the students have also collaboratively constructed a generalized frame of reference for how the failure event can relevantly be understood in and through the specific ways in which their accounts are put together. In critically assessing his own conduct, FAM invokes general issues of distinct "category-bound" responsibilities he had toward the patient as an assistant doctor. Occurring in the pragmatic context of FAM's generalized self-critique, FPM's feedback takes on a similar character. Furthermore, the accounting work done by FAM and FPM frames the problem in terms of their *relational* reasoning as socially considerate, ordinary persons. This particular logic is proposed by FPM and ratified by FAM. We believe this level of practical reasoning is important for understanding the instructor's subsequent remarks, as presented in Extract 2b.

Extract 2b

```
230   INS:    +@men va e de viktigaste+ i målet va e- va e de
              but what's the most important in the goal what's- what's
      fam:    +looks at INS----------+looks down---->
      fpm:    @looks at INS---->>
231   INS:    viktigaste för teamet (.) att uppnå i en sån här
              the most important thing for the team to achieve in such a
232   INS:    situation
              situation
233           (2.5)
234   INS:    +de e ju att (0.5) den samlade kompetensen+ förmågan
              it's (PRT) that (0.5) the collective competence the capacity
      fam:    +looks at INS----------------------------+looks in front---->
235   INS:    som teamet har (.) att de gagnar patienten så att den
              that the team has (.) that it benefits the patient so that it
236   INS:    får de mest optimala (0.3) omhändertagandet å då (0.2)
              gets the most optimal (0.3) care and then (0.2)
237   INS:    €då då +liksom får man kanske lägga und€an      [vilket uttryck]
              then then somehow one perhaps must set aside [what term     ]
      ins:    €leans forward looks at FAM-----------€looks up---->
      fam:            +looks at INS---->
238   FAM:                                                   [+m:        +]
      fam:                                                   +nods--------+
239   INS:    ska ja ha .ptk (0.4) finkänsligheten å kan €ja säga €[de här]
              shall I have .ptk (0.4) the tact and can I say       [this  ]
      ins:                                                  -->€looks
                                                    at FAM--€looks up->
240   FAM:                                                        +↑[m   ↑]!
      fam:                                                         ↑nods-↑
      fam:                                                         +looks at
                                                                   INS---->>
241   INS:    å så [vidare]
              and  [so on ]
242   FAM:         [m     ]
243   INS:    utan: (1) då har ju alla ett ansvar att se till
              but €(1) then everyone has (PRT) a responsibility to make sure
      ins:    €looks at FAM---->>
244   INS:    att man för[söker inom rimliga gränser  ]
              that one tri[es within reasonable limits]
245   FAM:               [+a just de (.) m:         +]
                         [yeah that's right (.) m    ]
      fam:               +nods--------------------->+
246   INS:    (att) upp↑nå °såna° ↑ELLER (.) va säger ni?
              (to) achieve °such° ↑OR (.) what do you say?
```

After both FPM and FAM have signaled the end of their turns in Extract 2a, the instructor enters the conversation with a question (lines 230–232). Prefaced with the disjunction marker "but", which signals an opposing stance, the question reframes the concerns about social relations raised in prior talk and instead highlights *professional* categories and priorities, asking what is most important for the "the team" to achieve in "such a situation". When the instructor begins to formulate the question, several of the students, including FPM and FAM, turn their attention toward her, but none of them make any attempt to respond, which suggests that they understand the question as rhetorical rather than as demanding an answer. After a longer pause of 2.5 seconds (line 233), during which the students continue looking at the instructor, she goes on to provide the answer. She begins by formulating *what* goal the team should strive for – to utilize their collective competence in a way that benefits the patient (lines 234–236) – and then provides a suggestion on *how* to achieve this, which involves setting aside tact and considerations of what is appropriate to say (lines 237–246). As in Extract 1, the instructor's suggestion here corresponds with one of the CRM principles for team behavior guiding the simulation training: *communicate effectively – speak up* (see e.g., Miller et al., 2014, p. 122).

The instructor's extended turn clearly indicates disaffiliation. At the same time, there is no indication that her assessment of the target performance differs from the concerns raised by FPM – that is, that FAM "could have provided support" (line 219). Quite to the opposite, in alluding to the *speak-up* principle, the instructor explicitly supports FPM's critique of FAM's passive behavior and further elaborates it by framing it as in line with a general model of team behavior. This means that the source of the disjunction must be sought elsewhere. We suggest that the instructor's remarks are directed at the practical reasoning evinced in the students' collaboratively produced accounts, possibly including FAM's prior self-critique, as much as responding to the target simulation performance.

In Excerpt 2a, we saw how the students collaborated in supporting the relevance of social-relational considerations as a frame of reference for the production of accounts. In affiliating with an account, the speaker also ratifies the relevance of the particular social and moral order the account invokes. Non-aligning responses may, by implication, target either the account itself as valid in relation to the suggested moral order or question the situated relevance of the latter. The instructor clearly leaves the individual accounts aside in favor of questioning the orientation to "tact" (Sw. "finkänslighet") that they index. As Buttny (1993) noted, there are often competing logics that may be applicable to a given situation, and a central question for speakers is to determine and negotiate this applicability. Here, the instructor introduces a competing moral order, populated by a different set of actors compared to the students' accounts. As indicated, the students are reasoning mostly in terms of social relations. The membership categories invoked include a nondescript generic "one" and, where professional categories are used, a highly asymmetrical and deferential social structure (where, for instance, "doctor in charge" is used interchangeably with "leader", whom one does not want to "disturb"). The instructor, by contrast, refers to "the team", "the patient", "optimal (0.3) care", "collective competence" (Extract 2b), and similar categories, explicitly placing this social structure and the moral order it embodies in opposition with the voiced concerns about tact. These elements clearly speak to the relevance of seeing the instructor's remarks as responsive not only to the simulator performance under discussion or to the assessments of it made in peer feedback, but also to the prior accounts and the practical reasoning they embody.

Discussion

Simulation-based training provides learners with practical experiences of (simulated) professional conduct and observers with the possibility of monitoring the performance in the simulated tasks. Through practical activities, "the body of the trainee is being socialized into the comportment and embodied skills of the expert" (Hindmarsh et al., 2014, p. 248). In addition, the embodied actions of the trainees provide observable grounds for assessment, feedback, and instruction. Our analyses have highlighted how the debriefing makes both the simulation *performance* and various *accounts* of this performance available for feedback discussion. This means that the instructor's comments might address the performance, various accounts of the performance, or both. Given the conditional relevancies set up by prior talk, instructors' contributions could, in many cases, be heard as part of a sequence and responsive to prior talk rather than to the performance in the simulated scenario as such.

In the analyzed extracts, the ties between instructors' contributions and prior talk feature an evaluative stance regarding the *accounts* produced in prior talk. The socialization of medical professionals involves what we have termed a *categorial shift*, whereby the particular "folk logic of action" set up in student accounts is replaced by one more fitted to the professional context. In the analyzed extracts, this shift has included downplaying an everyday social and moral order, and its typical designations of membership categories, in favor of an order where actors and actions are categorized in terms of the profession. We also identified the ways in which the accountability of simulation performances which was corrected by the instructor could be seen to reflect some of the CRM principles, the implementation of which was an important objective informing the analyzed simulation and debriefing sessions. For instance, when the students say that they do not want to disturb the doctor in charge or that they let someone do their own thing, they provide accounts of their actions that contrast with the principles of CRM. According to these principles, healthcare staff members "must advocate for the course of action that they feel is best, even if it involves conflict with others," and they should therefore "speak up and state their information with appropriate persistence until a clear resolution is achieved" (Powell & Hill, 2006, p. 188). While it is the obligation of each member of the interprofessional team to follow these principles, the guidelines on CRM also highlight the importance of integrating the principles in the organization, for instance, by encouraging and upholding a "challenge and response" environment (Powell & Hill, 2006).

As noted by Garfinkel, methods of practical reasoning are "organizationally situated and embody members' common sense knowledge of social structures" (Garfinkel, 1967, p. viii).[7] We can now see how the instructor's interventions serve to enforce a particular "organizational situatedness" of practical reasoning tied to professional understandings of emergency care teamwork. Seen in this light, student accounts are analyzable expressions of common-sense knowledge as they pertain to specific organizational contexts. This analyzability is an important resource for the instructor in producing follow-up responses. In the two episodes, we could see how instructors' interventions align with, depart from, or otherwise operate on prior talk, including the generalized claims and practical reasoning embodied in student accounts. Most centrally, the instructor analyzes what the students say with an orientation toward the fit between student accounting practices and "expectations of sanctionable performances" (Garfinkel, 1967, p. 199). These expectations, moreover, are formally tied to CRM principles, which we suggest can be characterized as *glosses* on some particularly salient aspects of how the socialization of practical reasoning breaks with everyday orientations to interpersonal relations and politeness, as well as with professional hierarchies. In conclusion, this shows how the instructional work addresses not only performance but also the ways in which performance is accounted for in student talk. The socialization of members thus entails an interplay between fostering performative competence through feedback on observable conduct and shaping professional, organizationally situated forms of accountability.

In relation to studies concerned with the evaluation and development of simulation and debriefing pedagogy, the present analyses cannot be easily translated into recommendations. They do point, however, toward the pedagogical value of allowing room for spontaneous student accounting talk, in that such talk is revelatory of operative "folk logics of action," which instructors may find a reason to address. Considering that one issue in the debriefing literature is the relative merits of tightly versus loosely structured debriefing formats (Keiser & Arthur, 2021), the present discussion at least highlights the possible value of accounting sequences whose presence in these recordings may hinge in part on a relatively permissive interactional structure. Obviously, the findings also speak to the relevance of facilitation by "a content domain expert" (Keiser & Arthur, 2021, p. 1012), through the ways in which the instructor may provide a professional frame of reference (see Waring, 2017; Hindmarsh et al., 2014) for the socialization of accountability practices, which the students, as learners, necessarily have limited access to.

Funding sources

This work was supported by the Swedish Research Council [project id: 2012-05450] and Riksbankens Jubileumsfond [P19-0667:1].

Notes

1 Interprofessional team training means that team members of two or more professions (e.g., physicians and nurses) train together to learn about each other's professions and to practice interacting with each other as a team (Salas et al., 2016).
2 The CRM principles are presented in Miller's *Anesthesia* 8th Edition (Miller et al., 2014). It should be noted, however, that the principles can be retrieved from a variety

of other sources and some variations in the formulation of the principles may occur. Moreover, while the principles serve as backdrop for the interprofessional simulation training, how the universities arranging this kind of training present them to the students varies.
3 The project involved three research teams that included both medical practitioners and educational researchers who worked in close collaboration to collect and analyse video-recorded data of simulation-based training. The first author of this chapter was part of one of these teams.
4 Transcription conventions are provided in the beginning of the volume (pp. 22–23).
5 A "patient monitor" is a bedside monitor that measures and displays the patient's vital parameters, such as blood pressure, heart rate, and mean arterial pressure.
6 In Extracts 2a and 2b, the acronym STX represents an unidentified student.
7 In introducing the notion of practical reasoning, Garfinkel (1967) states that "ordinary activities consist of methods to make practical actions, practical circumstances, common sense knowledge of social structures, and practical sociological reasoning *analyzeable*" (p. viii, emphasis added). For our purposes, we stress that this is an analyzability for members, rather than for the external observer.

References

Bolden, G. B. (2010). 'Articulating the unsaid' via and-prefaced formulations of others' talk. *Discourse Studies*, *12*(1), 5–32. https://doi-org.ezproxy.ub.gu.se/10.1177/1461445609346770

Buttny, R. (1987). Sequence and practical reasoning in accounts episodes. *Communication Quarterly*, *35*(1), 67–83. https://doi.org/10.1080/01463378709369671

Buttny, R. (1993). *Social accountability in communication*. Sage.

Buttny, R. (2004). *Talking problems: Studies of discursive construction*. SUNY Press.

Chiniara, G., Cole, G., Brisbin, K., Huffman, D., Cragg, B., Lamacchia, M., & Norman, D. (2013). Simulation in healthcare: A taxonomy and a conceptual framework for instructional design and media selection. *Medical Teacher*, *35*(8), e1380–e1395. https://doi.org/10.3109/0142159X.2012.733451

Copland, F. (2011). Negotiating face in feedback conferences: A linguistic ethnographic analysis. *Journal of Pragmatics*, *43*(15), 3832–3843. https://doi.org/10.1016/j.pragma.2011.09.014

Dieckmann, P., Reddersen, S., Zieger, J., & Rall, M . (2008). A structure for video-assisted debriefs in simulator-based training of crisis recourse management (pp. 667–676). In R. Kyle & B. W. Murray (Eds.), *Clinical simulation: Operations, engineering, and management* (pp. 667–676). Academic Press.

Eppich, W., Hunt, E. A., Duval-Arnould, J. M., Siddall, V. J., & Cheng, A. (2015). Structuring feedback and debriefing to achieve mastery learning goals. *Academic Medicine*, *90*(11), 1501–1508. https://doi.org/10.1097/ACM.0000000000000934

Evans, C. (2013). Making sense of assessment feedback in higher education. *Review of Educational Research*, *83*(1), 70–120. https://doi.org/10.3102/0034654312474350

Garfinkel, H. (1967). *Studies in ethnomethodology*. Englewood Cliffs, NJ: Prentice-Hall.

Glenn, P. (2003). *Laughter in interaction* (Vol. 18). Cambridge University Press.

Goffman, E. (1982). *Interaction ritual: Essays on face-to-face behavior* (1st ed.). Pantheon.

Hattie, J., & Timperley, H. (2007). The power of feedback. *Review of Educational Research*, *77*(1), 81–112. https://doi.org/10.3102/003465430298487

Heinemann, T., Lindström, A., & Steensig, J. (2011). Addressing epistemic incongruence in question-answer sequences through the use of epistemic adverbs. In T. Stivers, L.

Mondada, & J. Steensig (Eds.), *The morality of knowledge in conversation* (pp. 107–130). Cambridge University Press.

Heritage, J., & Sefi, S. (1992). Dilemmas of advice: Aspects of the delivery and reception of advice in interactions between health visitors and first time mothers. In P. Drew & J. Heritage (Eds.), *Talk at work: Interaction in institutional settings* (pp. 359–419). Cambridge University Press.

Hindmarsh, J., Hyland, L., & Banerjee, A. (2014). Work to make simulation work: 'Realism', instructional correction and the body in training. *Discourse Studies, 16*(2), 247–269. https://doi.org/10.1177/1461445613514670

Hontvedt, M. (2015). Professional vision in simulated environments—Examining professional maritime pilots' performance of work tasks in a full-mission ship simulator. *Learning, Culture and Social Interaction, 7*, 71–84. https://doi.org/10.1016/j.lcsi.2015.07.003

Issenberg, B. S., Mcgaghie, W. C., Petrusa, E. R., Lee, G. D., & Scalese, R. J. (2005). Features and uses of high-fidelity medical simulations that leads to effective learning: A BEME systematic review. *Medical Teacher, 27*(1), 10–28. https://doi.org/10.1080/01421590500046924

Issenberg, S. B., & Scalese, R. J. (2008). Simulation in health care education. *Perspectives in Biology and Medicine, 51*(1), 31–46. https://doi.org/10.1353/pbm.2008.0004

Jefferson, G. (1987). On exposed and embedded correction in conversation. In G. Button & J. R. E. Lee (Eds.), *Talk and social organisation* (pp. 86–100). Multilingual Matters.

Johansson, E., Lindwall, O., & Rystedt, H. (2017). Experiences, appearances, and interprofessional training: The instructional use of video in post-simulation debriefings. *International Journal of Computer-Supported Collaborative Learning, 12*(1), 91–112. https://doi.org/10.1007/s11412-017-9252-z

Keiser, N. L., & Arthur, W. Jr. (2021). A meta-analysis of the effectiveness of the after-action review (or debrief) and factors that influence its effectiveness. *Journal of Applied Psychology, 106*(7), 1007–1032. https://doi.org/10.1037/apl0000821

Keiser, N. L., & Arthur, W. (2022). A meta-analysis of task and training characteristics that contribute to or attenuate the effectiveness of the after-action review (or debrief). *Journal of Business and Psychology, 37*(5), 953–976. https://doi-org.ezproxy.ub.gu.se/10.1007/s10869-021-09784-x

Lindwall, O., & Lynch, M. (2021). "Are you asking me or telling me?": Expertise, evidence, and blame attribution in a post-game interview. *Discourse Studies, 23*(5), 652–669. https://doi.org/10.1177/14614456211016820

McGaghie, W. C., Issenberg, S. B., Petrusa, E. R., & Scalese, R. J. (2010). A critical review of simulation-based education research: 2003–2009. *Medical Education, 44*(1), 50–63. https://doi.org/10.1111/j.1365-2923.2009.03547.x

Miller, R. D., Eriksson, L. I., Fleisher, L. A., Wiener-Kronish, J. P., Cohen, N. H., & Young, W. L. (2014). *Miller's anesthesia e-book*. Elsevier Health Sciences.

Motola, I., Devine, L. A., Chung, H. S., Sullivan, J. E., & Issenberg, S. B. (2013). Simulation in healthcare education: A best evidence practical guide. *Medical Teacher, 35*(10), 1511–1530. https://doi.org/10.3109/0142159X.2013.818632

Nyström, S., Dahlberg, J., Edelbring, S., Hult, H., & Dahlgren, M. A. (2016). Debriefing practices in interprofessional simulation with students: A sociomaterial perspective. *BMC Medical Education, 16*(1), 1–8. https://doi.org/10.1186/s12909-016-0666-5

Park, I. (2014). Stepwise advice negotiation in writing center peer tutoring. *Language and Education, 28*(4), 362–382. https://doi.org/10.1080/09500782.2013.873805

Pomerantz, A. (1984). Agreeing and disagreeing with assessments: Some features of preferred and dispreferred turn shapes. In J. M. Atkinson & J. Heritage (Eds.), *Structures of social action* (pp. 57–101). Cambridge University Press.

Pomerantz, A., & Heritage, J. (2013). Preference. In T. Stivers & J. Sidnell (Eds.), *The handbook of conversation analysis* (pp. 210–228). Wiley Black.

Powell, S. M., & Hill, R. K. (2006). My copilot is a nurse—Using crew resource management in the OR. *Association of periOperative Registered Nurses Journal, 83*(1), 178–202. https://doi.org/10.1016/S0001-2092(06)60239-1

Rall, M., Manser, T., & Howard, S. K. (2000). Key elements of debriefing for simulator training. *European Journal of Anaesthesiology, 17*(8), 516–517. https://doi.org/10.1046/j.1365-2346.2000.00724-1.x

Roth, W. M. (2015). Cultural practices and cognition in debriefing: The case of aviation. *Journal of Cognitive Engineering and Decision Making, 9*(3), 263–278. https://doi.org/10.1177/1555343415591395

Roth, W. M., & Jornet, A. (2015). Situational awareness as an instructable and instructed matter in multi-media supported debriefing: A case study from aviation. *Computer Supported Cooperative Work (CSCW), 24*(5), 461–508. https://doi.org/10.1007/s10606-015-9234-5

Sacks, H. (1974). An analysis of the course of a joke's telling in conversation. In R. Bauman & J. Sherzer (Eds.), *Explorations in the ethnography of speaking* (pp. 337–353). Cambridge University Press.

Sadler, D. R. (2010). Beyond feedback: Developing student capability in complex appraisal. *Assessment and Evaluation in Higher Education, 35*(5), 535–550. https://doi-org.ezproxy.ub.gu.se/10.1080/02602930903541015

Sawyer, T., Eppich, W., Brett-Fleegler, M., Grant, V., & Cheng, A. (2016). More than one way to debrief: A critical review of healthcare simulation debriefing methods. *Simulation in Healthcare, 11*(3), 209–217. http://doi.org/10.1097/SIH.0000000000000148

Sellberg, C. (2018). From briefing, through scenario, to debriefing: The maritime instructor's work during simulator-based training. *Cognition, Technology and Work, 20*(1), 49–62. https://doi.org/10.1007/s10111-017-0446-y

Sellberg, C., Lindwall, O., & Rystedt, H. (2021). The demonstration of reflection-in-action in maritime training. *Reflective Practice, 22*(3), 319–330. https://doi.org/10.1080/14623943.2021.1879771

Svinhufvud, K. (2015). Participation in the master's thesis seminar. Exploring the lack of discussion. *Learning, Culture and Social Interaction, 5*, 66–83. https://doi.org/10.1016/j.lcsi.2014.12.002

Tannenbaum, S. I., & Cerasoli, C. P. (2013). Do team and individual debriefs enhance performance? A meta-analysis. *Human Factors, 55*(1), 231–245. https://doi.org/10.1177/0018720812448394

Van De Ridder, J. M., Stokking, K. M., McGaghie, W. C., & Ten Cate, O. T. J. (2008). What is feedback in clinical education? *Medical Education, 42*(2), 189–197. https://doi.org/10.1111/j.1365-2923.2007.02973.x

Vehviläinen, S. (2009). Problems in the research problem: Critical feedback and resistance in academic supervision. *Scandinavian Journal of Educational Research, 53*(2), 185–201. https://doi.org/10.1080/00313830902757592

Waring, H. Z. (2007). Complex advice acceptance as a resource for managing asymmetries. *Text and Talk, 27*(1), 107–137. https://doi.org/10.1515/TEXT.2007.005

Waring, H. Z. (2012). The advising sequence and its preference structures in graduate peer tutoring at an American University. In H. Limberg & M. A. Locher (Eds.), *Advice in discourse* (pp. 97–118). John Benjamins.

Waring, H. Z. (2017). Going general as a resource for doing advising in post-observation conferences in teacher training. *Journal of Pragmatics, 110*, 20–33. https://doi.org/10.1016/j.pragma.2017.01.009

Watson, R. (2015). De-reifying categories. In R. Fitzgerald & W. Housley (Eds.), *Advances in membership categorisation analysis* (pp. 23–50). Sage.
Waznonis, A. R. (2014). Methods and evaluations for simulation debriefing in nursing education. *Journal of Nursing Education*, *53*(8), 459–465. https://doi.org/10.3928/01484834-20140722-13

Index

accountability/accountable 1, 12–13, 50, 104, 113, 117, 127, 131, 141–142, 150, 160, 190, 239–242, 253–254; social accountability 249
accounts, feedback 247, 249–250, 253–254
adequacy *see* unique adequacy
affordances 207, 209–210; technological affordances 12, 212, 217
ALF (Announce, List, Find) 40
ambulance crews 10–11, 47–48, 53–62, 66; agreeing on coordination of priority tasks 63–66; agreeing on priority tasks based on patient's condition 60–63; identifying priority patients 55–60; timing for accomplishment of remaining tasks 66–67
aphasia 176; correcting and instructing speech sounds 178–180; instruction of speech-language therapy 177–178; *see also* speech-language therapy
apnea 4, 11, 130, 132–133, 135, 143–144, 147–148
apps for healthcare: introductions to 212–217, 231–234; Physitrack 207–208; use of in physiotherapy 211–212
asking questions (in operating room) 102–103, 125–127; creating opportunities for trainees to ask questions 107–117; experts initiate questions 117–120; expert's management of opportunities to ask questions 113–117; laparoscopic surgery as video training 105–106; surgeon's management of opportunities to ask questions 107–113; trainees initiating questions 120–125
assessable listening 160–161, 170; *see also* listening
assessments *see* evaluations
asymmetric: interaction 104, 178; settings 177–178; spatial positions 158

asymmetrical power relations 3, 5, social structure 252
asymmetry 43, 116, 126; of access 116–117, 126; in bodies' disposition and control 185; negotiation of asymmetry 178
audible features of urban settings 152
audible social order 153–154
audio recordings 1, 3, 5, 212; *see also* recordings; video recordings
audio-visual: cues 194, 196–197, 200; demonstrations 194; equipment 155, 172; hints 196, 200, 202; performance 201; recordings 1, 3, 5, 212; representations 200; *see also* video recordings

CA *see* conversation analysis
categorial shift 253–254
category-bound activities 225, 232
collecting recordings *see* data collection
collection (of cases, instances) 10–11, 27, 118, 130, 132, 152
competence 4–9; asking questions (in operating room) 117, 127; collective competences 252; embodied competences 5; of flight nurses 48–49, 52–54, 67–70; of members 2, 4–5, 8–10; non-competence 179; performative competences 254; vulgar competence 52; *see also* skills
conditional relevance/conditionally relevant 131, 135, 143, 149, 190, 244, 253
configurations: bodily configuration 185, 190–191, 196; interactional configurations 124; local configurations 171; mobile interaction configuration 73, 97–98; mutual gaze configuration 197, 200; participatory configuration 188, 194; senior member walks ahead, intern follows 96; spatial configurations

223; triangular configuration 207, 214, 217; urban configurations 155; walking behind 80–81, 83; walking-with-someone-following-them configuration 81, 83
context renewing/shaped 3
contingencies 12, 80, 102–113, 126, 130, 217, 241; identifying audible order in traffic 154, 166–169; in situ 207
conventions for transcriptions 16n1, 22–23, 76, 132–133, 181–182, 212, 255n4
conversation analysis (CA) 1, 24–26, 48, 102–104, 130, 152, 177, 179–180, 208, 240
cooperative labor *see* coordination
coordination 130–131; assessments and requests 137–139; between doctors and nurses in operating rooms 147–150; of priority tasks, flight nurses and doctors 63–66; *see also* interprofessional collaboration
corpus: of audio-recorded physician-patient encounters 5; of speech-language therapy sessions 180; of surgical laparoscopic operations 105; of video-recorded sessions 12
correcting speech sounds 178–180; through labeling activities 182–184
corrective demonstrations 179
corrective instructions 8, 155, 163, 179, 196, 201
corridors (of a clinic) *see* interns, walking with senior staff
cross a street *see* identifying audible order in traffic
cultural dope 4, 74

data collection 14–15, 132, 181, 243
debriefing (simulation training) 239–244, 253–254; generalizing character of accounts 247–253; peer-feedback talk 244–247
deference rules 11, 73, 96
deficiency model 7
demonstration 104; anatomical demonstration 112; bodily demonstrations 177; corrective demonstrations 179; embodied demonstrations 8, 154; instructional demonstrations 122; laparoscopy 105–106; speech-language therapy 193–196, 201

design: in collaboration 15; of educational interventions 14; education-oriented interventions 13; questions 32–34; repetition 195; of talk 163; for trainees 108
diagnosis 4, 28, 34, 38, 177
digital tools: interactive organization of instructional sequences 210–211; physiotherapists embodied organization of instructions 217–231; use of in healthcare 209–210
digitization in healthcare 208–209
disaffiliation 252
doctor-patient encounters/interactions 2–3, 10, 43
doctors 3, 42, 242; assisting doctors 248, 250; in charge doctor 252–253; *see also* flight doctors; physicians
domains of scrutiny 170–171
double bind 25
driver training studies, instructional sequences 153–155
dual projects, assessments and requests 137–139

ecological huddles, guiding selective listening to traffic 157–158
educational setting 6, 154, 210, 216
education-oriented activities 7
education research 3, 6–7, 9
educators 6, 14–15, 77, 82
eHealth literacy 207–209
EM *see* ethnomethodology
embodied demonstrations 8, 154; speech-language therapy 193–196, 201
embodied interactions 10, 179
embodied organization of physiotherapists' introduction task 217–231
EMCA *see* ethnomethodology and conversation analysis
emergency call centers 14
Emergency Medical Unit, flight nurses 53–54
empirical research 1
empirical studies 10, 24
endodontic surgery 7
ethnographic material 11
ethnography 73
ethnomethodological (studies) 14, 26, 50, 73–74, 79, 97, 102, 130, 169, 208
ethnomethodological and conversation analytic (EMCA) studies 50, 102, 130, 152, 208

ethnomethodological indifference 14
ethnomethodologists 52–53, 70
ethnomethodology (EM) 1–5, 7–10, 13, 15–16, 48–50, 102–104, 130, 147, 152, 154–155, 177, 179, 208, 211
evaluations/assessments 154, 241; self-evaluations 170; third-turn evaluations 178
excerpts: how to use a mobile app 213, 215–216, 218–221, 223–231; identifying audible order in traffic 159–160, 162, 164–169
exchange of preferences 30–31
experts 11, 102; interventions 119; laparoscopy surgery 104–106, 110–125; management of opportunities to ask questions 113–117
extracts: asking questions (in operating room) 107–115, 118–119, 121–124; interprofessional collaboration 55–57, 60–61, 64, 66; senior staff walking ahead of interns 82, 84, 86–89, 91–94; socialization and accountability 245, 248–249, 251; socializing patients in language therapy 183–199; when neurologists solicit preferences 29–32, 34–38

feedback 239–242; peer-feedback talk 244–247
flight doctors: agreeing on priority tasks based on patient's condition 60–63; coordination of priority tasks 63–66; identifying priority patients 55–60; timing for accomplishment of remaining tasks 66–67
flight nurses 47–48; agreeing on priority tasks based on patient's condition 60–63; competences 67–70; coordination of priority tasks 63–66; Emergency Medical Unit 53–54; identifying priority patients 55–60; practical management of prehospital care 54; in prehospital care setting 48–49; setting for 51–54; timing for accomplishment of remaining tasks 66–67; video recordings 51–52
four-step model of shared decision-making 41
fragments, soliciting absent requests 133, 136–140, 143, 145–146
'from within' 4–5, 8; contributing to research 9
full-form option-listing 40–41

gaze 5, 176–177, 179
generalizing character of accounts, debriefings 247–253
gesturing, speech-language therapy 189–190
guidance, identifying audible order in traffic 166–169
guidelines 54; for flight nurses 48–49; for prehospital care 51

healthcare: digitization in 208–210; policy 2, 9, 14; settings, collaboration in 49–51
hearable/hearably 34, 36, 126, 153, 164–165, 167, 170
heterotechnic cooperation 149
hospitalists 51
hybridity/hybrid study of work 14, 52, 70, 233; criterial properties 14

identifying audible order in traffic 171–172; assessable listening 160–161; guidance and contingencies 166–169; guiding selective listening 156–160; instructional sequences 160–164, 169–171; orienting to traffic as a continuous flow 164–166; settings for study 155–156
identifying priority patients, flight nurses 55–60
"if-then" declarative format 34
initiation of repair 180
in-passing activities 97
in situ: contingencies 207; laparoscopic surgery as video training 105–106; learning-by-doing introductions 207–208; patient-initiated questions 5; training, surgery 103–105
instructed action 154–155, 163–164, 166, 170, 196, 210–211, 222, 225–226
instructing: patient to gaze at therapist's mouth 189–196; speech sounds 178–180
instructional: activities 103, 106, 161, 179, 212–213; chains 216, 221, 224, 226–227, 232; corrections 241; demonstrations 122; expansions 242; function 241; interventions 244, 247, 253–254; response 225–226
instructional sequences 12, 153–155; guiding selective listening to traffic 158–160; of healthcare apps 214–217; identifying audible order in traffic 160–164, 169–171; interactive organization of 210–211

instructions 8–9, 154–155; about embodied conduct 201; clear-cut instructions 201; concerning digital tools 210; embodied instructions 217, 219, 222, 226; of embodied skills 179; following 169–170, 217, 232; giving 178; instructional activities 103, 161, 179, 212–213; instructions as teaching 233; physiotherapists embodied organization of instructions 217–231; related to technology 210
instructors 13, 48, 52, 156; socialization and accountability 239–240, 242–248, 251–254; teaching how to identify an audible order in traffic 156–171; teaching how to use mobile apps 210–211, 216, 222, 225
interns, walking with senior staff 77–79; behind senior staff 96–97; keeping the way clear 81–86; mill position 81–86; minding the distance 91–95; pushing through and going first 86–91; yielding the right-of-way 81–86
interprofessional collaboration 48–51, 69–70, 243; in healthcare settings 49–51; prehospital care 48
interprofessional teams 242, 253; training 254
interrogative format 34
interventions 10, 210, 213; expert's interventions 119; instructional interventions 244, 247, 253–254; training interventions 13
interviews 5, 9, 49, 52, 104, 211–212
introduction activities 212–213
introduction to healthcare apps 214–217, 231–234
I-R-E device 8, 154; *see also* instructional sequences

joint tasks, coordination 133–135
joint understanding 4

keeping the way clear while walking 81–86
"key-hole surgery" *see* laparoscopy

labeling activities 12, 176, 178, 182–189, 200
laparoscopy (key-hole surgery) 11, 105; experts 110–125; as video training 105–106
learning-by-doing activities 207, 222, 226, 232
learning-by-doing introductions 207–208; in face-to-face physiotherapy consultations 212–214; interactive organization of the introduction to apps 214–217; physiotherapists embodied organization of instructions 217–231
learning disabilities: aphasia *see* aphasia; mobility and instructions sequences 153–155
listening 12, 152, 155–156; assessable listening 160–161; guiding selective listening to traffic 156–160; orienting to traffic as a continuous flow 164–166
local: achievement 233; circumstances 161; configurations 171; contingencies 126; mobility 73–74, 98–99n1; relevance of audio-visual hints 200, 202; use of video 103–104
locally oriented and particularized feedback 242

management of requests 136–137
medical/healthcare education 6, 9, 16
membership categories 81, 154, 210–211, 244, 252–253
members of the field 6, 10, 13–15, 52
members' perspectives 4, 14–15, 48, 52, 177; of complex surgery procedures 15; investigating 4; on therapeutic process 181
members' phenomenon 8
mill position 81–86
minding the distance, walking 91–95
missing requests 142–147
mobile eHealth tool 12, 207
mobility 152; formations-in-action 80, 96; identifying audible order in traffic 156–160; instructional sequences for those with learning disabilities 153–155; local mobility 73–74, 98–99n1
mobility practices *see* walking
monitoring 8; interns, walking with senior staff 77, 86, 88; surgical procedures 133–134, 137, 141; traffic 157; when requests are given but not heard 131, 139–142
moving features of urban settings 12
multiactivity: parallel order 118; of surgical work and training 103–105

naturally occurring interactions 2–3, 5, 9, 15, 132, 207, 231
navigational problem, of walking 80
negative framing 25
negative observations 148
negotiation of face 241

Index 263

neurologists: patient view elicitors (PVEs) 26–27; post-recommendation position 27–33; pre-recommendation position 33–39; shared decision-making 39–43; soliciting preferences 24–25
not-yet-fully-competent 7–9
nurse anesthetist: assessments and requests 137–139; coordination 132–135; missing requests 142–147; requests in action 135–137; when requests are given but not heard 139–142
nurses, senior nurses 11, 78–79; *see also* flight nurses; nurse anesthetist
nursing interns *see* interns, walking

operating theater 102, 104–105, 148
opportunities for questions: expert's management of 112–117; surgeon's management of 107–113
option-listing 28
orderly management of requests 136–137
orientation and mobility (O&M) 153–154
orienting to traffic as a continuous flow 164–166
other-repair 4, 145
outpatient clinics 11, 73–74
outpatient neurology consultations 10

parallel crossing technique 158
passive resistance, to treatment recommendations 29–31
patient-centered care 2–3, 5, 43, 132
patient choice 26
patient-initiated questions 5
patient participation, in speech-language therapy 178
patient-related information, gathering of 67–68
patients: embodied and situated organization of instructions 217–231; identifying priority patients, flight nurses 55–60; preferences 25; *see also* treatment preferences
patient status 133, 135, 137, 144, 148
patient view elicitors (PVEs) 26–27; full-form option-listing 40–41; post-recommendation position 27–33; pre-recommendation position 33–39
peer feedback 241–242
peer-feedback talk 244–247
person with aphasia 8, 180–181
perspicuous phenomenon 12
perspicuous setting 6, 81, 207, 210, 212

physicians 5, 49, 51, 74; *see also* doctors; surgeons
physiotherapy 179, 207; eHealth literacy 208–209; interactive organization of the introduction to apps 214–217; introductions to apps 231–234; use of apps in 211–212
Physitrack 207–208
post-recommendation position, soliciting preferences 27–33
practical reasoning 154, 156, 244, 251–254, 255n7
praxeological validity 14
precedence rules, among the Burundi 96
preference: dispreference 5; organization 193, 227; preferred response 27, 144; for recognitionals/minimization 119
preferences: communicating about preferences 149; preferred option 33, 40; preferred way 63; *see also* treatment preferences
prehospital care 47–48, 53–54; activities 60, 67; competences of flight nurses 67–70; flight nurses 48–49; identifying priority patients 55–60
prehospital setting 47–48, 54
primary care 2–3, 10
priority tasks based on patient's condition 60–63
professional: categorical order 247; conduct 148; practice 247; socialization 239, 253; vision 103–104, 106, 120, 126–127
proof procedure 4–5
PVE *see* patient view elicitors (PVEs)

questions during introductions to the app 227–230; *see also* asking questions (in operating room)

radiologists 11, 130, 132, 148
recipient-oriented (recipient-designed) 108, 111, 167
recommendations 4–5; clinician's recommendations 25–27; post-recommendation position 27–33; pre-recommendation position 33–39; treatment recommendations 2
recommending and resisting treatment 31
recordings *see* audio recordings; data collection; video recordings
rehabilitation: for aphasia 178; speech-language therapy 177–180; telerehabilitation 208

remote: audiences 210; chat/video coaching 207, 214; education 15, 105; learning 105; settings 208–209
repair 4, 115; initiation 36, 116, 121, 124, 142; other-initiated repair 4, 145; preference organization 193; self-repair 4, 31, 139, 148, 180, 183–188, 193, 198–199, 224, 246
requestion-confirmation pair 135
requests in action 135–136; absence of timely requests 148; missing requests 142–147; orderly management of requests 136–137; when requests are given but not heard 139–142; when requests are missing 142–147
respecify 6–7, 80
right-of-way, yielding while walking 81–86
routine 8, 11, 30, 43, 50, 65, 104, 118, 130–132; coordination 136–137, 147

safety 4, 11, 130–132, 142, 147, 149–150, 209, 242
scaffolding 9, 12, 161–162, 171–172, 176, 178, 189, 196, 201
scrub nurse 140–142
scrutiny, domains of 170–171
SDM *see* shared decision-making
seen but unnoticed 16, 97
self-repair 4, 31, 139, 148, 180, 193, 198–199, 224; feedback 246; in speech-language therapy 183–184; speech-language therapy 185–189; *see also* repair
senior nurses 11, 78–79
sense-making methods 7
sequence, initiating 119
sequences for speech-language therapy 179, 189–196
sequencing: labeling activities 182; shared decision-making 41
sequential organization 149–150, 244; of ordinary conversation 96; soliciting absent requests 149; speech-language therapy 178–182, 201; of surgical operation 102, 110
sequential placement of trainees initiating questions 120–125
serial order 97; of instructional sequences 233; of senior member walks ahead, intern follows 11, 79, 81, 86, 91, 95
shared decision-making (SDM) 2–3, 5, 24, 39–43; ALF (Announce, List, Find) 40; four-step model 41; full-form option-listing 40; patient view elicitors (PVEs) 41–42; sequencing 41
simulation training 239, 242–243; debriefing *see* debriefing; identifying audible order in traffic 160–161
single-case analysis 12
situated: achievements/accomplishment 2–3, 80; actions 50, 70, 103, 185; contingencies 103; interactions 10, 16n1; learning 207, 212, 232–233; organization of instruction 217–218, 233; practice of talk 25; repair actions 4; teaching and learning opportunities 12
situatedness 102, 126, 254
skills 6, 67, 154; eHealth literacy 208–209; embodied skills 9, 179, 253; listening 12, 152, 155–156; required by healthcare members 9, 208–210; selective listening to traffic 156–160
socialization 6–9, 48, 150, 176, 201–202, 232; asking questions 102; collaboration 49–51; debriefing 254; and learning 179; of members 254; of novices 102, 128; opportunities for 48, 50; physiotherapy 208; professional socialization 239, 253; speech-language therapy 179–180; of those with aphasia 176–177; of trainees 103–106; training/instruction 120
social order 147; audible social order 153–154; walking 97
social status, walking 96
soliciting preferences from patients: neurologists 26–27; post-recommendation position 27–33; pre-recommendation position 33–39
speak-up principle 252
speech-language therapy 200–202; correcting and instructing speech sounds 178–180; corrections 178; gaze 176–177, 179, 188–189
speech sounds 12, 176–179, 189, 200–201
speech therapists 176; gesturing 189–190; verbal instructions 189–190
status; patient status 133, 135, 137, 144, 148; professional status 73; social status 96; visual status 145
street crossings *see* identifying audible order in traffic
student feedback 241
summons, sequencing 119
supervisors 8, 241
surgeons: coordination on surgical procedures 133–135; management of

opportunities to ask questions 107–113; *see also* physicians
surgery 15, 50, 102–103, 111; coordination between professionals 132–133, 147–150; embeddedness of work and training 103–105; endodentic surgery 7; laparoscopy (key-hole surgery) 11, 105–106; misunderstanding 147; surgical procedures and joint tasks 133–135; *see also* soliciting absent requests
surgical procedures, coordination 133–135
surgical teams 4, 105–106, 127, 132
surveys 9

talk: as social action 10, 24; and walking 81
target words 176, 178, 180, 182–187, 190–192, 194, 195, 198, 200–201
task coordination, identifying and agreeing on, flight nurses 60–63
teacher feedback 241
teachers *see* instructors
technological affordances 12, 207, 212, 217
technology: in healthcare 209–210; interactive organization of instructional sequences 210–211; *see also* digitization in healthcare
timing for accomplishment of remaining tasks, flight nurses and doctors 66–67
topical relevance/topically relevant 14–15, 52, 70, 211, 233–234
traffic: assessable listening 160–161; audible social order 153–154; selective listening 156–160; *see also* identifying audible order in traffic
trainees: creating opportunities for questions 107–117; initiating questions 120–125; socialization of 103–104
training 3–4, 6–8, 155–156: communication 40, 43, 132; driver training 154; flight nurses 47–49, 51, 70; interns 83, 97; interventions 13; laparoscopic surgery as video training 105–106; O&M 155; on-the-job 6, 97; in surgery 103–105; settings 6, 14, 16, 154; technology and 209–210; *see also* simulation training
transcription conventions *see* conventions for transcription
treatment preferences: post-recommendation position 27–33; pre-recommendation position 33–39

treatment recommendations, passive resistance to 29–31
triangular configuration 207, 214, 217
turn: allocation 241; design 26, 167; mobility turn 80; multi-unit turns 160, 171; spatial turn 73, 80; speech-language therapy 178; surgeons 126; surgeon's management of opportunities to ask questions 108–113; at talk 41, 81, 163; therapists 182, 193; trainees 121
tutors 6–8, 241

unique adequacy 9, 14–15, 52, 70, 156, 181, 211

video recordings 3, 14; coordination between professionals 132–133; of debriefings 243; of flight nurses 10, 48, 51–52; of how to use a mobile app 233; interaction in natural settings, traffic 153, 155–156; of interns, walking 75; or lessons to identify audible order in traffic 155–156; of naturally occurring interaction in physiotherapy consultations 207, 211–212; of simulation training 243; of speech-language therapy 180–182; of surgeries 132; for walking study 75–76; *see also* audio recordings
visual: bodily cues, speech-language therapy 180; phonemic cueing 180; status 145
visualization technologies, for surgical work and training 103–105
visually impaired persons *see* identifying audible order in traffic

walking 73–74; alone and with others 79–81; interns with senior staff 77–79; mill position 81–86; minding the distance 91–95; navigational problem 80; pushing through and going first 86–91; setting for study 74–76; social order 96–97; and talking 81; yielding the right-of-way 81–86
walking-behind 90, 97
"walking-with-someone-following them" interactional configuration 96–97
workplace study 207, 211

yielding the right-of-way while walking 81–86

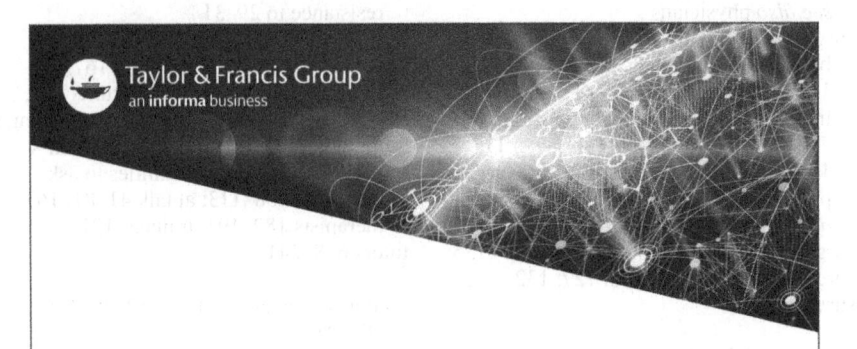